Lecture Notes in Artificial Intelligence   4565

Edited by J. G. Carbonell and J. Siekmann

Subseries of Lecture Notes in Computer Science

Dylan D. Schmorrow   Leah M. Reeves (Eds.)

Foundations
of Augmented
Cognition

Third International Conference, FAC 2007
Held as Part of HCI International 2007
Beijing, China, July 22-27, 2007
Proceedings

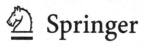 Springer

Series Editors

Jaime G. Carbonell, Carnegie Mellon University, Pittsburgh, PA, USA
Jörg Siekmann, University of Saarland, Saarbrücken, Germany

Volume Editors

Dylan D. Schmorrow
Office of Naval Research
875 N. Randolph Street, Suite 1448, Arlington, VA 22203-1995, USA
E-mail: schmord@onr.navy.mil

Leah M. Reeves
Potomac Institute for Policy Studies
901 N. Stuart Street, Suite 200, Arlington, VA 22203, USA
E-mail: lreeves@potomacinstitute.org

Associate Volume Editors

Michael B. Russo
U.S. Army Aeromedical Research Laboratory
Fort Rucker, Al 36362, USA
E-mail: schmord@onr.navy.mil

Martha Crosby
University of Hawaii at Manoa
Honolulu, HI 96823, USA
E-mail: schmord@onr.navy.mil

Library of Congress Control Number: 2007929545

CR Subject Classification (1998): I.2, I.4, J.3, H.2.8, H.3-5, C.2, I.4

LNCS Sublibrary: SL 7 – Artificial Intelligence

ISSN   0302-9743
ISBN-10   3-540-73215-2 Springer Berlin Heidelberg New York
ISBN-13   978-3-540-73215-0 Springer Berlin Heidelberg New York

Springer is a part of Springer Science+Business Media

springer.com

© Springer-Verlag Berlin Heidelberg 2007
Printed in Germany

Typesetting: Camera-ready by author, data conversion by Scientific Publishing Services, Chennai, India
Printed on acid-free paper   SPIN: 12080304   06/3180   5 4 3 2 1 0

Foreword

The 12th International Conference on Human-Computer Interaction, HCI International 2007, was held in Beijing, P.R. China, 22-27 July 2007, jointly with the Symposium on Human Interface (Japan) 2007, the 7th International Conference on Engineering Psychology and Cognitive Ergonomics, the 4th International Conference on Universal Access in Human-Computer Interaction, the 2nd International Conference on Virtual Reality, the 2nd International Conference on Usability and Internationalization, the 2nd International Conference on Online Communities and Social Computing, the 3rd International Conference on Augmented Cognition, and the 1st International Conference on Digital Human Modeling.

A total of 3403 individuals from academia, research institutes, industry and governmental agencies from 76 countries submitted contributions, and 1681 papers, judged to be of high scientific quality, were included in the program. These papers address the latest research and development efforts and highlight the human aspects of design and use of computing systems. The papers accepted for presentation thoroughly cover the entire field of Human-Computer Interaction, addressing major advances in knowledge and effective use of computers in a variety of application areas.

This volume, edited by Dylan D. Schmorrow and Leah M. Reeves, contains papers in the thematic area of Augmented Cognition, addressing the following major topics:

- Augmented Cognition Methods and Techniques
- Applications of Augmented Cognition

The remaining volumes of the HCI International 2007 proceedings are:

- Volume 1, LNCS 4550, Interaction Design and Usability, edited by Julie A. Jacko
- Volume 2, LNCS 4551, Interaction Platforms and Techniques, edited by Julie A. Jacko
- Volume 3, LNCS 4552, HCI Intelligent Multimodal Interaction Environments, edited by Julie A. Jacko
- Volume 4, LNCS 4553, HCI Applications and Services, edited by Julie A. Jacko
- Volume 5, LNCS 4554, Coping with Diversity in Universal Access, edited by Constantine Stephanidis
- Volume 6, LNCS 4555, Universal Access to Ambient Interaction, edited by Constantine Stephanidis
- Volume 7, LNCS 4556, Universal Access to Applications and Services, edited by Constantine Stephanidis
- Volume 8, LNCS 4557, Methods, Techniques and Tools in Information Design, edited by Michael J. Smith and Gavriel Salvendy
- Volume 9, LNCS 4558, Interacting in Information Environments, edited by Michael J. Smith and Gavriel Salvendy
- Volume 10, LNCS 4559, HCI and Culture, edited by Nuray Aykin
- Volume 11, LNCS 4560, Global and Local User Interfaces, edited by Nuray Aykin

- Volume 12, LNCS 4561, Digital Human Modeling, edited by Vincent G. Duffy
- Volume 13, LNAI 4562, Engineering Psychology and Cognitive Ergonomics, edited by Don Harris
- Volume 14, LNCS 4563, Virtual Reality, edited by Randall Shumaker
- Volume 15, LNCS 4564, Online Communities and Social Computing, edited by Douglas Schuler
- Volume 17, LNCS 4566, Ergonomics and Health Aspects of Work with Computers, edited by Marvin J. Dainoff

I would like to thank the Program Chairs and the members of the Program Boards of all Thematic Areas, listed below, for their contribution to the highest scientific quality and the overall success of the HCI International 2007 Conference.

Ergonomics and Health Aspects of Work with Computers

Program Chair: Marvin J. Dainoff

Arne Aaras, Norway
Pascale Carayon, USA
Barbara G.F. Cohen, USA
Wolfgang Friesdorf, Germany
Martin Helander, Singapore
Ben-Tzion Karsh, USA
Waldemar Karwowski, USA
Peter Kern, Germany
Danuta Koradecka, Poland
Kari Lindstrom, Finland

Holger Luczak, Germany
Aura C. Matias, Philippines
Kyung (Ken) Park, Korea
Michelle Robertson, USA
Steven L. Sauter, USA
Dominique L. Scapin, France
Michael J. Smith, USA
Naomi Swanson, USA
Peter Vink, The Netherlands
John Wilson, UK

Human Interface and the Management of Information

Program Chair: Michael J. Smith

Lajos Balint, Hungary
Gunilla Bradley, Sweden
Hans-Jörg Bullinger, Germany
Alan H.S. Chan, Hong Kong
Klaus-Peter Fähnrich, Germany
Michitaka Hirose, Japan
Yoshinori Horie, Japan
Richard Koubek, USA
Yasufumi Kume, Japan
Mark Lehto, USA
Jiye Mao, P.R. China
Fiona Nah, USA
Shogo Nishida, Japan
Leszek Pacholski, Poland

Robert Proctor, USA
Youngho Rhee, Korea
Anxo Cereijo Roibás, UK
Francois Sainfort, USA
Katsunori Shimohara, Japan
Tsutomu Tabe, Japan
Alvaro Taveira, USA
Kim-Phuong L. Vu, USA
Tomio Watanabe, Japan
Sakae Yamamoto, Japan
Hidekazu Yoshikawa, Japan
Li Zheng, P.R. China
Bernhard Zimolong, Germany

Human-Computer Interaction

Program Chair: Julie A. Jacko

Sebastiano Bagnara, Italy
Jianming Dong, USA
John Eklund, Australia
Xiaowen Fang, USA
Sheue-Ling Hwang, Taiwan
Yong Gu Ji, Korea
Steven J. Landry, USA
Jonathan Lazar, USA

V. Kathlene Leonard, USA
Chang S. Nam, USA
Anthony F. Norcio, USA
Celestine A. Ntuen, USA
P.L. Patrick Rau, P.R. China
Andrew Sears, USA
Holly Vitense, USA
Wenli Zhu, P.R. China

Engineering Psychology and Cognitive Ergonomics

Program Chair: Don Harris

Kenneth R. Boff, USA
Guy Boy, France
Pietro Carlo Cacciabue, Italy
Judy Edworthy, UK
Erik Hollnagel, Sweden
Kenji Itoh, Japan
Peter G.A.M. Jorna, The Netherlands
Kenneth R. Laughery, USA

Nicolas Marmaras, Greece
David Morrison, Australia
Sundaram Narayanan, USA
Eduardo Salas, USA
Dirk Schaefer, France
Axel Schulte, Germany
Neville A. Stanton, UK
Andrew Thatcher, South Africa

Universal Access in Human-Computer Interaction

Program Chair: Constantine Stephanidis

Julio Abascal, Spain
Ray Adams, UK
Elizabeth Andre, Germany
Margherita Antona, Greece
Chieko Asakawa, Japan
Christian Bühler, Germany
Noelle Carbonell, France
Jerzy Charytonowicz, Poland
Pier Luigi Emiliani, Italy
Michael Fairhurst, UK
Gerhard Fischer, USA
Jon Gunderson, USA
Andreas Holzinger, Austria
Arthur Karshmer, USA
Simeon Keates, USA
George Kouroupetroglou, Greece
Jonathan Lazar, USA
Seongil Lee, Korea

Zhengjie Liu, P.R. China
Klaus Miesenberger, Austria
John Mylopoulos, Canada
Michael Pieper, Germany
Angel Puerta, USA
Anthony Savidis, Greece
Andrew Sears, USA
Ben Shneiderman, USA
Christian Stary, Austria
Hirotada Ueda, Japan
Jean Vanderdonckt, Belgium
Gregg Vanderheiden, USA
Gerhard Weber, Germany
Harald Weber, Germany
Toshiki Yamaoka, Japan
Mary Zajicek, UK
Panayiotis Zaphiris, UK

Virtual Reality

Program Chair: Randall Shumaker

Terry Allard, USA
Pat Banerjee, USA
Robert S. Kennedy, USA
Heidi Kroemker, Germany
Ben Lawson, USA
Ming Lin, USA
Bowen Loftin, USA
Holger Luczak, Germany
Annie Luciani, France
Gordon Mair, UK

Ulrich Neumann, USA
Albert "Skip" Rizzo, USA
Lawrence Rosenblum, USA
Dylan Schmorrow, USA
Kay Stanney, USA
Susumu Tachi, Japan
John Wilson, UK
Wei Zhang, P.R. China
Michael Zyda, USA

Usability and Internationalization

Program Chair: Nuray Aykin

Genevieve Bell, USA
Alan Chan, Hong Kong
Apala Lahiri Chavan, India
Jori Clarke, USA
Pierre-Henri Dejean, France
Susan Dray, USA
Paul Fu, USA
Emilie Gould, Canada
Sung H. Han, South Korea
Veikko Ikonen, Finland
Richard Ishida, UK
Esin Kiris, USA
Tobias Komischke, Germany
Masaaki Kurosu, Japan
James R. Lewis, USA

Rungtai Lin, Taiwan
Aaron Marcus, USA
Allen E. Milewski, USA
Patrick O'Sullivan, Ireland
Girish V. Prabhu, India
Kerstin Röse, Germany
Eunice Ratna Sari, Indonesia
Supriya Singh, Australia
Serengul Smith, UK
Denise Spacinsky, USA
Christian Sturm, Mexico
Adi B. Tedjasaputra, Singapore
Myung Hwan Yun, South Korea
Chen Zhao, P.R. China

Online Communities and Social Computing

Program Chair: Douglas Schuler

Chadia Abras, USA
Lecia Barker, USA
Amy Bruckman, USA
Peter van den Besselaar,
    The Netherlands
Peter Day, UK
Fiorella De Cindio, Italy
John Fung, P.R. China
Michael Gurstein, USA
Tom Horan, USA
Piet Kommers, The Netherlands
Jonathan Lazar, USA

Stefanie Lindstaedt, Austria
Diane Maloney-Krichmar, USA
Isaac Mao, P.R. China
Hideyuki Nakanishi, Japan
A. Ant Ozok, USA
Jennifer Preece, USA
Partha Pratim Sarker, Bangladesh
Gilson Schwartz, Brazil
Sergei Stafeev, Russia
F.F. Tusubira, Uganda
Cheng-Yen Wang, Taiwan

Augmented Cognition

Program Chair: Dylan D. Schmorrow

Kenneth Boff, USA
Joseph Cohn, USA
Blair Dickson, UK
Henry Girolamo, USA
Gerald Edelman, USA
Eric Horvitz, USA
Wilhelm Kincses, Germany
Amy Kruse, USA
Lee Kollmorgen, USA
Dennis McBride, USA

Jeffrey Morrison, USA
Denise Nicholson, USA
Dennis Proffitt, USA
Harry Shum, P.R. China
Kay Stanney, USA
Roy Stripling, USA
Michael Swetnam, USA
Robert Taylor, UK
John Wagner, USA

Digital Human Modeling

Program Chair: Vincent G. Duffy

Norm Badler, USA
Heiner Bubb, Germany
Don Chaffin, USA
Kathryn Cormican, Ireland
Andris Freivalds, USA
Ravindra Goonetilleke, Hong Kong
Anand Gramopadhye, USA
Sung H. Han, South Korea
Pheng Ann Heng, Hong Kong
Dewen Jin, P.R. China
Kang Li, USA

Zhizhong Li, P.R. China
Lizhuang Ma, P.R. China
Timo Maatta, Finland
J. Mark Porter, UK
Jim Potvin, Canada
Jean-Pierre Verriest, France
Zhaoqi Wang, P.R. China
Xiugan Yuan, P.R. China
Shao-Xiang Zhang, P.R. China
Xudong Zhang, USA

In addition to the members of the Program Boards above, I also wish to thank the following volunteer external reviewers: Kelly Hale, David Kobus, Amy Kruse, Cali Fidopiastis and Karl Van Orden from the USA, Mark Neerincx and Marc Grootjen from the Netherlands, Wilhelm Kincses from Germany, Ganesh Bhutkar and Mathura Prasad from India, Frederick Li from the UK, and Dimitris Grammenos, Angeliki Kastrinaki, Iosif Klironomos, Alexandros Mourouzis, and Stavroula Ntoa from Greece.

This conference could not have been possible without the continuous support and advise of the Conference Scientific Advisor, Prof. Gavriel Salvendy, as well as the dedicated work and outstanding efforts of the Communications Chair and Editor of HCI International News, Abbas Moallem, and of the members of the Organizational Board from P.R. China, Patrick Rau (Chair), Bo Chen, Xiaolan Fu, Zhibin Jiang, Congdong Li, Zhenjie Liu, Mowei Shen, Yuanchun Shi, Hui Su, Linyang Sun, Ming Po Tham, Ben Tsiang, Jian Wang, Guangyou Xu, Winnie Wanli Yang, Shuping Yi, Kan Zhang, and Wei Zho.

I would also like to thank for their contribution towards the organization of the HCI International 2007 Conference the members of the Human Computer Interaction Laboratory of ICS-FORTH, and in particular Margherita Antona, Maria Pitsoulaki, George Paparoulis, Maria Bouhli, Stavroula Ntoa and George Margetis.

Constantine Stephanidis
General Chair, HCI International 2007

HCI International 2009

The 13th International Conference on Human-Computer Interaction, HCI International 2009, will be held jointly with the affiliated Conferences in San Diego, California, USA, in the Town and Country Resort & Convention Center, 19-24 July 2009. It will cover a broad spectrum of themes related to Human Computer Interaction, including theoretical issues, methods, tools, processes and case studies in HCI design, as well as novel interaction techniques, interfaces and applications. The proceedings will be published by Springer. For more information, please visit the Conference website: http://www.hcii2009.org/

General Chair
Professor Constantine Stephanidis
ICS-FORTH and University of Crete
Heraklion, Crete, Greece
Email: program@hcii2009.org

Preface

This 3rd edition of the Foundations of Augmented Cognition (FAC) represents the latest collection of diverse and cross-disciplinary research and development (R&D) efforts being performed by international scientists, engineers, and practitioners working in the field of Augmented Cognition. Since the first edition published in 2005, the FAC texts have become the leading science and technology (S&T) references for those working in this burgeoning new field and for those simply aiming to gain a better understanding of what Augmented Cognition R&D truly represents.

The goal of Augmented Cognition research is to create revolutionary human-computer interactions that capitalize on recent advances in the fields of neuroscience, cognitive science, and computer science. Augmented Cognition can be distinguished from its predecessors by the focus on the real-time cognitive state of the user, as assessed through modern neuroscientific tools. At its core, an Augmented Cognition system is a 'closed-loop' in which the cognitive state of the operator is detected in real time with a resulting compensatory adaptation in the computational system, as appropriate (Kruse & Schmorrow, FAC, 1st edition).

Being able to non-invasively measure and assess an operator's cognitive state in real time and use adaptive automation (mitigation) techniques to modify and enhance that user's information processing capabilities in any application context is a goal that could substantially improve human performance and the way people interact with 21st Century technology. Such a goal is now possible thanks in large part to the Augmented Cognition pursuits of numerous government, academic and industrial laboratories and businesses, and the continued investments from agencies such as: the National Science Foundation (NSF), National Research Council (NRC), the National Institutes of Health (NIH), and the Department of Defense (e.g., Defense Advanced Research Projects Agency [DARPA], Office of Naval Research [ONR], Air Force Research Laboratory [AFRL], Disruptive Technologies Office [DTO] and the Army Soldier Center). The aggressive goals and objectives in these funded programs have fostered the development of many neurophysiological-based tools and techniques that are maturing enough to become feasible toolsets for HCI researchers, designers and practitioners in their pursuit of improving human-computer system efficiency, effectiveness and general user accessibility.

The numerous and varied Augmented Cognition methods, techniques, and applications that are flourishing today range from basic academic research to industrial and military fielded operational and training systems to every day computing and entertainment devices. This edition provides a snapshot of such R&D and represents cross-disciplinary collaborations and contributions from more than 200 international Augmented Cognition researchers and developers of varied backgrounds, including psychology, neurobiology, neuroscience, cognitive neuroscience, mathematics, computer science and engineering, human-systems integration and training, and general human factors and ergonomics. To capture the essence of the S&T that is emerging from such cross-disciplinary collaborations, this edition is divided into two main sections. The first section is focused on general Augmented Cognition methods and techniques, including physiological and neurophysiological measures (e.g., EEG, fNIR), adaptive techniques, and sensors and algorithms for cognitive state estimation. The second section is devoted to discussions of various Augmented Cognition applications (e.g., simulation and training, intent-driven user interfaces, closed-loop command and control systems), lessons learned to date, and future directions in Augmented Cognition-enabled HCI.

The articles in this edition could not have been successfully compiled and edited without the due diligence in support received from the 2007 HCII Augmented Cognition Thematic Area paper session co-chairs and from the Associate Editors, COL Mike Russo of USAARL and Dr. Martha Crosby of the University of Hawaii at Manoa.

With each new FAC edition, I continue to be amazed at the quality and progress of the discoveries, innovations, and applications that Augmented Cognition scientists and technologists are cultivating because such discoveries, innovations, and breakthrough S&T solutions are no longer the exception—they have become the norm.

Dylan D. Schmorrow

Table of Contents

Part I: Augmented Cognition Methods and Techniques

Part II: Applications of Augmented Cognition

Part I

Augmented Cognition Methods and Techniques

Development of Gauges for the QinetiQ Cognition Monitor

Andy Belyavin, Chris Ryder, and Blair Dickson

QinetiQ Ltd, Farnborough, UK
ajbelyavin@qinetiq.com

Abstract. This paper describes the development of a new version of the calibration procedure for the QinetiQ Cognition Monitor so that it can be implemented to support the development of a cognitive cockpit at NAVAIR. A new signal cleaning procedure for processing the electro-encephalogram (EEG) automatically is outlined and the results from tests in the UK and US are summarized. It is concluded that estimates of the content of the EEG signal at high frequencies are important to gauges measuring verbal and spatial workload. The combination of results from UK and US tests suggests that the cleaning procedure is effective, although increased robustness of the verbal gauge is desirable.

Keywords: EEG, signal cleaning, calibration, cognitive workload.

1 Introduction

At the heart of an adaptive Augmented Cognition system there has to be a methodology for the conversion of information that reflects the physiological or psychological state of the operator(s) into a series of gauges that relate to key aspects of human performance. In the majority of systems it has been assumed that the most important gauges should measure aspects of task demand (workload) in the context of human capacity restraints, and there is an implicit assumption that other forms of performance degradation will be captured. A prototype version of the Cognition Monitor that was designed to achieve these objectives was described in 2005 [1]. The development of the gauges for the prototype was based on three principles:

- Gauges should be based on a model of cognitive workload to provide face validity;
- Gauges should be calibrated on relatively pure tasks involving few mental processes since this provides a clear test of sensitivity;
- Amplitude-invariant measures should be used as input to the state classifiers as this supports reproducibility.

The Prediction of Operator Performance (POP) workload model [2] was used as the basis of the construction of the gauges, although the results were corrected for individual task performance. A monitoring task with varying levels of workload was used as the basis of calibration [1] and the measures of the Electro-encephalogram (EEG) were coherences and gains between electrodes in defined frequency bands.

D.D. Schmorrow, L.M. Reeves (Eds.): Augmented Cognition, HCII 2007, LNAI 4565, pp. 3–12, 2007.

This system was effective, but there were problems with porting it to a generic platform. So that the Cognition Monitor could be incorporated in a new version of the Cognitive Cockpit at NAVAIR the calibration procedure was redesigned to be executed reliably and rapidly with minimal operator intervention. In addition, the system was extended to include the development of distinct verbal and spatial gauges.

To meet the extended requirements of the Cognition Monitor a number of modifications to the overall approach were made. New calibration tasks were selected so that distinct verbal and spatial gauges could be calibrated. An automatic system for cleaning the data was developed and calculation of the gauge equations was standardized. The complete procedure was implemented in a single application to simplify execution. The new calibration tasks are described in Section 2. The cleaning procedure is outlined in Section 3 and the fitting procedure is described in Section 4, including the results from trials at QinetiQ and NAVAIR.

2   Calibration Tasks and Workload

The selection of tasks to serve as the basis of the calibration was a central component of the procedure. For the purposes of calibration it was decided that the tasks should satisfy three criteria:

- It should be possible to vary the task load in a controlled manner, so that a number of levels of workload could be defined;
- The task workload should be dominated by either verbal or spatial activity;
- The POP workload should be readily calculated.

There was substantial previous experience with two tasks that met all three criteria: the two-dimensional compensatory tracking task and the Bakan vigilance task [3]. Previous work indicated that compensatory tracking was dominated by spatial workload and that the Bakan task was dominated by verbal workload.

The spatial load was calibrated using the two-dimensional compensatory tracking task. The joystick provided first-order (velocity) control in both x and y directions and the disturbances were applied to the velocities of the cursor in both dimensions. The forcing function was constructed from separate combinations of six sinusoids for x and y, selected so that the pattern appeared random and the disturbance repeated only after a long interval. The frequency content of the forcing functions determines workload by affecting the frequency of operator interventions. This content was controlled through a single parameter, defined as *Dwork*, and the amplitudes were adjusted so that the root mean square error (RSME) of the cursor position in the absence of a participant response was independent of the value of *Dwork*, maintaining task difficulty.

A visual version of the Bakan vigilance task was used to generate verbal workload. Single digits in the range 0–9 were displayed in the middle of the screen for 500 milliseconds and successive stimuli were displayed at fixed inter-stimulus intervals. The target demanding participant response was a three-digit sequence of odd–even–odd digits. The rate at which targets appeared in the sequence was controlled at 5% of presentations. The Bakan task was displayed on the same screen as the compensatory tracking task, so that it was possible to choose either task alone or both together.

The cognitive workload associated with the compensatory tracking task was estimated using the POP model in the Integrated Performance Modelling Environment (IPME). The results were compared with experimental observations and a good match was found for *Dwork* set to 0.75 [2]. The model was used to estimate workload and RMSE for a range of values of *Dwork*, and the results for RMSE were compared with a small experimental test sample as displayed in Figure 1. There was good agreement between observed and predicted changes in RMSE and it was concluded that the estimates of workload for the tracking task could be used in the calibration.

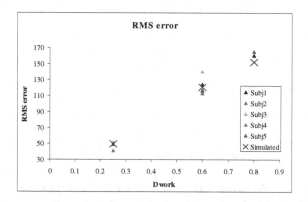

Fig. 1. Observed RMSE (Subjects 1–5) and predicted RMSE changes with *Dwork*

Previous work with the visual Bakan task established a simple relationship between the inter-stimulus interval and POP workload [2]. These results were incorporated in the IPME model so that estimates of workload for the dual-task case could be calculated and used in the calibration. The model indicated that there should be slight interference between the tracking and Bakan tasks, resulting in small increments in verbal or spatial workload in the dual-task case, and these were applied in the calibration procedure. The final version of the calibration procedure comprised 10 tests each of 150 seconds' duration:

- Single tracking task: *Dwork* = 0.25, 0.5 and 0.75;
- Single Bakan task: ISI = 0.75, 1.25, and 2.0 seconds;
- Simultaneous tracking/Bakan task: *Dwork* = 0.25/ISI = 2.0, *Dwork* = 0.25/ISI = 0.75, *Dwork* = 0.75/ISI = 2.0, and *Dwork* = 0.75/ISI = 0.75.

3 Pre-processing the EEG Data

The electro-encephalogram (EEG) was recorded from fourteen silver/silver chloride electrodes applied at the sites of the international 10-20 electrode placement system as indicated in Figure 2 [4]. All signals were amplified with respect to linked electrodes applied to the mastoid processes and vertical and horizontal derivations of the electro-oculogram (EOG) were recorded from electrodes placed above and below the right eye and lateral to the outer canthus of each eye respectively. A ground electrode was applied to the mid-forehead. Data were digitized at a rate of 1024 samples/second, with a 500 Hz low pass filter and a high pass of 0.01Hz.

The recorded signals were analyzed in blocks of 4 seconds' length for tests using a single tracking task and blocks of length corresponding to the nearest multiple of the inter-stimulus interval for tests involving a Bakan task. The workload value assigned to a test is assumed to be uniform for the period and it is important to ensure that the activities within each analysis block are as uniform as possible.

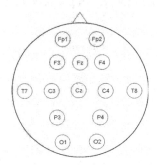

Fig. 2. Scalp placement of electrodes

For each block, multivariate kurtosis [5] was calculated using the data from the fourteen scalp electrodes. The contracted kurtosis tensor, C, was calculated where C is defined as

$$C_{ij} = k_{ijkl}\, \delta_{kl} \tag{1}$$

where summation is implied over repeated suffices, δ is the Kronecker delta and k_{ijkl} is the kurtosis tensor.

The eigenvalues and eigenvectors of C were calculated. If either the value of multivariate kurtosis or the largest eigenvalue of C did not support the rejection of the hypothesis of multivariate normality at 99%, no further analysis of the sample was conducted. If normality was rejected, a mixture of two normally distributed populations with a common zero mean but different variances was fitted to the one-dimensional projection of the sample onto the first eigenvector. Those observations for which the likelihood of belonging to the population with larger variance exceeded 0.5 were then corrected by projecting the sample value orthogonal to the first eigenvector. The procedure was then repeated for the second and third eigenvectors if the corresponding eigenvalues exceeded the 99% point for the largest eigenvalue. If any observations were corrected the complete procedure was repeated for the whole sample. If the sample was swept 12 times and there was still evidence for non-normality the block was rejected from the subsequent analysis.

The output from the pre-processing procedure is displayed in Figure 3. The dashed trace is the raw data and the superimposed solid trace is the "cleaned" data. From the data displayed in Figure 3 it is clear that the procedure correctly detects the effect of the blink visible on the EOG channel and provides a plausible correction to the observations. Apart from the major correction for the blink, the other adjustments in this block are relatively slight. For many blocks the adjustments include high-frequency corrections that are probably associated with temporalis muscle action. The procedure was compared with direct regression on the EOG channels as a method of removing eye movement effects [6]. The kurtosis-based method did not prove completely effective at correcting for all eye movements, but it was found that the regression method occasionally *introduced* anomalies into the data and that on balance the current procedure is more satisfactory.

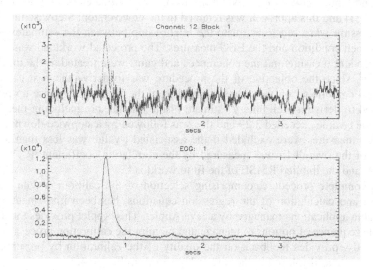

Fig. 3. Cleaned and raw data for a single 4 second block

Following data cleaning, the spectrum was calculated in each of the nine frequency bands defined in Table 1. The cross spectra between the 14 scalp electrodes in the nine bands were derived to yield estimates of the coherence between electrode pairs and the gains of one electrode relative to another, providing 1629 inter-correlated variables describing the EEG in each block.

Table 1. Frequency bands selected for spectral analysis

Band	Range UK analysis[1] (Hz)	Range US analysis[2] (Hz)
Delta	0.0 – 3.5	0.0 – 3.5
Theta	3.5 – 8.0	3.5 – 8.0
Alpha1	8.0 – 10.2	8.0 – 10.2
Alpha2	10.2 – 14.1	10.2 – 14.1
Beta1	14.1 – 20.0	14.1 – 20.0
Beta2	20.0 – 30.0	20.0 – 30.0
Gamma Low	30.0 – 47.0	30.0 – 47.0
Gamma Mid	53.0 – 70.0	47.0 – 57.0
Gamma High	70.0 – 100.0	63.0 – 100.0

---

[1] The bands exclude a small region around 50Hz.
[2] The bands exclude a small region around 60 Hz. These exclusions were made to disregard the predominant source of electromagnetic interference introduced from the mains power supply.

4   Calibration Procedure

4.1   Fitting the Calibration Equations

The prototype version of the Cognition Monitor used linear combinations of coherences and gains between electrode pairs to provide estimates of workload based on the EEG [1] and this approach was retained in the new version. Stepwise multiple linear regression was used to estimate the relationship between the estimates of workload in each condition and the EEG measures. The projected workload was treated as the dependent measure and the coherences and gains were treated as the independent measures, since the objective of the procedure was to derive the best estimates of workload conditional on the values derived from the EEG. A stepwise-up procedure was used to derive a preliminary estimate of the relationship including measures for which the t-value exceeded 3.29 and this was followed by a stepwise-down procedure in which measures were excluded if the associated t-value was less than 3.29. The quality of the overall fit was measured by the correlation coefficient, R^2, for the regression and the implied RMSE of the fit to workload.

The complete procedure, comprising selection of the calibration data files, data cleaning and calculation of the regression equations, has been implemented as two executable applications managed by a Java Applet. This Applet provides the user with a simple sequence of options to manage and monitor the calibration process and, more importantly, provides feedback on the quality of the calibration by presenting summary findings as displayed in the screenshot shown in Figure 4.

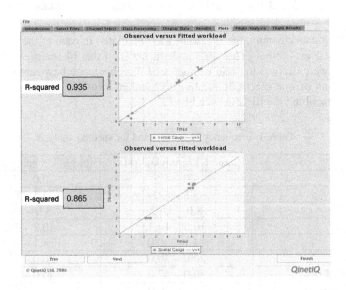

Fig. 4. Screenshot from the Java Applet showing the plots of observed and fitted workload

The points displayed in Figure 4 correspond to the means for observed and fitted values for each 150-second condition. The R^2 value *includes* the variation between 4-second blocks within the period in the values calculated from the EEG, since the calibration is calculated at the level of the individual blocks. A high R^2 value implies both a good fit to the differences in mean values between the conditions and a relatively constant value within each condition, corresponding to good discrimination between workload levels.

4.2 Testing the Calibration Procedure

The complete calibration procedure was tested in the UK using a designed experiment. Eight participants were tested on two days. On both experimental days an extended calibration procedure of 15 test sessions was applied at the start of the experimental period, which included all the conditions of the standard calibration defined in Section 3, extended to cover all possible pairs of the six single-task conditions. After completion of the calibration, there was a short rest period, followed by three 5-minute tests in the Cognitive Cockpit with graded flying difficulty. Three test sessions of 150 seconds' duration with a different verbal logic task were recorded with controlled levels of inter-stimulus interval. The logic task involved reading statements concerning the status of a hypothetical vehicle system and then choosing an action that is consistent with the apparent state of the vehicle. Finally, the participant was tested for 10 minutes in the Cognitive Cockpit in which the logic task was executed for 30 seconds out of each minute.

The data were recorded for all sessions at a frequency of 1024 Hz. The calibration data were analyzed using the full procedure and estimates were made for Verbal and Spatial workload gauges. The data from the test sessions were cleaned using blocks with 4-second durations and the gauges applied to the cleaned data to derive estimates of the workload. The R^2 values were recorded for each calibration for Verbal and Spatial gauges. The estimates of the Verbal and Spatial gauges were collated for the flight and logic task sessions and were assessed for sensitivity using repeated-measures Analysis of Variance (ANOVA) treating Experimental Day (D), Task type (T), and Level of Workload (L) as fixed factors.

The final stage of the assessment of the overall procedure was conducted at NAVAIR. A single participant was tested using the basic calibration procedure described in Section 3 on 10 occasions. On a subset of the runs the participant was also tested in the cockpit and with the logic task. The R^2 values for the calibrations were recorded and, when available, the estimated workload gauges for the tests. No systematic analysis was conducted on the US results.

4.3 Results

The R^2 values generally exceeded 0.650 for both verbal and spatial calibrations in the UK and US, consistent with reasonable fits for the gauges. A plot of the values for the two gauges is displayed in Figure 5. As can be seen from the plot the majority of the values for spatial gauges are larger than the corresponding values for verbal gauges. In addition, the lower values mainly corresponded to earlier trials (Day 1 in the UK; earlier tests in the US).

The set of independent variables is clearly inter-correlated from the way it is constructed and there is considerable variation in the set of variables fitted in the calibration equations on each occasion. A count of the incidence of variables by electrode and band was conducted for both verbal and spatial gauges and it was concluded that more than half the independent variables for the verbal gauge depended on measures in frequency bands 8 and 9 and more than a third for the spatial gauge were from the same source.

The analysis of the UK experiment indicated that there was a difference for both verbal and spatial gauges between the logic task and the flying task – F = 7.32, df = 1,32 p < 0.05 for the verbal gauge; F = 10.76, df = 1,32 p < 0.01 for the spatial gauge. In addition there was evidence for an effect of Day in the spatial gauge – F = 9.30, df = 1,6 p < 0.05. The means are displayed in Table 2. The residual error terms in both analyses indicate the level of variation for 4-second blocks in terms of their prediction – 1.821 for the verbal gauge and 0.911 for the spatial gauge.

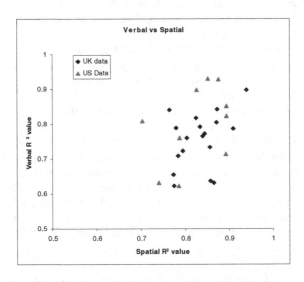

Fig. 5. Plot of the R^2 values for verbal gauges against spatial gauges for UK and US tests

Table 2. Means for the verbal and spatial gauges for the tasks in the UK experiment

		Verbal gauge		Spatial gauge	
		Day 1	Day 2	Day 1	Day 2
Low workload	Flying Task	3.18	3.88	6.24	4.92
	Logic Task	3.80	4.50	5.68	4.36
Medium workload	Flying Task	3.19	3.90	6.42	5.10
	Logic Task	3.81	4.52	5.86	4.54
High workload	Flying Task	3.43	4.13	6.40	5.07
	Logic Task	4.05	4.75	5.84	4.51

5 Discussion

For both the UK and US calibrations the EEG signal in the high frequency bands is an important component of both verbal and spatial gauges. There are problems in the use of signals at these frequencies as they are vulnerable to contamination from electromagnetic interference from the mains supply, computer displays, EOG artefact (especially blinks) and temporalis muscle action. The cleaning procedure has been tested on signals that include known artefacts of this kind and it appeared to be effective at detecting and removing the majority of artefacts if applied to blocks of 4-second length.

Investigation of variation in the selected block length for cleaning and analysis indicated that the verbal gauge calibrated most successfully if the block length selected for cleaning and calibration was a multiple of the Bakan task inter-stimulus interval. Initial tests in the US employing a conventional analogue notch filter at 60 Hz to condition the signal prior to digitization almost completely eliminated any relationship between the EEG and verbal workload. On the basis of this evidence it is argued that the calibrations of verbal and spatial workload that use the high-frequency content in the EEG appear to be using content in the signal that relates to verbal or spatial activity. The main problem with the use of the high frequencies is the forced difference between UK and US analyses due to the different mains power supply frequencies. On the basis of the results obtained to date, it appears that the procedure works as well in the US as it does in the UK, despite the change in the banding of medium and high gamma activity.

The analysis of the UK designed experiment indicates that it is possible to distinguish the flying task from the logic task using the calibrated gauges. Analysis of individual runs in the US reveals that on most occasions the same result holds for similar patterns of flying task and logic task, although some calibrations of the verbal gauge appear to fail this test. The analysis of the UK data indicates substantially greater residual variability in estimates of verbal load than spatial load. It is not clear whether this pattern reflects true variability in verbal activity or failure of the calibration procedure. It is worthy of note that it is extremely difficult, perhaps impossible, to model very low verbal workloads due to the continual verbalisation that humans perform.

The revision of the procedure has provided a systematic and reproducible method for calibrating verbal and spatial workload gauges based on the EEG in a reasonable period of time. It is desirable that the procedure be extended to include other signals with different characteristics such as cortical blood oxygenation levels assessed using a Functional Near Infrared (fNIR) methodology to complement the EEG analysis and increase the robustness of the procedure. The use of high-frequency EEG signals is relatively novel and further work is needed to demonstrate that the overall procedure is robust.

References

1. Belyavin, A.J.: Construction of appropriate gauges for the control of Augmented Cognition systems. In: Proceedings of the 1st International Conference on Augmented Cognition, Las Vegas, NV (2005)
2. Belyavin, A.J., Farmer, EW.: Modeling the workload and performance of psychomotor tasks. In: 2006 Conference on Behavior Representation in Modeling and Simulation (BRIMS)-022. Baltimore (2006)

3. Bakan, P.: Extraversion–introversion and improvement in an auditory vigilance task. Br. J. Psychol. 50, 325–332 (1959)
4. Jasper, H.H.: The ten-twenty electrode system of the international federation. Electroencephalography and Clinical Neurophysiology 10, 371–375 (1958)
5. Mardia, K.V.: Measures of multivariate skewness and kurtosis with applications. Biometrika 57, 519–530 (1970)
6. Gratton, G., Coles, MG., Donchin, E.: A new method for off-line removal of ocular artifact. Electroencephalography and Clinical Neurophysiology 55(4), 468–484 (1983)

Quantitative EEG Changes Under Continuous Wakefulness and with Fatigue Countermeasures: Implications for Sustaining Aviator Performance

Carlos Cardillo[1], Michael Russo[2], Patricia LeDuc[2], and William Torch[3]

[1] Navigator Development Group, Inc. - US Army Aeromedical Research Laboratory
Fort Rucker, AL 36362
[2] US Army Aeromedical Research Laboratory, Fort Rucker, AL 36362
[3] Washoe Sleep Disorders Center and Eye-Com Corporation, Reno, NV

Abstract. Sleep management, naps, and pharmacological countermeasures may be combined to assist operators requiring around the clock tasks. We used QEEG methodologies to elucidate the CNS effects of stimulants (caffeine, modafinil, and dextroamphetamine) combined with sleep deprivation. Thirty-two UH-60 pilots were tested during 87 hours of continuous wakefulness using frequency analysis to quantify eight EEG channels for up to 20 frequency bands. Data were analyzed using brain mapping techniques and repeated measure analysis of variance. After 50 hours awake, all groups showed the sleep deprivation effects: increases in slow-waves and decreases in alpha activity. Caffeine and modafinil groups appeared to have the greatest degree of effect, producing delays on the electrophysiological deterioration for up to 46 hours into the sleep deprivation cycle. Additional analysis of these data could systematically correlate cognitive tasks and QEEG data for each pharmacologic intervention.

Keywords: QEEG, CNS, Brain Mapping, Artifact, Epoch.

1 Introduction

Military operations require Army aviation units to operate around the clock during time of conflict. The success of military operations, particularly in special operations units, depends on maintaining the speed and momentum of continuous day-night operations [1]. To achieve optimal cognition, sustain judgment and decision-making, and enhance performance, we need to understand how to best manage personnel and missions involving acute total sleep deprivation, partial chronic sleep deprivation, and demanding cognitive workloads. To this end, sleep management, naps, and pharmacological fatigue countermeasures may be combined to assist in achieving successful military outcomes.

Amphetamine-like stimulants and caffeine are known to increase wakefulness, and their effects on the brain are well reported. Modafinil, unlike amphetamines, ameliorates sleep deprivation effects without generally stimulating the central nervous system (CNS).

D.D. Schmorrow, L.M. Reeves (Eds.): Augmented Cognition, HCII 2007, LNAI 4565, pp. 13–22, 2007.

The most direct indicator of CNS functionality is the electroencephalogram (EEG). The validity and reliability of quantitative electroencephalography (QEEG) methodologies in the classification of psychotropics were demonstrated based on retrospective and prospective studies [2, 3]. Itil [4] discovered psychotropic properties of new drugs that could not be predicted by animal pharmacology and biochemistry. Additionally, EEG signals are clearly influenced by sleep deprivation [5, 6].

In the context of such research, a large number of studies have employed different approaches in efforts to detect and classify patterns of EEG changes associated with pharmacological interventions or with total sleep deprivation. In the present study, QEEG methodologies were used in an effort to elucidate the CNS effects of the study drugs combined with the sleep deprivation factor. To determine the electrophysiological effects and help reveal the performance enhancing modes of action of the study drugs (caffeine 200 mg, dextroamphetamine 5 mg, and modafinil 100 mg) on sleep deprived pilots, the following neurophysiological hypotheses are stated: a) sleep deprivation of up to 68 hours will fragment awake EEG patterns, producing an increase on slow wave activities (1.3 – 7.5 cps) and a decrease on alpha and faster activities (7.5 – 14 cps) and b) caffeine, dextroamphetamine, and modafinil will generate predictable and significant improvements on the EEG patterns when compared to placebo.

2   Methods

2.1   EEG Recording and Processing

EEG was continuously recorded from scalp electrodes in a standard unipolar setting (F7-A1, F8-A2, C3-A1, C4-A2, FZ-A1, CZ-A2, O1-A1, and O2-A2). The EEG isolated amplifier low and high filter was set at 1.3Hz and 70Hz respectively. To accomplish the analog to digital conversion of the EEG signal, a 12 bit, 16 channels A-D board was used.

All EEG channels were processed and quantified using frequency analysis, where up to 20 frequency bands on each channel can be analyzed on-line using time-domain [7]. The resulting variables are average amplitude, amplitude variability, average frequency, and frequency deviation, along with twenty frequency bands (1.3-2.5, 2.5-3.5, 3.5-4.5, 4.5-5.5, 5.5-6.5, 6.5-7.5, 7.5-8.5, 8.5-9.5, 9.5-10.5, 10.5-11.5, 11.5-12.5, 12.5-13.5, 13.5-15.0, 15.0-17.0, 17.0-20.0, 20.0-26.0, 26.0-32.0, 32.0-38.0, 38.0-48.0, 48.0Hz and up.). The selected epoch size for all channels was 5 seconds. Automatic online artifact detection was used during EEG recording, followed by an off-line visual inspection of the EEG to further select artifact free epochs for the analysis.

2.2   Procedures

QEEGs were performed for 10 minutes, awake and with eyes closed. Each period was divided into two sub-periods, with a 1-2 minute break between. During the first five minutes, standard eyes closed, resting EEG was performed and no attempt was made to control the subject's vigilance level (resting recording labeled RR). During the second sub-period, a random acoustic stimulus was presented at 7-45 second intervals and subjects were asked to respond to the stimulus by raising their thumb (simple reaction time task labeled RT). The RT task was not intended to measure performance but rather to keep the vigilance at a relative constant level (control of spontaneous drowsiness).

Thirty-two subjects were scheduled for a full week at the Laboratory in groups of two and under the same drug condition. Due to technical mishap, data from two pairs of subjects (on placebo and caffeine) could not be included in the analysis. Thus, data presented represents six subjects on caffeine, eight on dextroamphetamine, eight on modafinil, and six on placebo. Among several other tests performed on this study, participants completed three QEEG training sessions during the first three days to adapt to the procedure and also to compare their QEEGs to a normative database to ensure that there were no significant deviations from normative patterns. Subsequent testing took place on 13 additional QEEG sessions (Fig. 1).

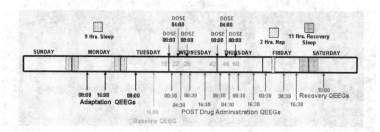

Fig. 1. Timeline for drug and QEEG administration. Green numbers indicate hours awake at the dose time. QEEGs were recorded 30-40 minutes after drug administration.

3   Results

3.1   Multi-lead Evaluation

To determine the effects on multiple areas of the brain, a dynamic brain map system was used. With dynamic brain mapping, it is possible to view delta, theta, alpha, and beta activities of a multichannel QEEG recording in the form of a brain map. This way, the average amounts of activities are displayed by color coding on an anatomically correct brain image. The QEEG data are displayed on the brain image in the exact location where the recording electrodes were placed and the areas between electrode locations are interpolated using blending algorithms that depict the regional spread of the brain's electrical activity. The means of delta (1.3-3.5 Hz), theta (3.5-7.5 Hz), alpha (7.5-13.0 Hz), and beta (13.0 Hz and up) activity, over all subjects, for each session and for each drug group were averaged. Fig. 2 shows maps for the baseline QEEGs for each group.

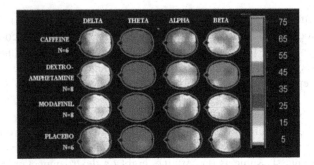

Fig. 2. Frequency bands and drug groups represented as brain maps. As expected for baseline QEEGs all groups showed similar average power (color code) on each frequency band. The dextroamphetamine group showed a slight different alpha and beta activities when compared to caffeine, modafinil, and placebo.

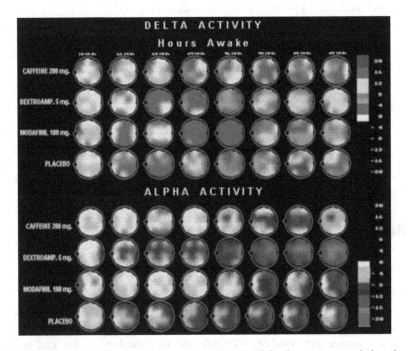

Fig. 3. Dynamic brain map changes from baseline for each of the drug groups tended to show a systematic increase of delta activity and a decrease of alpha activity in all time periods

The percentage of delta, theta, alpha, and beta bandwidths in the recorded time periods were calculated before- and after- drug administrations, and the changes in each of the time periods (18, 22, 26, 34, 42, 46, 50, and 58 hours awake) were compared with baselines. To measure the absolute difference before and after drug, the pre-drug (baseline) was subtracted from each post-drug brain map to obtain a change from baseline state. Accordingly, any changes in brain map can be attributed to the effect of drug, sleep deprivation, or both combined. In this way, the effects of caffeine, dextroamphetamine, modafinil and placebo could be visualized as independent factors, as depicted in Fig. 3.

Caffeine, modafinil and dextroamphetamine, in that order, showed less increases of delta activity over all areas of the brain up until 42 hours of sleep deprivation (after three doses). Although alpha activity had the tendency to decrease as the number of hours awake increased, modafinil and caffeine groups showed virtually no changes from baseline until 46 hours of sleep deprivation, suggesting a delay in the deterioration or decrease of alpha activity. Dextroamphetamine and placebo, however, produced a systematic decrease of alpha activity after the second dose (22 hours awake) with the highest increases shown on dextroamphetamine rather than placebo.

A systematic but slight increase of theta after the fourth session is seen in all drug groups with the least increase in the caffeine group. However, no marked changes for any of the drug groups were seen in the theta activity levels. Beta activity showed a systematic but slight increase in all sessions and in all drug groups, with modafinil having the least changes from baseline. The placebo group had a decline in beta activity after 46 hours, which produced a marked decrease of the activity after 50 and 58 hours of SD.

3.2 Detection of Drug Effects

Measures of the 20 frequency bands were collapsed into 4 frequency bands to generate delta, theta, alpha, and beta activities for an occipital (O2), central (CZ), and frontal (FZ) electrode. To remove variability among subjects in the same group and to determine performance trends over the sleep deprivation cycle, a repeated measures analysis of variance (ANOVA) was carried out for each frequency band. We used the four drug groups (caffeine 200 mg, dextroamphetamine 5 mg, modafinil 100 mg, and placebo) as between-subjects factors, and the eight QEEG sessions (18, 22, 26, 34, 42, 46, 50, and 52 hours) as a repeated measure. Each of these QEEGs was subtracted from the baseline QEEG to create score changes on delta, theta, alpha, and beta bandwidths at O2, CZ, and FZ. The analysis was performed on the overall recording time using both RR and RT segments. In checking assumptions, Box's M and Mauchly's test of sphericity were used. To circumvent the compound symmetry violation in all variables, we used lower-bound epsilon adjustment which represents the most conservative approach.

Delta Activity. The different pharmacological conditions resulted in distinct changes in delta activity. Drug main effects and Session effects were present at the three electrodes. The drug effects at O2, $F(3, 52) = 3.01$, $p = 0.038$; CZ, $F(3, 52) = 7.51$, $p = 0.0002$; and FZ, $F(3, 52) = 3.56$, $p = 0.020$ were tested using Tukey HSD post-hoc comparisons. This test revealed significant differences between modafinil and placebo at O2 and CZ and between caffeine and placebo at CZ and FZ. Caffeine was also discriminated with dextroamphetamine at CZ. The session effects at O2, $F(1, 52) = 6.39$, $p = 0.015$; CZ, $F(1, 52) = 26.81$, $p < 0.0001$; and FZ, $F(1, 52) = 52.49$, $p < 0.0001$ were primarily due to a significant linear increase in delta activity from the first to the last sessions of the sleep deprivation cycle. In addition, there was a session by drug interaction at CZ, ($F = 3.36$, $p = 0.026$). The mean score changes for the three leads are shown in Fig. 4.

Alpha Activity. There was no drug main effect in the frontal electrode, FZ. However, alpha activity showed significant drug effects at O2, $F(3, 52) = 3.12$, $p = 0.034$ and CZ, $F(3, 52) = 3.61$, $p = 0.019$. Post-hoc analysis disclosed that dextroamphetamine is significantly different from modafinil at O2 and significantly different from caffeine at CZ. There were significant session effects at O2, $F(1, 52) = 27.14$, $p < 0.0001$; CZ, $F(1, 52) = 34.90$, $p < 0.0001$; and FZ, $F(1, 52) = 44.94$, $p < 0.0001$, produced by significant linear and quadratic decreases in all leads. The session by drug interactions at CZ, $F = 3.51$, $p = 0.022$ and at FZ, $F = 2.39$, $p = 0.042$ were essentially the result of high variability over time among the four groups. Fig. 5 depicts the score changes for alpha over the sessions.

Theta Activity. Theta activity did not show drug effects or interactions at any of the three leads. The only significant change was a session effect at O2, $F(1, 52) = 4.84$, $p = 0.032$, due to a constant linear increase across all sessions. Fig. 6 shows mean changes.

Beta Activity. Similar to theta activity, beta did not produced drug effects or interactions at any electrode. There were, however, session effects at CZ, $F(1, 52) = 4.35$, $p = 0.042$ and FZ, $F(1, 52) = 9.89$, $p = 0.003$, due to a significant linear decrease in both leads. Beta activity is shown in Fig. 6b.

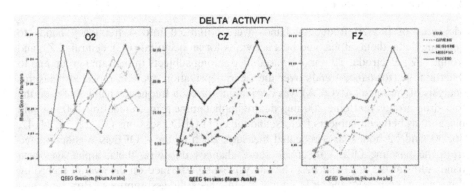

Fig. 4. Mean score changes for delta activity at O2, CZ, and FZ

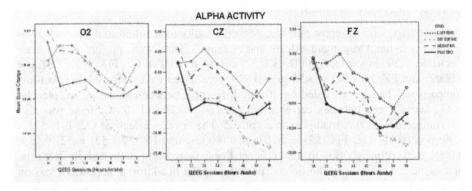

Fig. 5. Mean score changes for alpha activity at O2, CZ, and FZ

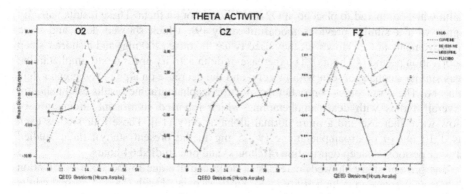

Fig. 6. Mean score changes for theta activity at O2, CZ, and FZ

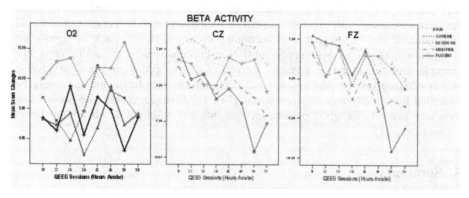

Fig. 6b. Mean score changes for beta activity at O2, CZ, and FZ

4 Discussion

The results from the repeated measure ANOVA during the drug sessions tend to confirm the trends observed on the multi-lead evaluation using brain mapping. Theta and beta activities were not sensitive to pilot fatigue due to sleep deprivation or drug effects. The most predominant changes were established in delta and alpha activities showing session effects at all electrodes with linear increase on delta and linear and quadratic decrease on alpha. Delta activity showed significant between-subject responses at the three leads and alpha at the occipital and central leads. Also, all three significant interactions were produced at these activities mainly in the central and frontal regions.

Caffeine produced less significant changes from baseline and was clearly differentiated from placebo and dextroamphetamine. Caffeine attenuated the slow waves and slightly increased beta activity, consistent with a recent study on the effects of caffeine on the brain [8]. Similar to caffeine, modafinil produced fewer changes from baseline on the slow activities during the first 34 hours and on alpha activity during the first 42 hours of wakefulness. Modafinil showed virtually no changes on beta activity throughout the entire cycle and showed improvement on delta when compared to placebo at O2 and CZ but not on theta. These results partially agree with a similar previous modafinil study [9], which showed delta and theta improvements at CZ. However, they used twice the dose (200 mg) and a shorter sleep deprivation period (40 hours). The increase of delta activity under dextroamphetamine was similar to changes seen with placebo and the decrease on alpha even greater than placebo. These outcomes contradict the electroencephalographic results established in several studies with dextroamphetamine which reported significant attenuation of slow-wave increase and a more normal alpha activity [10]. These four studies each used 10 mg of dextroamphetamine (vs. 5 mg in the present study); three studied shorter periods of sleep deprivation (40 hours) and one studied 64 hours.

The present study showed increases in delta activity due to the sleep deprivation factor; an increase in delta activity is primarily associated with sleep in normal adults [11]. It is also known that sleepiness and fatigue elevates slow-wave activities [6]. However, this study revealed virtually no increases in theta activity across the sleep deprivation cycle, for all groups, including placebo. An increase in theta activity alone has been associated with generalized performance decrements on cognitive tasks [12] and reduced speed of response to incoming stimuli [13]. The lack of significant changes in theta activity may represent effort levels consistently across all groups. For example, motivation can counteract the effect of sleep deprivation, since the adverse effects of sleep loss on performance and behavior are very labile and can easily be cancelled by suitably arousing conditions [14]. Furthermore, it was also shown that monetary rewards for good performance maintained baselines levels for 36 hours without sleep [15].

5 Summary

We identified the extent and distribution of electrophysiological changes induced by sleep deprivation and three different wake promoting agents. We found that after 50 hours, the groups showed EEG signs of sleep deprivation: increases in slow-waves (mainly delta) and decreases in alpha waves. The electrophysiological effects of sleep deprivation are reversed during the initial 42 hours with smaller increases in delta activity by caffeine, modafinil, or dextroamphetamine, and less deterioration of alpha activities for caffeine and modafinil when compared to baseline levels. Caffeine and modafinil appeared to have the greatest degree of effect with respect to producing delays on alpha activity deterioration. Alpha activity remained close to baseline levels for the first 46 hours. A marked deterioration of alpha after the second dose (22 hours awake) was observed in the dextroamphetamine and placebo groups.

The multi-lead evaluation shows that the dynamic brain mapping of subjects from all drug groups had similar (normal) QEEG patterns when well rested and without drugs (baseline QEEGs)., We can confirm that sleep-deprived subjects have different QEEG spectrums (profiles) than those not sleep-deprived. Interestingly, those QEEG profiles for the sleep-deprived subjects are opposite to the QEEG changes induced by psychostimulants in well rested healthy volunteers. Based on this, we hypothesize that QEEG differences between non sleep-deprived and sleep-deprived subjects are due to quantifiable changes in the brain produced by sleepiness and fatigue. Correct doses of psychostimulants would reverse that imbalance, so that the drug-induced changes of the QEEG would be toward the normalization of function of the sleep deprived brain.

In order to determine the best adaptability to sustained operations, future studies are needed to establish the CNS effective doses for the drugs, based on the magnitude of the deprivation. Individual differences that exist for personality features, physiological reasons, and circadian typology may be accounted for by titrating drug dose to both performance and electrophysiological measures. Additional analysis of this study data could systematically correlate cognitive tasks and QEEG data for each pharmacologic intervention. Through QEEG, measures are available that may be used to directly relate the brain effects of the drug to the performance effects.

Acknowledgements. We would like to recognize the team effort of all personnel within the U.S. Army Aeromedical Research Laboratory and all volunteer helicopter pilots who made possible this study. This research was supported by SOCOM, USAMRMC and by the EyeCom Eye-tracker Congressional Research Program. The research work reported in this paper and involving human subjects follows the MRMC / HSRRB A-13257 human use protocol. The opinions expressed herein are those of the authors do not reflect the policy of the Army or the DoD.

References

1. DA, Army Aviation Operations. FM 1-100. Washington DC: Department of the Army (1997)
2. Herrmann, W.M., Fichte, K., Itil, T.M., Kubicki, S.: Development of a classification rule for four clinical therapeutic psychotropic drug classes with EEG power spectrum variables of human volunteers. Pharmakopsychiat. 12, 20–34 (1979)
3. Itil, T.M., Shapiro, D.M., Herrmann, W.M., Schulz, W., Morgan, V.: HZI System for EEG parameterization and classification of psychotropic drugs. Pharmakopsychiat. 12, 4–19 (1979)
4. Itil, T.M.: The use of computerized bio-electrical potentials (CEEG) in the discovery of psychotropics. Drug Develop. Res. 4, 373–407 (1981)
5. Lorenzo, I., Ramos, C.A., Guevara, M.A., Corsi-Cabrera, M.: Effect of total sleep deprivation on reaction time and waking EEG activity in man. Sleep 18, 346–354 (1995)
6. Pigeau, R.A., Heselgrave, R.J., Angus, R.G.: Psychological measures of drowsiness as estimators of mental fatigue and performance degradation during sleep deprivation. Electric and magnetic activity of the central nervous system: Research and clinical applications in aerospace medicine. In: Proceeding of the North Atlantic Treaty Organization Advisory Group for Aerospace Research and Development, vol. 432(21), pp. 1–16 (1987)
7. Itil, T.M., Eralp, E., Itil, K., Manco, A., Akman, A.: CEEG dynamic brain mapping, a new method to evaluate brain function in different psychological and drug conditions. Electric and Magnetic Activity of the CNS; Research and Clinical Applications in Aerospace Medicine, Trondheim, Norway May 25-29, Organized by the Advisory Group for Aerospace Research and Development, North Atlantic Treaty Organization (AGARD) Medical Panel (1987)
8. Hammond, D.C.: The Effects of Caffeine on the Brain: A Review. J Neurother 7(2), 79–89 (2003)

9. Caldwell, J.A., Caldwell, J.L., Smythe, N.K., Hall, K.K.: A double-blind, placebo-controlled investigation of the efficacy of Modafinil for sustaining the alertness and performance of aviators: a helicopter simulator study. Psychopharmacology (Berl) 150(3), 272–282 (2000)

10. Caldwell, J.A., Hall, K.K.: Placebo-controlled studies sustaining the alertness and flight performance of aviators with Dexedrine®. RTO Lecture Series 232. Sleep/Wakefulness Management in Continuous/Sustained Operations, pp. 7–5 (2001) RTO-EN-016 AC/323(HFM)-064) TP/39

11. Ray, W.: The electrocortical system. In: Cacioppo, T., Tassinary, L.G. (eds.) Principles of Psychophysiology: Physical, social, and inferential elements, pp. 385–412. Cambridge University Press, Cambridge, England (1990)

12. Belyavin, A., Wright, N.A.: Changes in electrical activity of the brain with vigilance. Electroencephalographic Clinical Neurophysiology 66, 137–144 (1987)

13. Ogilvie, R.D., Simons, I.: Falling asleep and waking up: A comparison of EEG spectra. In: Broughton, R.J., Ogilvie, R.D. (eds.) Sleep, arousal, and performance, pp. 73–87. Birkhauser, Boston (1992)

14. Wilkinson, R.T.: The measurement of sleepiness. In: Broughton, R.J., Ogilvie, R.D. (eds.) Sleep, Arousal and Performance, pp. 254–265 Birkhauser: Boston (1992)

15. Horne, J.A., Pettitt, A.N.: High incentive effects on vigilance performance during 72 hours of total sleep deprivation. Acta Psychologica. 58, 123–139 (1985)

Exploring Calibration Techniques for Functional Near-Infrared Imaging (fNIR) Controlled Brain-Computer Interfaces

Peter Wubbels[1], Erin Nishimura[1], Evan Rapoport[1], Benjamin Darling[2], Dennis Proffitt[2], Traci Downs[1], and J. Hunter Downs, III[1]

[1] Archinoetics, LLC. 700 Bishop St. Ste 2000. Honolulu, HI 96813
[2] Proffitt Perception Lab. University of Virginia. 102 Gilmer Hall, Box 400400. Charlottesville, VA 22904

Abstract. Functional near-infrared sensing (fNIR) enables real-time, non-invasive monitoring of cognitive activity by measuring the brain's hemodynamic and metabolic responses. We have demonstrated the ability for non-vocal and non-physical communications through detecting directed changes in cognitive tasks. Building upon past research, this paper reports methods that allow the calibration of the fNIR oxygenation signal to better be used in more complex communicative and selection tasks. This work is then discussed in the context of a faster, continuous fNIR brain-computer interface framework.

Keywords: Functional Near-Infrared Imagining, Brain-Computer Interface, fNIR, BCI.

1 Introduction

Near-infrared technology uses optical imaging in the near-infrared spectrum to monitor relative changes in oxy- and deoxy-hemoglobin in human tissue based on the scattering response of light in these wavelengths [1]. Functional near-infrared (fNIR) sensing monitors relative oxygenation in the tissue of specific brain regions during cognitive activity. Lagging several seconds after the onset of neuronal activity, a hemodynamic and metabolic response leads to increases in blood flow and an increase in the concentration of oxy-hemoglobin in the area of the brain required for that activity. These regional rises in oxygenation can be detected as activations through fNIR sensing in that area, and then used to control software applications, such as brain-computer interfaces [5].

State of the art fNIR brain-computer interfaces (BCIs) use binary selection, or the process of choosing between two options, to control an interface or communicate. While researchers have shown that this method can be up to 95 percent accurate, it is slow, requiring upwards of two minutes to select an item from a list of eight possibilities [7].

D.D. Schmorrow, L.M. Reeves (Eds.): Augmented Cognition, HCII 2007, LNAI 4565, pp. 23–29, 2007.

In an attempt to address this speed bottleneck, researchers are exploring the feasibility of more complex selection schemes. This study specifically looked at the controllability of gradient selection interface with an fNIR system. A gradient selection can be understood as analogous to moving a cursor in one-dimension over a series of "bins" or choices. Eventually, a user will stop their cursor over a particular "bin," signalling the selection of the option it represents. However, using fNIR to control this new type of interface is not trivial or straightforward. Whereas in current systems selection blocks are post-processed, to truly take advantage of gradient selection interfaces, a user will need to control the system in real-time. This goal and the fact that the selection algorithm is no longer limited to a single yes or no distinction, point to a need for a new framework for calibration, thresholding and interface control. The algorithms used for post-processed binary selection need to be updated and applied in a new, more adaptable and dynamic manner.

This paper aims to address the first step in bringing more continuous selection methods to fNIR controlled BCIs by testing three calibration methods used to transform relative oxygenation data into a more meaningful and immediately controllable signal. This initial calibration stage is vitally important to an fNIR controlled BCI because the physiological process being measured can vary drastically from trial to trial, and even on an hourly basis. Calibration thus serves to provide not only a more useful derived signal, but also a current range for operation. Among other things, the current range can also function as an indicator of signal quality, or even a user's level of control. Once research into the calibration of the fNIR signal for gradient interfaces matures, the results can be used to significantly improve fNIR BCI speed and selection rate.

2   Methods

The OTIS system, developed by Archinoetics, LLC, is a continuous-wave fNIR system that was used in this study to monitor regional oxygenation changes due to cognitive activity. This system, shown below in Figure 1, is a portable device with up to two sensors that allow for sensing over areas of the scalp with hair, a distinct feature of this fNIR sensing system. The system uses three wavelengths of NIR light and has a sampling frequency of 34.8Hz [4].

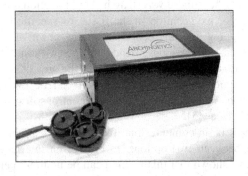

Fig. 1. The OTIS system with a two-channel sensor

2.1 Study Design

For this study, three calibration techniques (explained below) for transforming relative oxygenation data derived from an fNIR system into a gradient interface control signal were tested. All techniques were themselves initialized through the analysis of two, ten second periods of data. In the first period, the test subject was asked to generate an active response, whereas in the second, the subject was asked to relax. Since the fNIR sensor was placed over Broca's area, the designated active task was subvocal counting and the inactive task was nonsense syllable repetition; these tasks were selected because the former task strongly activates Broca's area whereas the latter task does not. The two blocks were designed to give a realistic expected range of values for the particular technique and they were recorded separately before each of the three trials. A ten second recording period was chosen based on previous analysis of two trials, each with the same subject and each containing an active and rest task. These data showed all calibration techniques stabilized at or around six seconds (Figure 2).

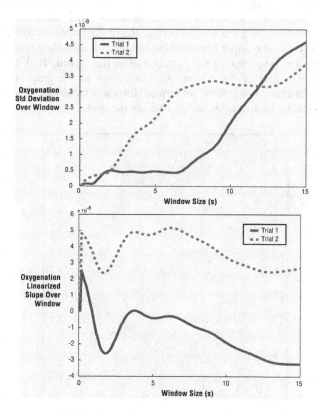

Fig. 2. Window size versus value derived from calibration technique over two trials. *Technique 2 (Standard Dev.)* is shown on the top, while *Technique 3 (Best Fit Line Slope)* is shown at bottom. The graph for *Technique 1 (Simple Max/Min)* is not provided because it requires no stabilization time.

After the initialization was completed, one of three calibration techniques was used to establish an expected range for subsequent data. The range was calculated in the following manner:

- *Technique 1(Simple Max/Min):* Global maximum and minimum oxygenation values were pulled from the initialization data. These specify the limits for subsequent data points.
- *Technique 2 (Standard Dev.):* Using a moving window of six seconds (192 data points), the standard deviation was calculated for the windowed data. The maximum and minimum observed values were recorded and used as the range for later data.
- *Technique 3 (Best Fit Line Slope):* Using a moving window of six seconds (192 data points), the best fit line was calculated using the least squares method for the windowed data. The maximum and minimum observed slope for this line were recorded and used as the range for subsequent data.

Once the range was calculated, testing proceeded with a series of activation trials. A user was shown a graph of their current data, as calculated by one of the three techniques, and then asked to make the signal move to either the upper or lower half of the screen by the end of a ten second period. Responses were classified into one of four groups: 1) Above the upper bound of the range. 2) Below the lower bound of the range. 3) Within the range and in the correct half of the screen. 4) Within the range, but in the incorrect half of the screen. An illustration of the graph is provided in Figure 3. Ten selection tasks were performed for each technique, and the targeted selection half was not known to the subject before the trial.

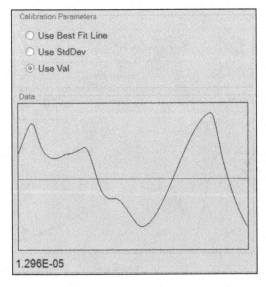

Fig. 3. The calibration screen. Currently, *Technique 1 (Simple Max/Min)* is being used. The horizontal line on the graph denotes the division between the upper and lower halves used in the trials. The value in the bottom left corner is the current data point as calculated by the calibration technique. For *Technique 1*, the value is a representation of the relative oxygenation values in the blood.

2.2 Data Analysis

The data gathered was logged in raw optical form with timestamps and state information. Relative oxy-hemoglobin concentrations were calculated using a modified Beer-Lambert equation. This oxygenation signal was then ideally filtered with zero phase distortion using a low-pass filter to remove higher frequency noise and normalized to the mean and standard deviation of the filtered signal over each trial. This derived data stream was then used as the source for all calibration techniques. Finally, the output of each calibration technique was graphed in the interface for the subject to monitor.

2.3 Subjects and Environment

For this case study we used one male subject with experience using an fNIR system. The subject was seated in a comfortable chair in a dark, quiet room with only the light from the computer monitor. The subject's eyes were closed throughout the initialization periods, but open during the testing phase to allow feedback. Each selection task was performed over ten seconds, followed by a five second rest period.

3 Results

Ten trials per technique, each conducted with the same subject, had accuracy rates of 10%, 80% and 90% for *Techniques 1, 2,* and *3* respectively. A detailed chart of the trial results is presented in Table 1.

Table 1. Trial Results. Accuracy for each response target (upper or lower half) is provided, as well as data addressing "nearly correct" responses. These include responses that were out of range, but adjacent to the target half.

Accuracy	Technique 1 (Simple Max/Min)	Technique 2 (Standard Dev.)	Technique 3 (Best Fit Slope)
Total	**10%**	**80%**	**90%**
Lower Half	20%	80%	80%
Upper Half	0%	80%	100%
Out of Range	**90%**	**10%**	**10%**
Correct Half	40%	10%	10%
Adj. Total	50%	90%	100%

Researchers noticed that the trials run for *Technique 1* were affected by a downwards trend that overwhelmed any activations. In this case, the range initially set was too limited, and the values fell below the lower bound soon after the first trial was run. To make this technique more robust, a new range would need to be recalculated every few minutes. This would assure the current values would stay within range and be usable as a control signal for a BCI.

Also of note is the final row in Figure 4. This row specifies the number of trials during which the user managed to move the oxygenation values towards the correct half, but ended with a value outside of the preset range. This can be understood as slightly overshooting a target, and still indicates a "nearly correct" response for that trial. If these trials are counted as correct responses, then *Technique 2* and *Technique 3* would have accuracy levels of 90% and 100% respectively.

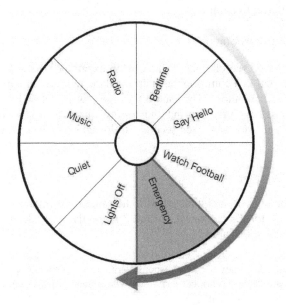

Fig. 4. A wheel interface. Each division of the circle represents a different idea or action that can be communicated or enacted by a user of the BCI. The highlighted section travels around the circle in the direction indicated by the arrow as a user increases their activation level. When it stops, the action designated in the highlighted section is executed.

4 Discussion

This exploratory study was designed to evaluate the feasibility of three different calibration methods by examining their real-time controllability. This work serves to validate both *Technique 2* and *Technique 3* as potential calibration options for an fNIR BCI. This is the vital first step in creating a continuously controlled BCI framework for assistive or augmentative purposes.

To further develop this calibration stage, more will be done on fine-tuning the parameters of each calibration algorithm. *Technique 1* in particular could benefit significantly from a more dynamic approach to the maximum and minimum value calculation.

As the calibration process for continuous and gradient BCIs advances, work can begin to proceed on the next steps in the BCI pipeline. In the meantime, however, because this new continuous control signal is available, more complex interfaces with many more choices can be presented to a user. This will significantly increase the speed and bit-rate of a BCI. These new interfaces will also be more intuitive, allowing direct selection of an item, rather than a binary narrowing down of a list.

The authors have already prototyped a number of ideas for more continuous BCIs, including a wheel interface that consists of a circle, divided into many "slices" that a user can select. The interface translates the fNIR control signal into "force" that spins the wheel until it rests on a selection (see Figure 4). Small increases in the control signal cause small rotations of the wheel, while a larger increase can lead to a full revolution.

Once perfected, these interfaces will open up a new world of possibilities for both disabled and able-bodied users. For the severely disabled, such as those suffering from amyotrophic lateral sclerosis (ALS), or Lou Gehrig's disease, a BCI offers a means of communication after all other physical means have failed. ALS patients, in the later stages of their illness, often lose all motor control and a BCI is one of their only options for continued linguistic interaction [2], [3]. For able-bodied users, a faster and more robust BCI offers a different kind of benefit. It allows for non-verbal communication, monitoring of cognitive load and perhaps even control of a remote or wearable system [7].

References

1. Cope, M.: The development of a near-infrared spectroscopy system and its application for non-invasive monitoring of cerebral blood and tissue oxygenation in the newborn infant, Ph.D. Thesis, Dept. of Medical Physics and Bioengineering, University College London (1991)
2. Feldman, M.H., M.D.: Physiological observations in a chronic case of locked-in syndrome. Neurology 21(5), 459–478 (1971)
3. Leon-Carrion, J., Van Eeckhout, P., Dominguez-Morales, M.R, Perez-Santamaria, F.J.: The locked-in syndrome: a syndrome looking for therapy. Brain Injury 16(7), 571–582 (2002)
4. Nishimura, E.M., Stautzenberger, J.P., Robinson, W.J., Downs, T.H., Downs III, J.H.: A New Approach to fNIR: the Optical Tomographic Imaging Spectrometer (OTIS). In: HCI International 2005 (2005)
5. Nishimura, E.M., Darling, B.A., Rapoport, E.D., Zadra, J.R., Downs, T.H., Proffitt, D.R., Downs III, J.H.: Functional Near-Infrared Sensing for Brain-Computer Interface Control By a Locked-In Individual. In: Augmented Cognition International 2006 (2006)
6. Rapoport, E.D., Downs, T.H., Proffitt, D.R., Downs III, J.H.: First Investigations of an fNIR-Based Brain-Computer Interface. In: HCI International 2005 (2005)
7. Rapoport, E.D., Nishimura, E.M., Darling, B.A., Zadra, J.R., Downs, T.H., Proffitt, D.R., Downs III, J.H.: Brain-Computer Interface for Communications Using Functional Near-Infrared Imaging (fNIR). In: Augmented Cognition International 2006 (2006)

A Sensor Positioning System for Functional Near-Infrared Neuroimaging

Ping He[1], Betty Yang[1], Sarah Hubbard[2], Justin Estepp[1], and Glenn Wilson[2]

[1] Department of Biomedical, Industrial and Human factors Engineering,
Wright State University, Dayton, OH, U.S.A.
[2] Air Force Research Laboratory, Wright-Patterson Air Force Base, U.S.A.

Abstract. In cognitive studies using functional near-infrared (fNIR) techniques, the optical sensors are placed over the scalp of the subject. In order to document the actual sensor location, a system is needed that can measure the 3D position of an arbitrary point on the scalp with a high precision and repeatability and express sensor location in reference to the international 10-20 system for convenience. In addition, in cognitive studies using functional magnetic resonance imaging (fMRI), the source location is commonly expressed using Talairach system. In order to correlate the results from the fNIR study with that of the fMRI study, one needs to project the source location in Talairach coordinates onto a site on the scalp for the placement of the fNIR sensors. This paper reports a sensor positioning system that is designed to achieve the above goals. Some initial experimental data using this system are presented.

Keywords: 10-20 system, brain mapping, fNIR, neuroimaging, Talairach.

1 Introduction

Recent advancements in the functional near-infrared (fNIR) technique have expanded its potential applications in mapping the human brain's hemodynamic response to various cognitive tasks. In most studies reported in the literature, the optical sensors were placed over the forehead [1-3]. However, in many functional neuroimaging studies, the location nearest to the activation area in the brain may not be on the forehead [4]. In such cases, the optical sensors need to be placed at various locations on the scalp in order to optimize the reception of fNIR signals. In order to document the actual sensor location in a study, a device is needed that can measure the 3D position of an arbitrary point on the scalp with a high precision and repeatability. In addition, in cognitive studies using functional magnetic resonance imaging (fMRI), the source location is commonly expressed using the Talairach coordinate system. In order to correlate the results from the fNIR study with that of the fMRI study, one needs to project the source location in Talaraich coordinates onto a site on the scalp and then place the fNIR sensors over that site. Finally, since the most recognized standard for scalp electrode localization is the international 10-20 system used in the EEG studies [5], it may be convenient to express the fNIR sensor location in reference to the international 10-20 system, but a much higher spatial resolution is required (the typical 10-20 system has only 19 electrode locations). This paper reports a sensor

D.D. Schmorrow, L.M. Reeves (Eds.): Augmented Cognition, HCII 2007, LNAI 4565, pp. 30–37, 2007.

positioning system that is designed to achieve the above goals. Some initial experimental data using this system are presented.

2 Method

2.1 The Three-Dimensional (3D) Sensor Positioning System

The sensor positioning system is built upon an electromagnetic tracking device manufactured by Polhemus (3SPACE® FASTRAK®, Colchester, Vermont). The device has a system electronics unit, a transmitter, and four receivers numbered as Receiver 1 to Receiver 4. Receiver 1 is a hand-held stylus which is used to point to a location for position measurement. Receivers 2, 3, and 4 have the same shape of a small cube that will be attached to the subject's head to form a reference coordinate system. Upon receiving a reading command, each receiver reports its real-time position and orientation with reference to the transmitter. For the current application, only the 3D position coordinates are used.

Since the head of the subject can move during an experiment, the goal of the sensor positioning system is to define the location of a point in a head system (HS) that is unique to a particular subject, a method similar to EEG channel localization in the 10-20 system. This goal is achieved by establishing three coordinate systems and suitable transformations of coordinates between the systems. The following is a description of the three coordinate systems as shown in Fig. 1.

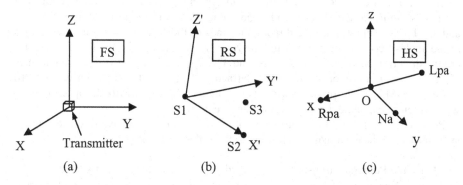

Fig. 1. (a) The fixed coordinate system (FS). (b) The reference coordinate system (RS) where S1, S2, S3 are three reference receivers which form the X'-Y' plane of RS. (c) The head system (HS) where Na is the nasion, and Lpa and Rpa are left and right pre-auricular points. These three points define the x-y plane of HS.

1) The fixed system (FS, the X-Y-Z system): which is defined by the fixed Polhemus transmitter. The real-time positions of the four receivers are all expressed in this fixed system (Fig. 1(a)).
2) The reference system (RS, the X'-Y'-Z' system): which is defined by the three cubic receivers. The centers of these three receivers (S1, S2, S3 in Fig. 1(b)) form the X'-Y' plane of RS. The origin is the position of Receiver 2. The line

from Receiver 2 to Receiver 3 defines the X'-axis. The position of Receiver 4 indicates the positive direction of the Y'-axis. The Z'-axis and the actual Y'-axis are defined by the right hand rule of convention (Fig. 1(b)).

3) The head system (HS, the x-y-z system): which is established using the following three points of the subject's head: the left pre-auricular point (Lpa), the right pre-auricular point (Rpa), and the nasion (Na). These three points form the x-y plane of HS. The origin O is the middle point of the line connecting Lpa and Rpa. The line from O to Rpa defines the x-axis. The Na indicates the positive direction of the y-axis. The z-axis and the actual y-axis are defined by the right hand rule of convention (Fig. 1(c)).

Notice that RS and HS both move with respect to FS during an experiment, but the relation between these two systems is fixed as long as the three receivers attached to the subject's head do not move relatively to the subject's head.

The position of a location pointed by the stylus receiver is originally expressed by the 3D coordinates in FS. These coordinates are first transformed to the coordinates in RS, and then to that in HS. The general method of transformation of coordinates involving translation and rotation can be described by the following matrix equation:

$$\begin{pmatrix} X' \\ Y' \\ Z' \end{pmatrix} = \begin{bmatrix} T_{11} & T_{12} & T_{13} \\ T_{21} & T_{22} & T_{23} \\ T_{31} & T_{32} & T_{33} \end{bmatrix} \begin{pmatrix} X - X_0 \\ Y - Y_0 \\ Z - Z_0 \end{pmatrix} \tag{1}$$

where: X-Y-Z are the coordinates in the old system; X'-Y'-Z' are the coordinates in the new system that has an origin O' whose coordinates in the old system are X_0, Y_0 and Z_0; T_{11}, T_{12} and T_{13} are the direction cosines of the X' axis which are the cosines of the angles between the X' axis and the X, Y, Z axes, respectively; T_{21}, T_{22}, and T_{23} are the direction cosines of the Y' axis; and T_{31}, T_{32}, and T_{33} are the direction cosines of the Z' axis. For a coordinate system defined by three points, as shown in Fig. 1(b) and 1(c), a MATLAB program <points2cosines>, which is available upon request, was written to calculate the T-matrix of the direction cosines.

Prior to actual position measurement in an experiment, the above three coordinate systems need to be established according to the following procedures.

- Place the Polhemus transmitter to a fixed location near the subject's head.
- Attach Receivers 2, 3, and 4 to the subject's head using an elastic bandage near the line of the ears but not to cover any standard 10-20 channel locations.
- Using the stylus receiver (Receiver 1) to point to the left pre-auricular point (Lpa), and then send a reading command. The Polhemus system always provides the positions of all four receivers. Thus, at each reading, a real-time RS is formed, and the position of Lpa originally expressed in FS is mapped to a point in RS.
- The same procedure is repeated for the right pre-auricular point (Rpa) and nasion (Na). At each reading, a new, real-time RS is formed and a corresponding point of Rpa (or Na) in RS is determined.
- The HS can then be established and the transformation between RS and HS is established.

For every new subject, the positions (3D coordinates in HS) of the standard 19 channels are measured and saved according to the following procedures. The locations of the standard 19 channels of the subject are marked by an experienced operator according to the method described by Jasper [5]. After performing the procedures for establishing coordinate systems described above, the operator moves the stylus receiver to each of the 19 channels. At each location, the coordinates of that channel are first mapped to the real-time RS, and then to HS. In the end, the coordinates of all 19 channels in HS are stored in a file which will be used in future experiments with that subject.

2.2 Several Utility Programs for Use with the Above Sensor Positioning System

2.2.1 Display the 19 Channel Positions on a 2D Round Head Model

The locations of the standard 19 channels for a particular subject are originally expressed in three dimensions. To present this location information on a computer screen, one choice is to display a 3D head model with the 19 channels shown on the surface of the head [6]. A disadvantage of such an approach is that the operator usually cannot see all the channels at once and often needs to rotate the head model to see different channels. Since the purpose of model display is to observe the position of a particular point on the head in reference to the 10-20 system, we chose to display a 2D head model. A custom 3D to 2D conversion is written that maps Cz to the center of the head model and maps all other 18 channels proportionally. Fig. 2(a) shows an example of the displayed 19 channels for a particular subject. The figure also shows the position of an arbitrary point P measured by this system and consequently displayed on the model. Alternatively, the operator can enter the 3D coordinates of a reference point and display that point on the head model for sensor placement.

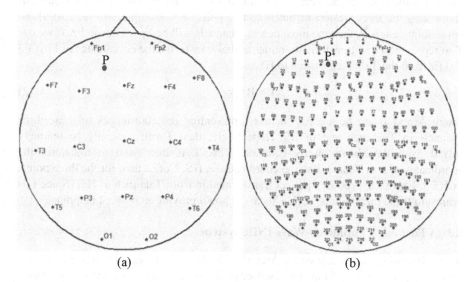

(a)   (b)

Fig. 2. (a) 2D display of the 19 channel locations of the 10-20 system for a particular subject. P is an arbitrary point on the scalp. (b) 2D display of a dense grid containing 217 points that are expanded from the original 19 channel locations. P is the same point as in (a).

2.2.2 Generate a Dense Grid for Displaying Expanded 10-20 Channel Positions

In order to be able to express the location of a point in the 10-20 system more precisely, we expand the locations of the 19 channels by generating a dense grid using curvilinear interpolation. Fig. 2(b) shows the expanded 10-20 system based on the one shown in Fig. 2(a). For this particular expansion, a total of 217 points are generated, numbered, and displayed. This grid of points allows a more precise localization of a point on the scalp in reference to the 10-20 system.

2.2.3 Convert the Position of a Point on the Cortical Surface from the Talairach System to the Head System

There is a rich literature of functional neuroimaging studies using fMRI. In these studies, the area of activation in the brain is often expressed in Talairach coordinates. In order to correlate the results from the fNIR study with that of the fMRI study, one needs to project the source location in Talairach coordinates onto a site on the scalp of a particular subject so that the fNIR sensor can be placed over that site for the fNIR study. A MATLAB program is written to perform a transformation from the given Talairach coordinates to the coordinates in the head system (HS) of a particular subject. This program uses the data provided by Okamoto et. al. [Table 3 in 6] that list the average Talairach coordinates of the cortical projection points of the 19 channels of the 10-20 system based on the measurements performed on 17 healthy subjects. The program first loads the coordinates of the 19 channels in HS of a particular subject that were previous measured and stored (see section 2.1). We now have two sets of the coordinates of the 19 channel locations: a set in Talairach and a set in HS. The operator is prompted to enter a set of Talairach coordinates that represents a particular point of interest on the cortical surface. The program then calculates the distance between this point to each of the 19 channels (in Talairach) and selects the three nearest channels to this point. For example, in Fig. 2(a), if the point of interest is P, then the three nearest channels will be Fp1, F3, and Fz. If we use **T** to represent a 3x3 transformation matrix that transforms the coordinates of Fp1, F3 and Fz from the Talairach system to HS:

$$AT = B . \tag{2}$$

where A and B are both a 3x3 matrix representing the coordinates of these three channels in Talairach and in HS, respectively, then T can generally be uniquely solved from the above matrix equation. This T is then used to transform the coordinates of P in Talairach to the coordinates in HS. Notice that, for the three points Fp1, F3, Fz, this T produces perfect transformation from Talairach to HS. Since P is nearest to these three points, such a 'local' T should provide an optimal mapping.

2.3 A Portable Continuous-Wave fNIR System

An fNIR system manufactured by Archinoetics (Honolulu, Hawaii) was used in this study to test the utility of the above sensor positioning system. The fNIR system uses an optical probe consisting of a photo-emitter and two photo-sensors. The miniature emitter and sensors are each installed on a slender, spring-loaded leg which can easily penetrate the subject's hair to reach the scalp surface. The system operates at three wavelengths (760, 810, and 850 nm) and provides relative changes in blood oxygenation.

3 Preliminary Test Results with the System

3.1 Repeatability of the System for Position Measurement

To test the practical repeatability of the sensor positioning system, we marked three sites on one subject's scalp near C_z, F_3 and F_4, and repeated five times the entire procedure of position measurement; that includes attachment of the three reference receivers to the subject's head, establishment of the three coordinate systems, and measurement of the positions of the three sites. During the measurements, the head of subject was free to move. The standard deviation of the measurement at each site is 0.85 mm, 1.09mm, and 1.05 mm, respectively.

3.2 Hemodynamic Response to Three Mental Tasks Measured Near F_7

It has been reported that the frontal cortex corresponding to Brodmann area 45 is often activated in response to an N-back working memory task [4]. In this experiment, we place the optical sensor near channel F_7 and let the subject to perform three kinds of cognitive tasks: silent number counting, a verbal N-back task in which a series of letters are used as the stimuli, and a spatial N-back task that used a set of four squares to form different spatial patterns. Fig. 3 shows an example of the relative change in oxygenation in a test where the three tasks were performed in the following sequence: number counting, spatial 3-back task, and verbal 3-back task. It is evident that, during each cognitive task, the blood oxygenation increases.

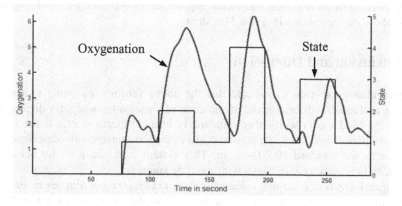

Fig. 3. Relative oxygenation level measured at a location near F_7. State indicator: 1. – relaxed, 2 – silent counting, 3 – verbal 3-back task, 4 – spatial 3-back task.

3.3 Topographic Map of Hemodynamic Response to a Mental Task

In this study, the locations of the standard 19 channels of a subject were first measured, and a dense grid of 217 points was generated. The fNIR sensor was systematically moved to each of the points located in the front half of the head to record the relative change in tissue oxygenation during a verbal 3-back task and a spatial 3-back task. For each task, a color-coded topographic map was derived that showed the level of activation (increase in oxygenation, red color) and deactivation (decrease in oxygenation, blue color) over the front half of the scalp. The results of the verbal task are presented in Fig. 3(a) and the results of the spatial task are presented in Fig. 3(b). Both figures show that the strongest activation takes place near F_7 and F_8.

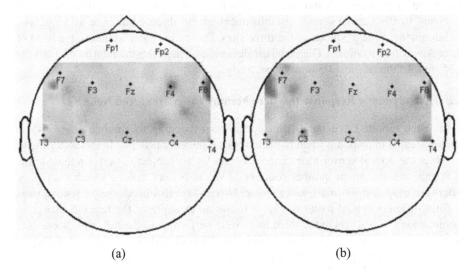

(a)   (b)

Fig. 4. (a) Topographic map of hemodynamic response in verbal 3-back test. (b) Topographic map of hemodynamic response in spatial 3-back test.

4 Conclusion and Discussion

Our preliminary experiences indicate that the above sensor positioning system can precisely and reliably determine the 3D position of a site on the scalp. By displaying a background head model with either standard 19 channel locations or a dense grid of expanded channel locations, the sensor position can be conveniently described with reference to the standard 10-20 system. This system could be used for sensor re-positioning in repeated experiments with multiple subjects.

The transformation from the Talairach coordinates to the coordinates in the head system allows for correlating the source location in the fNIR study on a particular subject with that reported in the fMRI literature. The numerical values used for deriving the transformation matrix in this study are solely based on the data provided by Okamoto et. al. [Table 3 in 6], which have not been corroborated by other studies.

Due to the variation in the coordinates reported in the fMIR literature, the result of transformation may also show some degree of variation. For example, Okamoto et al. gave Talairach xyz coordinates (in mm) of the cortical projection point of Fp1 as (21.3, 68.0, -3.0). But in Table II of [4], three different sets of Talairach coordinates are given for the region of the frontal pole (Brodmann area 10 corresponding to Fp1): (-36, 44, 20), (-38, 44, 20), and (-32, 42, 10). If one enters these three sets of coordinates, our program will produce three points that are all closer to F_3 than to Fp1. We are currently investigating the source and scope of this discrepancy. We also plan to conduct more experiments with several subjects to fully test the capability and limitations of the system.

Acknowledgments. This work was supported in part by the AFRL/DAGSI Ohio Student-Faculty Research Fellowship Program and the Air Force Summer Faculty Fellowship Program.

References

1. Hoshi, Y., Tamura, M.: Detection of dynamic changes in cerebral oxygenation coupled to neuronal function during mental work in man. Neuroscience Letters 150, 5–8 (1993)
2. Takeuchi, Y.: Change in blood volume in the brain during a simulated aircraft landing task. Journal of Occupational Health 42, 60–65 (2000)
3. Izzetoglu, M., Izzetoglu, K., Bunce, S., Ayaz, H., Devaraj, A., Onaral, B., Pourrezaei, K.: Functional near-infrared neuroimaging. IEEE Trans. Neural Syst. Rehab. Eng. 13, 153–159 (2005)
4. Owen, A., McMillan, K., Laird, A., Bullmore, E.: N-back working memory paradigm: A meta-analysis of normative functional neuroimaging studies. Human Brain Mapping 25, 46–59 (2005)
5. Jasper, H.: The ten-twenty electrode system of the International Federation. Electroencephalogr. Clin. Neurophysio. 10, 367–380 (1958)
6. Okamoto, M., Dan, H., Sakamoto, K., Takeo, K., Shimizu, K., Kohno, S., Oda, I., Isobe, S., Suzuki, T., Kohyama, K., Dan, I.: Three-dimensional probabilistic anatomical cranio-cerebral correlation via the international 10-20 system oriented for transcranial functional brain mapping. NeuroImaging 21, 99–111 (2004)

Ad-Hoc Wireless Body Area Network for Augmented Cognition Sensors

Curtis S. Ikehara, Edoardo Biagioni, and Martha E. Crosby

University of Hawaii at Manoa - Information and Computer Sciences Department
1680 East-West Road, POST 317, Honolulu, Hawaii, 96822, USA
cikehara@hawaii.edu, esb@hawaii.edu, crosby@hawaii.edu

Abstract. There is a "spaghetti" of wires when physiological sensors are used for augmented cognition tying a user down to a fixed location. Besides being visually unappealing, there are practical issues created by the "spaghetti" that have a negative impact on the adoption of sensor based augmented cognition technologies. A wireless sensor network can support sensors commonly used in augmented cognition. This paper describes the benefits and issues of implementing an ideal wireless network of physiological sensors using Bluetooth and other related types of networking approaches.

Keywords: *Ad hoc* network, wireless, biosensor, augmented cognition.

1 Introduction

Augmented cognition uses ". . . scientific tools to determine the 'in real time' cognitive state of the individual and then adapts the human-system interaction to meet a user's information processing needs based on this real-time assessment.[1]" The physiological sensors system is the primary tool used to determine the cognitive state of the individual. The authors of this paper will discuss the issues regarding the implementation of a wireless augmented cognition sensor system based on their experience with health monitoring sensors, sensors for augmented cognition and *ad hoc* wireless networks.

Dr. Curtis Ikehara, one of the authors, has recently completed a project for a Waterproof 24/7 Data Recording Biosensor Patch (see Figure 1). The device is a waterproof continuous wear seven day recording biosensor patch to provide physiological vital signs of the wearer and environmental data. The biosensor patch is a thin flat rectangle worn continuously like a bandage for several days and continuously collects vital signs and environmental data while retaining the last seven days of data, like an aircraft black box. The biosensor suite records blood flow (pulse rate), motion, gun fire sound level, skin temperature and ambient temperature. Data from different biosensor patches, individually or in combination, can be used to assess a variety of conditions. The biosensor patch will allow the detection of injury onset and shock while allowing the assessment of fatigue, environmental stress exposure and explosive ordnance exposure. The biosensor patch uses IRDA communications to control the device and to download data.

D.D. Schmorrow, L.M. Reeves (Eds.): Augmented Cognition, HCII 2007, LNAI 4565, pp. 38–46, 2007.

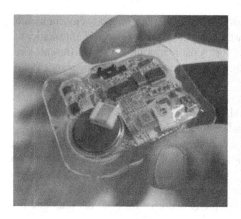
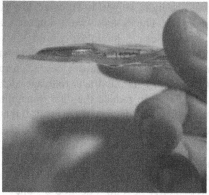

Fig. 1. Two perspective views of the Waterproof 24/7 Data Recording Biosensor Patch

Dr. Edoardo Biagioni, one of the authors, is an associate professor in the department of Information and Computer Sciences at the University of Hawaii at Manoa. His research interests include networking protocols, particularly routing and data transfer protocols for wireless sensor networks and for wireless ad-hoc networks. In 2000-2003 he was co-PI on a DARPA grant, "PODS: A Remote Ecological Micro-Sensor Network"[2], designed to collect information to aid in the preservation of endangered plant species. He has worked on the design and development of a wireless sensor network designed for the long-term study of rare and endangered plant species. These species are monitored in their environment via high-resolution cameras and temperature, rainfall, wind, and solar radiation sensors. Sensor units are part of a large network, the largest deployment having at least 60 nodes. The nodes consume very little power and can operate from batteries for multiple months, and indefinitely long from solar panels. The network uses specialized routing algorithms over 802.11 (adapted to run over Bluetooth, but not tested in the field) to allow communication beyond the range of any individual transmitter. Sensor units exploit transmission path redundancy to compensate for network transmission problems using the wireless routing protocol Multipath On-demand Routing (MOR) [3], which computes multiple optimal routes to avoid depleting the energy at any given node, to recover faster from interference, and to obtain overall higher performance. Other protocols developed as part of this project include Geometric Routing, which scales to large networks, and Lusus, which is useful for networks made up of very simple nodes.

Dr. Martha Crosby, one of the authors, has worked for decades evaluating cognitive performance with a large variety of techniques. She has extensive expertise in the development and use of eye tracking as an indicator of cognitive states and performance. Recently, she has been doing research with Dr. Ikehara on the use of low cost physiological sensors to assess cognitive performance [4], [5], [6], [7].

2   The Ideal Physiological Sensor Network

The ideal physiological sensor network would have a sensor suite so comfortable that the user can wear it for long periods without being tied to a location. The modules would be light weight, low power, low cost and operate under various environmental conditions. The system would support a large number of sensors, would automatically add new sensor modules, would allow for sensor modules with different data characteristics, and would not interfere with nearby users with a similar sensor system or with other electronic devices. Sensor modules would have on-board processing and memory to: extract relevant data using signal processing, perform data compression to reduce the data transmitted, store data if re-transmission is required, time stamp the data, and perform diagnostics to alert the data collection system of problems. The sensor modules would exceed the data transmission requirements, correct for data transmission problems, tolerate sensor module faults, and have an operation time exceeding mission time. Also, the sensor suite would be easy to interface with standard computer equipment, have data encryption and have low detect ability beyond a desired distance to improve security for both the data and the wearer.

The previous paragraph paraphrases some of the characteristics of a 2006 Small Business Innovative Research (SBIR) request, OSD06-H01, for a Bidirectional Inductive On-body Network (BIONET) for Warfighter Physiological Status Monitoring (WPSM). The paragraph also includes characteristics that would be ideal for an augmented cognition physiological sensor suite. The wireless networked health monitoring physiological sensor suite will be coming in the near future. There will be many benefits for an augmented cognition sensor suite that can be compatible with this new wireless health monitoring technology, but there are several issues that need to be addressed.

2.1 Human Factors – "So Comfortable That the User Can Wear It for Long Periods"

Having a comfortable wireless sensor network (WSN) that the user voluntarily wears throughout the work day has many advantages. A few of the advantages are described in this paragraph. First, placement and calibration of the WSN is done once per day, instead of every time the user operates the augmented cognition enabled systems (ACE). The repetitive placement and calibration of the WSN is a major impediment to wider use of the ACE system. Second, knowing the user's cognitive state before using the ACE system allows the ACE system to compensate for pre-existing conditions, such as a racing heart rate caused by running back from lunch. The ACE system would know that heart rate will soon drop and stabilize. Third, knowing the user's cognitive state after performing work will allow the determination of how long a user takes to mentally recover from the previous cognitive task and when the user will be ready to continue working. Fourth, the user can move around and work at several different types of ACE work stations without having to plug into each of the separate stations.

One of the human factors lessons learned by Dr. Ikehara when he was developing the health monitoring biosensor patch was that for the user, a thin large sensor is more desirable than a small and thick sensor. Subjects using the thin sensor, which is approximately 2.5 inches square (65x65mm) commented that after application they couldn't feel it. Where the small 1.25 inches square (30x30mm) sensor was felt and interacted with clothing more. The thin sensor also flexed better with the skin and did not protrude.

The aesthetics would also make the WSN more wearable. One subject who wore the biosensor patch would not wear it again unless the color was blended into the skin so that it wouldn't draw so much attention.

2.2 "Light Weight, Low Power, Low Cost and Operate Under Various Environmental Conditions"

A light weight WSN improves user comfort and allows for multiple sensors to be comfortably worn, but there are several factors that contribute to a sensor's weight. Among the major contributing factors are the size of the power source required for the desired operational duration, the fabricated weight of the electronics and the weight of the encapsulating medium. Low power electronics is desired since less power consumed means longer operational life, a lighter weight battery or the potential for alternate power sources. With very low power electronics, it becomes possible to use alternate power sources including a Peltier device to convert body heat into electricity or a piezoelectric device to convert body motion into electricity [9]. Using the human body as a power source would allow the augmented cognition sensor system to operate for indefinite periods.

To have a low cost augmented cognition sensor system, one approach would be to make the augmented cognition sensor system compatible with mass manufactured health sensor networks. A separately designed augmented cognition sensor network is likely to be more expensive since it will not benefit from the cost saving obtained from large scale production.

The augmented cognition sensor system should operate under various environmental conditions. Environmental conditions fall into two general classes: external factors and conditions that are related to the device as applied to the user's skin. External factors include weather (e.g., water, sun & heat) and chafing (e.g., clothing, carried equipment or between moving body parts). Skin related conditions include skin motion caused by flexing muscles, perspiration, itching and body hair. To address these issues, Dr. Ikehara's biosensor patch encapsulated the electronics using medical grade silicone to repel external factors and medical grade adhesive with perspiration channels. The device was placed on areas of the skin with minimal hair and away from flexing muscles. With improved sensor technology, the sensors could be part of the clothing or a cap, but would still need to operate in various environmental conditions.

2.3 Network Issues

The ideal physiological sensor network should support a large number of sensors, should automatically add new sensor modules, should allow for sensor modules with different data characteristics, and should not interfere with nearby users with a similar sensor system or with other electronic devices. Interference avoidance is accomplished by using low power devices (which also helps reduce energy requirements) and by operating them in a frequency range where they are unlikely to interfere.

Bluetooth is particularly suitable since some Bluetooth devices can transmit as little as 1mW of RF power, and the RF is in the 2.4GHz worldwide ISM band, the same frequency as used by microwave ovens. Bluetooth also uses frequency-hopping, which lessens the likelihood of interference from other devices. Bluetooth is a general-purpose protocol which can support a variety of communication schemes, including those needed by most existing physiological sensors. While unintended communication among Bluetooth nodes can happen, this can be avoided with proper node configuration and programming. The major constraint concerns the maximum data rate, which is limited to anywhere between 700Kb/s and a theoretical maximum of 3Mb/s depending on the version of Bluetooth. In addition, Bluetooth requires a moderate duty cycle, which has higher power consumption than lower-duty cycle technology. Finally, a Bluetooth master device is limited to communicating with at most seven slave devices at any given time, though standards are under development to override this limitation. Overall, Bluetooth provides good quality of service and low data latency.

Two other technologies suitable for use in physiological sensor networks are Zigbee (based on IEEE 802.15.4) and 802.11/WiFi. While some long-distance sensor networks employ 802.11/WiFi, its relative bulk, high power, and high latency makes it unsuitable for physiological sensor networks in spite of its higher overall throughput. In contrast, Zigbee was designed specifically for wireless sensor networks. Zigbee typically uses more power than Bluetooth but can have lower duty cycles, leading to lower overall power consumption. In addition, Zigbee typically has longer range than low-power Bluetooth, allowing communication across a room and at least part way across a building. Finally, Zigbee networks have low data latency and can have up to 65,000 nodes. Golmie, Cypher and Rebala [10] when using Zigbee for ECG found a goodput rate of approximately 50% for 1 to 3 channels of ECG data declining to 5% for 16 channels of ECG data. Bluetooth may be a better choice given the higher data rate requirements of multi-channel electroencephalogram (EEG) data.

Table 1. Salient properties of the three technologies (Bluetooth, Zigbee & WiFi)

	Bluetooth [11], [12], [13], [14], [15]	Zigbee [10], [11]	WiFi® (WLAN) [14], [15]
IEEE Std	802.15.1	802.15.4	802.11
Modulation	FHSS	DSSS	DSSS/OFDM
Frequency	2.4 GHz	2.4 GHz	2.4 GHz / 5GHz
Channels	79 frequencies	16	11
Maximum network speed	3 Mbit/s	250 kbit/s	54Mbps
Range	10 or 100 meters	10-100 meters	50-150 meters
Security	Three security modes	Three security modes	WPA and WPA2 encryption
Approximate Cost	$3	$3	$9
Power Range	0.3-350ma	Can last for years	480-700ma

It is important to recognize that although health monitoring sensors and augmented cognition sensors overlap in function, there are several types of augmented cognition sensors that fall outside of health sensor data requirements. Both health and augmented cognition measure heart rate, heart rate variability, electrocardiogram (EKG/ECG), temperature, blood oxygen, and respiration [16]. Sensors more specific to augmented cognition include: EEG [17], [18], electromyogram (EMG), galvanic skin response (GSR) [16], eye movement and body acceleration [19].

During the normal course of the day health monitoring sensors do not have a high sensor data rate. Although photoplethysmography data is sampled at 16 Hz (i.e., blood flow light sensor), the derived heart rate can be recorded once per minute, while other sensors may need to be recorded less frequently. During intensive care, the data sampling rate for an EKG can be in the 512 Hz range with an accuracy of 12 bits [20]. That would be a 32 times increase in data over the previous sample rate of 16 Hz used to collect heart rate. Augmented cognition sensors like EEG would require more channel capacity given that the sensor uses 128 channels, sampled at 1000 Hz, with 16 bits of accuracy, for a total of about two megabits per second [17]. he previous comparison of EKG and EEG show that health and augmented cognition sensors can have significantly different requirements.

Intermediate Wireless Solutions. Current wireless solutions connect physiological sensors to a single radio frequency wireless transmitter. The signal is received by a nearby device that is connected to a computer. Problems occur when there is another transmitter causing interference, the user moves out of range of the receiver, or ambient electrical noise causes data loss. Also, since the transmission is unidirectional, when a transmission error occurs, there is no method to request retransmission of the data. Another intermediate approach is to use IEEE 802.11/WiFi to transmit the data to an internet-connected access point. Since data delivery time is not guaranteed, sensor synchronization or time stamping is required. Data from multiple sources will need to be synchronized. This occurs even with wire based data collections using the internet [21]. The TCP/IP protocol is most efficient for large blocks of data and much less efficient when transmitting small amounts of data. The latency between data collection and data storage can exceed the system response requirements. Attempts to improve efficiency by collecting large amounts of data before transmitting can further increase latency, whereas using timestamps can substantially increase throughput requirements.

The augmented cognition sensor suite that transmits unprocessed data is likely to tax the health monitoring sensor network, if not overload it with too much data. For the augmented cognition sensor to work within the health monitoring sensor network, it is likely that the data needs to be heavily preprocessed and transmission of the results should be compressed to reduce transmitted data. That would mean that the sensor module may require digital signal processing components to facilitate the signal analysis and data compression.

The augmented cognition sensors create high channel capacity demands on the wireless sensor network. This suggests Bluetooth may be a better choice than Zigbee given the higher data rate requirements of multi-channel EEG data.

Degradation in performance of personal area networks (PAN) can occur because of signal noise and interference from another similar PAN operating nearby. Also, the user may be wearing a wireless health monitoring network that may interfere with the augmented cognition wireless network. Should the augmented cognition sensor network be independent of the health monitoring sensor, it should not interfere with the health monitoring sensor network, since the user's health data should have priority.

Each of the standard wireless approaches, Bluetooth, Zigbee, or WiFi, has its problems. It is likely that a modification of one of the approaches will be necessary. The table below lists some of the issues that need to be considered if a modification or new network protocol is developed assuming all sensor nodes have processing capacity and memory for temporary data storage.

Table 2. New wireless network protocol considerations

How do the sensor network nodes identify themselves as belonging to a user?
How many sensor nodes can be handled?
How is self-diagnosis performed and how is a fault reported?
How do the sensor network nodes communicate with the ACE system?
How will data security be handled?

Initialization of the sensor network
  How do sensors initialize in the network?
  How to re-establish communications after a break in communications.
  How to identify missing or faulty sensors.
  How are new sensor nodes added to or removed from the system?

Data
  What is the minimum quality of service?
  What type of pre-processing of the data can occur at the node?
  How is data compression implemented?
  How to synchronize or timestamp all data.
  How to prioritize data transmission.
  How to change sensor data transmission rates on demand.

Data loss   Retransmission of data protocol
How does a node break communications if it decides to power down.

An *ad hoc* network with the appropriate multi-hop transport protocol and redundant wireless nodes can have redundant communication pathways to the nearest wireless node of the ACE system [2], [3]. With low cost sensor nodes, increasing the number of redundant nodes can create a more robust communications network and provide redundant sensor nodes that can take over the function of a faulty sensor node and improve the overall reliability of the augmented cognition sensor system.

2.4 Additional Network Benefits

The sensor network itself could be used to detect body motion of the user such as appendage movement and the position of the user in a room. To detect body motion, it may be possible to use changing transmission signal strength or the travel time of radio signals from the sensors placed on the user, though both of these techniques suffer in varying degrees from reflections (e.g. from walls and furniture) and self-interference of the radio signal.

3 Conclusion

Wireless sensor networks for health monitoring are almost certain to appear in the next few years. Whether the augmented cognition sensor network is integrated into the health monitoring system or is a separate system, going wireless will be part of the future of augmented cognition.

This paper discussed the benefits and issues relating to an ideal wireless augmented cognition data acquisition sensor system. The benefits of the ideal system will ultimately result in improved user task performance and increase satisfaction with task performance.

Acknowledgements. We thank the Hawaii Technology Development Venture, a project of the Pacific International Center for High Technology Research and funded by the Office of Naval Research for funding the Waterproof 24/7 Data Recording Biosensor Patch. We also thank the Defense Advanced Research Projects Agency (DARPA) SensIT program for funding the Pods project.

References

1. Schmorrow, D.D.: Augmented Cognition: Past, Present, and Future. In: Schmorrow, D.D., Stanney, K.M., Reeves, L.M. (eds.) Augmented Cognition: Past, Present, and Future. xi (2nd edition, 2006)
2. Biagioni, E., Bridges, K.: The Application of Remote Sensor Technology to Assist the Recovery of Rare and Endangered Species. Special issue on Distributed Sensor Networks for the International Journal of High Performance Computing Applications 16(3) (2002) http://www2.ics.hawaii.edu/ esb/prof/pub/ijhpca02.html
3. Biagioni, E., Chen, S.: A Reliability Layer for Ad-Hoc Wireless Sensor Network Routing. In: The Hawaii International Conference on Systems Sciences, Waikoloa, Hawaii (January 2004) http://www2.ics.hawaii.edu/ esb/prof/pub/hicss37chen.pdf
4. Crosby, M.E., Ikehara, C.S.: Using Physiological Measures to Identify Individual Differences. In: Schmorrow, D.D., Stanney, K.M., Reeves, L.M. (eds.) Response to Task Attributes, Augmented Cognition: Past, Present, and Future, 2nd edn. (2006)
5. Ikehara, C., Crosby, M.E., Chin, D.N.: A Suite of Physiological Sensors for Assessing Cognitive States. In: 11th International Conference on Human-Computer Interaction (July 2005)
6. Ikehara, C., Crosby, M.E.: Assessing Cognitive Load with Physiological Sensors. In: Proceedings of the Hawaii International Conference on System Sciences, Kona, Hawaii (January 2005)
7. Ikehara, C., Chin, D.N., Crosby, M.E.: A Modeling and Implementing an Adaptive Human-Computer Interface Using Passive Biosensors. In: Proceedings of the Hawaii International Conference on System Sciences, Kona, Hawaii (January 2004)

8. SITIS Archives, OSD06-H01, Bidirectional Inductive On-body Network (BIONET) for Warfighter Physiological Status Monitoring (WPSM) http://www.dodsbir.net/SITIS/archives_display_topic.asp?Bookmark=29641
9. Baard, E.: People Power: Capturing The Body's Energy For Work On and Off Earth (November 28, 2001), Space.com, http://www.space.com/businesstechnology/technology/body_power_011128-1.html
10. Golmie, N., Cypher, D., Rebala, O.: Performance analysis of low rate wireless technologies for medical applications. Computer Communications 28(10), 1266–1275 (2005)
11. Wexler, J.: Bluetooth and ZigBee: compare and contrast. Network World: Mobility & Wireless Briefings (March 16, 2005) http://www.techworld.com/mobility/features/index.cfm?FeatureID=1261
12. Bluetooth SIG, Inc., How Bluetooth Technology Works, http://www.bluetooth.com/Bluetooth/Learn/Works
13. Bluetooth SIG, Inc., Compare with Other Technologies, http://www.bluetooth.com/Bluetooth/Learn/Technology/Compare/
14. Knutson, C.D., Brown, J.M.: IrDA Principles and Protocols: The IrDA Library, vol. 1, MCL Press, Salem, UT, 24
15. Zahariadis, T.: Evolution of the Wireless PAN and LAN standards. Computer Standards & Interfaces 26(3), 175–185 (2004)
16. Orasanu, J.M., Kraft, N., Tada, Y.: Psychophysiological Indicators of Task Stress in a Team Problem Solving Task. In: Schmorrow, D.D., Stanney, K.M., Reeves, L.M. (eds.) Augmented Cognition: Past, Present, and Future, 2nd edn. (2006)
17. Shelley, J., Backs, R.W.: Categorizing EEG Waveform Length in Simulated Driving and Working Memory Dual-tasks using Feed-forward Neural Networks. In: Schmorrow, D.D., Stanney, K.M., Reeves, L.M. (eds.) Augmented Cognition: Past, Present, and Future, 2nd edn. (2006)
18. Mathan, S., Ververs, P., Dorneich, M., Whitlow, S., Carciofini, J., Erdogmus, D., Pavel, M., Huang, C., Lan, T., Adami, A.: Neurotechnology for Image Analysis: Searching for Needles in Haystacks Efficiently. In: Schmorrow, D.D., Stanney, K.M., Reeves, L.M. (eds.) Augmented Cognition: Past, Present, and Future, 2nd edn. (2006)
19. Auguslyn, J.S., Lieberman, H.R.: Robust Methods for Assessing Cognitive State in the Dismounted Warfighter: Leveraging the Power of Social Cognition. In: Schmorrow, D.D., Stanney, K.M., Reeves, L.M. (eds.) Augmented Cognition: Past, Present, and Future, 2nd edn. (2006)
20. Raju, M.: Heart Rate and EKG Monitor using the MSP430FG439, Technical document, SLAA280, Texas Instruments (October 2005), http://focus.ti.com/lit/an/slaa280/slaa280.pdf
21. Aschwanden, C., Stelovsky, J.: Measuring Cognitive Load with EventStream Software Framework. In: Hawaii International Conference on System Sciences (HICSS) (January 2003)

Integrating Innovative Neuro-educational Technologies (I-Net) into K-12 Science Classrooms

Ronald H. Stevens[1], Trysha Galloway[1], and Chris Berka[2]

[1] UCLA IMMEX Project, 5601 W. Slauson Ave. #255, Culver City, CA 90230
immex_ron@hotmail.com,
tryshag@gmail.com
[2] Advanced Brain Monitoring, Inc, Carlsbad, CA 92008
chris@b-alert.com

Abstract. With the U.S. facing a decline in science, math and engineering skills, there is a need for educators in these fields to team with engineers and cognitive scientists to pioneer novel approaches to science education. There is a strong need for the incorporation problem solving and emerging neuroscience technologies into mainstream classrooms, and for students and teachers to experience what it means at a very personal level, to engage in and struggle with solving difficult science problems. An innovating and engaging way of doing this is by making the problem solving process visible through the use of real-time electroencephalography cognitive metrics. There are educational, task, and measurement challenges that must be addressed to accomplish this goal. In this paper we detail some of these challenges, and possible solutions, to develop a framework for a new set of Interactive Neuro-Educational Technologies (I-Net).

Keywords: EEG, Problem solving, Skill Acquisition, Cognitive Workload.

1 Introduction

Science educators are increasingly being pressured to make their efforts more effective, efficient and relevant to the needs of today's workforce. Promoting "...an individual's capacities to use cognitive processes to confront and resolve real, cross-disciplinary situations where the solution path is not immediately obvious" is a worldwide educational priority (National Research Council, 2005, OECD, 2004). As tasks and problems become more complex, students face greater demands to hold and manipulate many forms of data in working memory. The burden placed on working memory (i.e., cognitive load) in these situations can have a significant impact on students' abilities to perform learning tasks and to benefit from them, because working memory capacity is limited (Baddeley, 2003, Sweller, 1989, 1994). Given the increasing consolidation of job functions within the workforce, the reality is that students will be assuming more responsibility for learning and decision making in the future, and will be increasingly confronted by data / information overload.

While students are individually struggling with increased mental demands, it is becoming more difficult for teachers to support their learning in meaningful cognitive

D.D. Schmorrow, L.M. Reeves (Eds.): Augmented Cognition, HCII 2007, LNAI 4565, pp. 47–56, 2007.

ways. With limited training resources and staff size, rapid identification of students who are / are not developing problem solving skills has remained elusive (National Research Council, 2004). Part of the challenge is cognitive. Strategic problem solving is complex with skill level development being influenced by the balance of the task and the experience and knowledge of the student. Another challenge is observational. Assessment of problem solving requires real-world tasks that are not immediately resolvable and require movement among structural, visual and auditory representations. Lastly, there are challenges of how rapidly valid inferences of the cognitive state of a student can be made and reported from the performance data.

Application of neurophysiologic solutions, especially electroencephalography (EEG) to education offers cutting-edge approaches to these educational challenges. First, with a temporal resolution of seconds or milliseconds the goal of real-time feedback could optimize engagement and cognitive workload during learning. As EEG data collection occurs without interfering with normal task-driven cognition, it can provide an assessment of cognitive load that is not confounded by strong measurement effects. Further on the horizon would be the use of brain-computer interfaces to drive learning in ways that remain in the domain of science fiction.

With today's technologies, classroom-wide application of EEG during educational tasks could individualize the learning experience in specific ways. For example: Existing monitoring devices could detect situations where the student is simply not ready to learn. This could arise through sleep deprivation, a common occurrence among pre-teens and teens (Meijer et al, 2000), or excessive stress / poor stress management. Under these situations classroom instruction may fail, and errors in the learning process will increase

There may also be situations where the task exceeds the individual's immediate ability to mentally model the problem due to the difficulty of the task with respect to content / language and the student cannot be adequately engaged in the learning process although they are motivated to do so. This would be evidenced either by disengagement or 'thrashing', (acquiring excessive data while not engaged or while not processing it), conditions that could lead to poor decision making. Finally there are conditions where distractions and constraints in the environment combine to make a task that a student would normally easily learn, difficult. Such constraints include time pressure, noise, distraction and/or peer pressure. Were these situations quickly recognized and corrected then learning could become accelerated and more personalized.

Throughout education, there is a wide gap in translating the findings of cognitive neuroscientists into everyday educational practice (Goswami, 2006). The challenges are multi-factorial involving issues of diffusion of innovations, disconnects between scientists and educators, and issues of technology and turf. In this paper we draw from multiple perspectives of technology and education to explore possible pathways for taking I-NET into the messy world of real tasks and classroom environments. We first outline the major challenges along the way and close with a near vision of what these approaches can contribute to improving the learning of students.

Our starting framework for situating I-NET tools in education includes the:

- Parameters for measures and devices
- Approaches for situating neurophysiologic measures in education,

- Specifications for the design and delivery of meaningful tasks, and guidelines regarding the capture of cognitive measurements and reporting of findings.

In doing so, we draw from programmatic lessons of the initial DARPA Augmented Cognition Program which emphasized the need for these technologies to "extract meaningful cognitive measures for identified periods of interest", as well as to "situate themselves within environments where they demonstrate high visibility effects that satisfy near as well as long-term needs" ("The End of the Beginning", Washington DC, 1/26/07).

2 EEG as a Neurophysiologic Method of Choice

For routine use in classroom settings I-NET instrumentation should be non-obtrusive for the students and the classroom environment, easy for students to apply, applicable to multiple task formats, inexpensive, and easy to collect meaningful data from. Real-time EEG monitoring satisfies many of these requirements. Technically, EEG-based cognitive load measurements offer the advantage of extremely high temporal resolution. Electrophysiological data is collected at a grain-size of tenths of a second, in contrast to the tens or hundreds of seconds required for traditional measures. This opens the possibility for effective monitoring of workload fluctuations during very rapid decision-making processes that are unobservable using traditional methods. Although there is a large and growing literature on the EEG correlates of attention, memory, and perception (Fabiani, 2001) there is a relative dearth of EEG investigations of the process skill acquisition and learning in classrooms (Smith,1999). Recording and analysis of EEG has traditionally been confined to laboratory settings and training to criterion tasks due to the technical obstacles of recording high quality data and the computational demands of real-time analysis.

Advances in electronics and data processing set the stage for ambulatory EEG applications. A recently developed wireless EEG sensor headset facilitates easy acquisition of high quality EEG combining battery-powered hardware with a sensor placement system to provide a lightweight, easy-to-apply method to acquire and analyze six channels of high-quality EEG. These headsets have been developed by Advanced Brain Monitoring, Inc. and are useful for in-the-field studies where the setup and acquisition of high quality recordings can be obtained by the user without technical assistance. Such units capture EEG data and provide real-time reports of (a) working cognitive load (EEG-WL), (b) distraction (EEG-DT) and (c) engagement (EEG-E). Quantification of the EEG in real time, referred to as the B-Alert system, is achieved using signal analysis techniques to identify and decontaminate eye blinks, and identify and reject data points contaminated with electromyography, amplifier saturation, and/or excursions due to movement artifacts (Berka et al., 2004). The EEG sensor headset requires no scalp preparation and provides a comfortable and secure sensor-scalp interface for 12 to 24 hours of continuous use.

Recent validation studies that included tests of forward and backward digit span, 3-choice vigilance, standard image recognition, verbal paired associate recognition, etc suggest that EEG-E reflects information-gathering, visual scanning and sustained attention. EEG-WL increases with increasing working memory load and during problem-solving, integration of information, analytical reasoning and may be more reflective of executive functions. Inspection of EEG on a second-by-second timescale has revealed associations between workload and engagement levels when aligned with specific task events providing preliminary evidence that second-by-second classifications reflect parameters of task performance (Berka et al., 2004). These associations have been demonstrated with adults in tasks such as driving and weapons training simulation. We have extended this approach to investigate the role of cognitive effort (workload, distraction, and engagement) in high school students' math and science learning.

3   Challenges in the Educational System

An innovation has to be important to the teachers and administrators of a school system if it is going to be used; if it is just based on pure research protocols it probably won't be (Rogers, 1995). A proposed educational innovation should align with existing educational activities and practice; or be used to extend or expand the existing curriculum. Our interactions with educators have approached these challenges from both perspectives.

Maximizing the benefits of EEG technologies, involves developing an understanding of what students and teachers are looking at. Developing a firm grounding in the basic neuroscience and in the clinical neurology of EEG is needed. One approach for expanding the curriculum is through the development of a Brain, Mind and Learning Tool-kit for high school science teachers that features systems and software for acquisition, analysis, and interpretation of the EEG. Introducing brain monitoring into the classroom creates the opportunity for content-rich training in neuroscience, psychology, and a hands-on experience for students and teacher to observe their brain activity in real-time and understand how different states of mind are reflected in the electric fields of the brain. Study of EEG can contribute to a better understanding of the physics of energy, electricity, and waves, as well as the chemistry of biosynthetic pathways and signaling cascades. These workshop / hands-on activities build awareness and understanding of the science and the goals of the project including broad issues of investigation and experimentation.

An alternative method of providing value to the educational system is to incorporate tools that complement existing curricular activities and extend them by providing fast, accurate and more detailed information to support student learning. Using second-by-second EEG and detailed descriptions of cognitive events during the performance of complex tasks provides models for mediating the tasks, and/or the stress on an individual when workload exceeds an optimal threshold. By studying the dynamics of cognitive patterns within different classroom environments new insights are gained about complex problem solving, collaborative learning tasks and hands-on and minds-on science activities.

Example questions that could be approached include:

- What are the ranges and dynamics of cognitive workload and engagement with students demonstrating different levels of problem solving proficiency? Are these features stable, or do they change with experience, various domains and the acquisition of skills?

- What would be the likely classroom impacts if a teacher were able to monitor a graphic display tracking the engagement, distraction and workload of an entire class in real time?
- How do cognitive workload and engagement levels differ for students performing a simulation vs. observing a simulation?

4 IMMEX™ Scientific Problem Solving Tasks

From this spectrum of educational possibilities we have aligned our research activities with complex problem solving tasks that are being used extensively throughout school districts across this country and other nations such as China. This problem solving simulation system, termed IMMEX (Interactive Multi-Media Exercises) contains dozens of standards-based science simulations suitable for middle and high school classrooms. Over 600,000 student performances have been obtained on these simulations leading to the construction of probabilistic models of performance and skill acquisition (Stevens et al, 1999, Stevens & Casillas, 2006). IMMEX simulations are also cognitively complex and most student activities while engaged in problem solving can be mapped to specific elements of cognition (Chung et al, 2002). A final advantage of IMMEX is that simulations exist in many science domains and across grade levels; students will often perform over 100 simulations each year in domains as diverse as math, chemistry, earth science and health. Aligning I-NET tools into such an activity could provide high project visibility throughout the school district.

Deriving EEG measures during open-ended problem solving is not easy. The development of problem solving skills is a gradual process and not all novices solve problems in the same way, nor do they follow the same path toward understanding at the same pace. Given the diversity of the student population it can be difficult to assess what their relative levels of competence are when performing a task, making it difficult to accurately relate EEG measures to other measures of task skill. In real-world educational settings there is not anything approaching the control over the relevant experimental parameters like others studying the sensory and motor systems. There one knows exactly when light hits the retina; however, how does one determine when a memory has occurred on a millisecond timescale?

Complex problem solving activities can critically depend upon the student's motivational and emotional states, creating additional complexity and variability when compared with automatic behavioral responses, or even voluntary motor responses. The memory traces of learning are not necessarily formed with any reproducible temporal offset relative to the time the student demonstrates the memory behaviorally, and this temporal ambiguity makes the job of ascribing meaning to a particular firing correlate especially difficult as we are less sure of when to look, or indeed what a neural correlate of problem solving might look like.

Our approach decomposes problem solving into behaviorally relevant segments and is much like an exercise in situation awareness where data is continuously acquired and consolidated to provide a 'big picture' understanding of the problem. Components of such awareness include perception of the elements in the environment, comprehension of the elements, and prediction of future interaction and events. The analogous components in problem solving are <u>framing</u>, <u>navigation and investigation</u>, and <u>closure</u>.

Framing. The perception analog in IMMEX tasks is a framing event. Text or multimedia descriptions are presented describing a situation, and posing one or more challenges. For example, in the middle school problem set Phyto Phyasco the prologue describes a newspaper clip indicating that a local farmer's potato crop is mysteriously dying; the challenge for the student becomes to determine if this is due to pests, lack of nutrients, infection, etc.

Successful framing is critical for solving problems and experts often spend a disproportionate amount of time on framing. Similarly, in situation awareness, the majority of errors are based on errors in perception (Endsley, 1999). If the student reads the prologue too quickly or does not take notes, or does not sufficiently understand the terms then the framing process could fail. Occasionally students become so involved in the details of the problem solving itself that they forget what the question being asked is and need to reframe the problem. Currently it is very difficult to know if the student has correctly framed the problem without extensive verbal questions and answers. EEG can help illuminate the framing process by determining if the student is engaged or overwhelmed by the task being proposed. We have also observed that as the student gains problem solving experience on the tasks the level of workload needed for effective framing begins to decrease (Stevens et al, 2007).

Navigation and Integration. Once the problem is framed the next important step is the identification of the most relevant resources available to solve the problem. All IMMEX tasks contain a hierarchy of resources that students navigate while gathering information. Figure 1 shows the problem space for Phyto Phyasco which consists of 5 major categories, each containing multiple sub categories of information.

The top menus are mainly used for problem space navigation. The sub menu items to the left are more decision making points as there is a cost or risk associated with each. In the problem set Phyto Phyasco there are 38 choices. What results is a dynamic iterative process of data collection and integration from which the solution to the problem is derived.

This is a complex process as few students solve IMMEX problems using the same sequence of actions, and currently it is not possible to determine from the framing, navigation, and decision events alone whether the student will solve the problem. Some students may have the relevant information in hand but do not understand the significance of it in the context of the problem. Other students through either bias or poor framing will never acquire the most useful information. Still others will access all the available information in a non-discriminating way without a clear hypothesis. Probabilistic descriptions of navigation and integration can provide a proxy for student understanding, but the models often lack the precision and temporal updating needed for a global metric of student's situation awareness (Stevens & Casillas, 2006).

During efficient navigation and investigation, students often demonstrated a cycling of the B-Alert cognitive indexes characterized by relatively high workload and low engagement which then switched to lower workload and higher engagement. These cycle switches were often, but not always associated with selection of new data items.

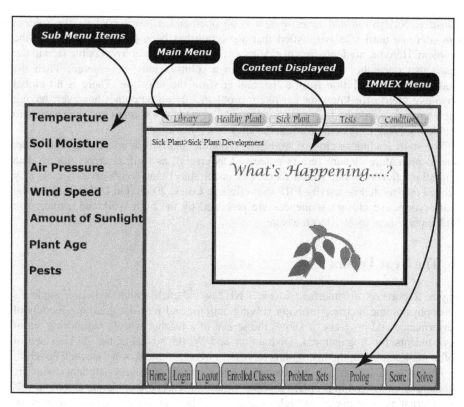

Fig. 1. Sample IMMEX™ simulation. In the Phyto Phyasco simulation, potato plants are dying and the student must identify the cause by examining weather conditions, nutrients, etc. Students navigate throughout the problem space using the Main Menu and select data to make decisions using the Sub Menu Items.

Multiple EEG correlates exist that are useful for understanding the navigation and integration events. On complex tasks, humans seem to use prior information to generate predictive codes for anticipated future events and continually compare incoming data with these codes (Summerfield et al, 2006). Perception-related evoked response potentials (ERP) similar to the auditory mismatch negativity (MMN) (Naatanen, 2001), may be observed when data is displayed that is not consistent with the current hypothesis. The absence of such signals could also be important if a deviant source of data was not recognized when presented.

It is also likely that there will be differences in engagement and workload when specific items of data are seen for the first time vs. subsequent times. The first time a piece of data is examined the student must categorize both the representation of the data, as well as associate the importance of the data to the context of the problem. Once the representation of the data is understood then the subsequent data viewing should only relate to the problem context and workload and engagement measures would be expected to be shorter or lower. At the level of ERP, a decrease in the latency of the P300 wave may be seen once the data representation is learned (Luck, 1998).

Closure. Navigation and investigation is an open-ended process where the student can continue until s/he is satisfied that a solution has been obtained and closes the problem. Here the students first decide to solve the problem, an irreversible step in the sense that once this decision is made then a solution must be entered. Then the students select a solution from a list, and confirm the selection. There is no global cognitive metric for knowing the likely problem solving outcome; however, having such a metric would be important for learning as student's success and approaches to problem solving can persist for months after initial learning.

The steps leading to closure are highly dynamic and rich in uncertainty and errors due to premature closure (errors perceived as errors), as well as errors due to data limitations (errors about which there was uncertainty) can be observed which may evoke error-related negativity ERP (Scheffers & Coles, 2000). On IMMEX tasks, the more productive closure sequences are preceded by the high workload, rather than high engagement by B-Alert measures.

5   The Near Future

Figure 2 portrays an interface to the I-NET workbench which will link student's neurophysiologic metrics, problem solving actions, and machine learning models of performance and progress. It shows the screen of a teacher who is monitoring six of her students for Engagement, Distraction and Workload using the B-Alert sensor software. Each bar in the histograms represents averaged metrics at 1-second epochs.

Panels A, C and to a lesser extend F most closely represents students who are productively engaged in problem solving; workload levels are moderate and the levels are alternating with cycles of high engagement. Many of these cycles are associated with navigation and interpretation events. Panel B illustrates a student who may be experiencing difficulties and may not be prepared to learn. The workload and engagement levels are low and distraction is consistently high. Under these conditions the student should be asked to terminate the task as productive learning is not likely to occur.

The student in Panel D has just encountered a segment of the simulation that induced 10-15 seconds of distraction (middle row) and decreased workload and engagement. By clicking on those EEG segments the teacher retrieved a view of the data that the student was looking at, which in this case is an animation of a plant growing. She could then make a note to discuss with the student to determine the source of the distraction and / or to see if others in the class have struggled with the same or similar issues.

Panel E shows a student who, while not distracted, appears to be working at beyond optimal capacity with workload levels consistently near 100%. The teacher then retrieved the artificial neural network performance assessment models for this student (Stevens et al, 2004, Stevens & Casillas, 2006) which shows that this student does not seem to be developing efficient strategies on his own. Utilizing this information, the instructor may suggest the adjustment of the difficulty of the task for this student and continue monitoring to see if more acceptable (in a learning sense) levels of workload and engagement result.

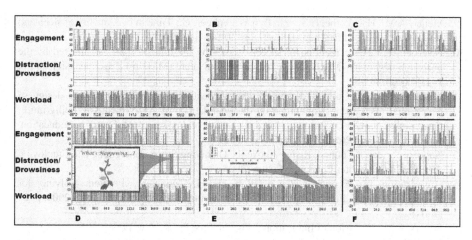

Fig. 2. Prototype I-NET interface for linking EEG measures of workload, distraction and engagement with details of the tasks and probabilistic models of problem solving performance and progress. While the interface itself is not yet functional, the tasks, EEG readings and machine learning model reports are actual student performance data.

Acknowledgements. This project has been funded by several grants from the National Science Foundation, (DUE- 01236050, REC-02131995, NSF-ROLE 0528840, HRD-0429156, DUE-0512526) whose support is gratefully acknowledged.

References

1. Baddeley, A.: Working Memory: Looking Back and Looking Forward. Nature Reviews I Neuroscience 4, 829–839 (2003)
2. Berka, C., et al.: Real-time analysis of EEG indexes of alertness, cognition and memory acquired with a wireless EEG headset. International Journal of Human-Computer Interaction 17(2), 151–170 (2004)
3. Berka, C., Levendowski, D.J., Cvetinovic, M., Petrovic, M.M., Davis, G.F., Lumicao, M.N., Popovic, M.V., Zivkovic, V.T., Olmstead, R.E.: Real-Time Analysis of EEG Indices of Alertness, Cognition and Memory Acquired with a Wireless EEG Headset. International Journal of Human-Computer Interaction 17(2), 151–170 (2004)
4. Chung, G.K.W.K, deVries, L.F., Cheak, A.M., Stevens, R.H., Bewley, W.L.: Cognitive Process Validation of an Online Problem Solving Assessment. Computers and Human Behavior 18, 669 (2002)
5. Endsley, M.R.: Situation awareness in aviation systems. In: Garland, D.J., Wise, J.A. (eds.) Handbook of aviation human factors. Human factors in transportation, pp. 257–276. Lawrence Erlbaum Associates, Mahwah (1999)
6. Fabiani, M., Gratton, G., Coles, M.G.: Event-related brain potentials. In: Caciooppo, J.T., Tassinary, L.G., Berntson, G.G. (eds.) Handbook of Psychophysiology, pp. 53–84. Cambridge University Press, Cambridge, England (2000)
7. Goswami, U.: Neuroscience and education: from research to practice? Nature Reviews Neuroscience 7, 2–7 (2006)
8. Luck, S.: Sources of dual-task interference: Evidence from human electro-encephalography. Physiological Science 9, 223–227 (1998)

 9. Meijer, A.M., Habekothe, H.T., van Den Wittenboer, G.: Time in bed, quality of sleep and school functioning of children. J. Sleep Res. 9, 145–153 (2000)
10. Naatanen, R.: The perception of speech sounds by the human brain as reflected by the mismatch negativity (MMN) and its magnetic equivalent (MMNm). Psychophysiology 38, 1–21 (2001)
11. National Research Council, Knowing what students know: The science and design of educational assessment. Committee on the Foundations of Assessment. In: Pelligrino,J., Chudowsky, N., Glaser, R. (eds.) Board on Testing and Assessment, Center for Education. National Academy Press, Washington. DC (2001)
12. National Research Council, Rising Above the Gathering Storm: Energizing and Employing America for a Brighter Economic Future (2005)
13. Organization for Economic Cooperation and Development, Problem Solving for Tomorrow's World, First Measures of Cross-curricular competencies from PIS 2004. p. 26 (2004)
14. Rogers, E.M.: Diffusion of Innovations, 4th edn. Free Press, New York (1995)
15. Scheffers, M.K., Coles, M.: Performance monitoring in a confusing world: Error related brain activity, judgments of response accuracy and types of errors. Journal of Experimental Psychology: Human Perception and Performance 26, 141–151 (2000)
16. Stevens, R., Casillas, A.: Artificial Neural Networks. In: Mislevy, R.E., Williamson, D.M., Bejar, I. (eds.) Automated Scoring, pp. 259–312. Lawrence Erlbaum, Mahwah (2006)
17. Stevens, R.H., Ikeda, J., Casillas, A., Palacio-Cayetano, J., Clyman, S.: Artificial neural network-based performance assessments. Computers in Human Behavior 15, 295–314 (1999)
18. Summerfield, C., Egner, T., Greene, M., Koechlin, E., Mangels, J., Hirsch, J.: Predictive codes for forthcoming perception in the frontal cortex. Science 314, 1311–1315 (2006)
19. Sweller, J.: Cognitive technology: Some procedures for facilitating learning and problem solving in mathematics and science. Journal of Cognitive Psychology 81(4), 457–466 (1989)
20. Sweller, J.: Cognitive load theory, learning difficulty, and instructional design. Learning & Instruction 4(4), 295–312 (1994)

The Impact of Direct Data Entry by Sensory Devices on EMR Systems

David Pager, Dennis J. Streveler, and Luz M. Quiroga

Department of Information & Computer Sciences, University of Hawaii,
1680 East-West Road, Honolulu, HI 96822, USA
pager@hawaii.edu

Abstract. This paper takes an interdisciplinary look at how the electronic record is likely to evolve in the future. From what new sources will data be drawn? Will such data be directly recorded from sensory devices and from one's personal "memex"? Will these data enable a new set of outputs to more fully interconnect patients with their health care system. The paper considers the combined impact of a host of emerging technologies:

1. the impact of the networking phenomenon
2. the impact of adding robust patient access to the EMR
3. the impact of the growing emergence of PHRs
4. the impact of emerging technologies on the usability of the EMR
5. the impact of direct sensory input devices
6. the impact of bioinformatics and genomics
7. the impact of the personal memex

Keywords: Electronic Medical Record, Sensory Devices, Human-Computer Interface Issues, Biomedical Technology.

1 Introduction

The EMR is very much a system in development. After a struggle of about 50 years[1], the notion of an Electronic Medical Record [EMR] has now finally begun to take firm root in the USA and elsewhere. Spurred by encouragement from the American government as a way to reduce medical errors[2] and to stem the inherent inefficiency of the paper-based record, most major healthcare institutions in the USA now have emerging EMR projects in various stage of implementation[3] .

---

[1] The first attempt at creating an electronic medical record may have occurred at Kaiser-Permanente circa 1956 [1].

[2] Perhaps the most dramatic moment occurred in the year 2000 when the Institute of Medicine published its now classic paper "To Err is Human" in which it postulated that perhaps as many as 98,000 lives are lost each year due to medical error in the United States [2].

[3] It is estimated that approximately 8% of health information is currently collected using EMR technology in the USA [3].

D.D. Schmorrow, L.M. Reeves (Eds.): Augmented Cognition, HCII 2007, LNAI 4565, pp. 57–64, 2007.

It is clear that the "electronification" of health datawill have impacts far beyond those of the immediate use of the data in direct clinical care. For the first time in human history, detailed patient-identified data will be digitally created on a massive scale. This availability will reduce the need for timely and costly chart audits which introduce significant error and bias into data analysis.

How will this massive amount of data be collected? Clearly the great bulk of this data will need to be entered from electronic sources. On a relatively small scale data from interfaced clinical laboratory equipment is already collected in this way. Is it, in addition, possible that in the not-so-distant future patient-specific data might flow directly to the EMR via sensory devices, and that one's genomic data might also directly populate one's EMR?

In this paper, we attempt to look at the future implications of the Electronic Medical Record – how it will likely evolve, how data is likely to be collected, the purposes to which the data will be put, and how a host of new emerging technologies may impact that progression.

2   The Impact of the Network Phenomenon

Like the progression of the personal computer itself, great synergy is created by linking stand-alone sites together in a network configuration. In the USA, the recent interest in the creation of RHIOs (Regional Health Information Organizations) has had some success in inter-linking EMRs at different institutions within a larger catchment area[4].

However, as with the RHIOs' predecessor, the CHINs[5] (Community Health Information Networks), the exact use and utility of this interlinking is still not clear.

The first use of the RHIO will likely be to improve the flow of "upward referrals" from lower levels of care (especially primary care) to tertiary hospitals and academic medical centers. This improvement will address many of the issues relating to the current paucity of data which is currently available to a receiving emergency room or super-specialist clinic.

After "upward referrals" are addressed, it is likely that we will finally begin to address a perhaps even more significant and vexing problem, that of "downward referrals", i.e. how to move the patient, along with his or her newly generated clinical information, back down to a more appropriate (and more cost-effective) level of care once the specialty treatment episode has concluded [6]. This return to lower-levels of care has been hampered by a litany of perverse economic, regulatory and social incentives which generally prize "holding on to a patient" as long as possible. Whether specialists can be cajoled into loosening up on this social grip remains to be seen.

---

[4] In Hawaii, for example, the Holomua Project [4] is underway to link 5 public Primary Care Clinics with 2 large tertiary urban health centers on the island of O`ahu.

[5] Most of the CHINs of the 1980's failed miserably to garner the support needed from the various competing stakeholders.

[6] In Hawaii it is estimated that only 30% of patients suffering their first Myocardial Infarction are adequately returned to primary care for long-term management of their Coronary Artery Disease [5].

After referrals, and authorizations for referrals, are fully automated, we may have the luxury of considering an even more dramatic change – can the electronic availability of patient data (via the EMR) actually allow full and virtual collaboration on treatment among institutions in a community?   With an MRI done in one institution, a super-specialist in another, and post-intervention therapies in yet another, could we remake our healthcare institutions to be less duplicative (read, requiring less capital expenditure) and more complementary and collaborative?[7]

Could, further, the emergence of the EMR be one of the missing pieces which finally makes telemedicine available on a broad scale? Telemedicine is yet another high-technology initiative which has engendered speculation since 1924[8] (!), but has languished largely because of the lack of "glue" to bind healthcare institutions together.[9]

The convergence of the EMR and initiatives in telemedicine may cause a major realignment and rethinking of the fundamental way that healthcare is provided across the continuum of care.   In these new circumstances important issues of security, confidentiality, privacy and access rights will have to be addressed. In this larger environment, these issues will dwarf those we face today as more and more institutions have some access to medical histories.

3   The Impact of Adding Robust Patient Access to the EMR

Given the general spread of computers and availability of broadband connections, people have become familiar with secure access via the web to their personal data, such as to their bank accounts, share holdings, etc.   There appears to be no good reason why they should not also have access to the bulk of their medical and

---

[7] We stress again the need to look at the vexing fragmentation problem in the context of a plethora of economic, legal, regulatory and social complexities.

[8]

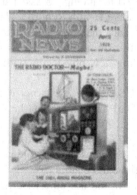

Radio News magazine, April 1924

[9] It can be reasonably argued that there are of course other pernicious reasons why the scope of telemedical practice has remained so limited relative to its long-touted potential. Among these in America are the statutory restriction of medical practice across state lines, perverse or non-existent economic incentives, and the general sense that telemedicine is often inconvenient and poorly orchestrated.

pharmaceutical records. As reported in [6] this facility is already under development in various forms at several sites in the US, such as at Kaiser-Permanente, the Group Health Cooperative in Seattle, Beth Israel Deaconess Medical Center in Boston, and the Cleveland Clinic. The various online services offered (by at least one of these institutions) include allowing patients to:

(a) View their own medical records, including lab. results, radiology reports, allergy results, with links to lay person explanations of procedures and tests (Physician office notes are however not included.)
(b) Make appointments
(c) Request referrals
(d) Post questions. Triage nurses are employed to answer these, making use of a library of customizable prewritten templates. Questions are forwarded on to physicians only where necessary
(e) Populate the database with their own family and social histories.

In addition to the explanation of diagnostic test results and optional therapies referred to in (a), broadband connection makes possible the explanation of medical conditions with graphics and video components. Furthermore, the emerging technologies of natural language processing and web searching will increase the potential of systems implementing computer-generated responses, and so relieve some of the burden and cost of answering patient in queries (see d). Just how far and how fast patients will be given such robust access to their medical information remains an open question.

4   The Impact of the Growing Emergence of PHRs

Patients will not only want/demand robust access to their EMRs, but will also want to make entries about their own personal health data. Already a large number of products have been developed (as listed e.g. in [7]) to attempt to assist users in the creation and maintenance of their own PHRs (Personal Health Reports). These PHRs are intended to serve as central depositories of data that may be spread over the medical records maintained by numerous health-care providers, and serve such functions as avoiding duplicate tests, and providing new physicians with additional medical history.

The fact of the matter is that, at least in the USA, there exists no ideal place to house one's (truly longitudinal) clinical data. The very nature of the fragmented healthcare system (or putting it more kindly of our independent mostly laisser-faire system) assures that no one point is ideal. In the USA, therefore, we will likely see the continued growth of institutionally owned EMRs (whose focus, logically enough, is to benefit that institution). Thus PHRs will continue to be attractive.

Patients can add to their PHRs information that would not otherwise be collected, e.g. their use of over-the-counter [OTC] medication, drug interactions, vital signs, nutritional data, signs and symptoms, etc.

There is clearly a close relationship between the EMR and the PHR. Patients will obviously want the ability to download material from their EMRs to their PHRs, and have links to their PHRs inserted into their EMRs. Will facilities for such cross-references indeed be incorporated into the EMR? If so, a number of important questions need to be addressed, including: (a) patients may not have enough medical knowledge to know what to put into their PHRs (b) most importantly, can a physician legally and reasonably act on information placed in the PHR by a patient without validating it?

For these reasons and more, the PHR has had a limited penetration into the "mainstream" of medical care. Certain hybrids have emerged which combine certain aspects of EMR and PHR[10]. These hybrids have thus far been less than satisfactory.

5   The Impact of Emerging Technologies on the Usability of the EMR

In addition to new data entry methods, new search techniques, and new paradigms of patient involvement, we will need to fundamentally assess the usability of our current practices. Might new technologies help in this regard?

Busy doctors and nurses resist having to resort to data access terminals in order to input or extract information. The integration of EMR with Wi-Fi mobile devices can go a long way to solving this problem. The technology for this is beginning to make an appearance [8] . Examples of such devices include:

a) *Pda's and tablet computers.* A number of hospitals, such as the Ohio State University Medical Center (OSU), have established access points through out their hospital for this purpose.

b) *Wireless wearable computers with LCD screen mounted glasses.* Devices of this kind go one step further than pda's as far as convenience is concerned. The cost and weight problems which have hindered their acceptance are being solved as a side-effect of Moore's law on the doubling of computer speed for a given cost. Some doctors at OSU have already begun wearing devices of this kind.

c) *Voice recognition* which can add a significant convenience factor for many input chores. The technology involved is improving. It is one of those technologies which benefits from increased raw computer power[11]. Radiology transcription systems, for instance, are now quite good, given that they use a relatively small specialized vocabulary, but they still suffer from occasional almost comical blunders.   A much larger vocabulary will be required for robust diverse description in Internal Medicine, which is now beyond the reach of today's computing power, but this limitation will likely gradually fade over time.

d) *Hand-held scanners.* We are all familiar with the use of these devices by car-rental companies and your friendly Fedex delivery man, and they have begun to find their way into hospitals. Such scanners can also be put to use on a large scale to keep track of medication dispensed to patients. For instance on administering medication to a patient, the nurse involved scans the bar codes on

---

[10] Experiments at Kaiser-Permanente, Oakland, for example have given the patient "views" of her clinical data and limited ability to add "patient-entered" data, but these data are not fully integrated with "institution-entered" data.

[11] For instance the recent introduction of multi-core processors will have an immediate impact on the capability of voice recognition systems.

the medication, the patient's wristband and her own badge. Together with the timestamp, the information can immediately be posted to the Medication Administration Record (MAR).

The full adoption of these devices might spur further progress in data collection. Of course with this opportunity comes the now familiar battle between confidentiality and accessibility. In order to be HIPAA-compliant[12], robust encryption and authentication protocols need to be employed, e.g. using WEP or other encryption schemes (as well as the usual security needs such as user id's, passwords, etc). Other important problems that require attention include network reliability (particularly critical in this case), access point placement, and (today's relatively short) battery lives. Finally, interference can be caused by radio devices inside a medical institution which can potentially have dangerous effects on telemetry, and even on patient-imbedded devices such as pacemakers.

6   The Impact of Direct Sensory Input Devices

If one accepts the premise that the world (and the "healthcare world" specifically) will soon be highly interconnected, that patient's will have/demand robust access to that world, and that in fact the PHR might become an umbrella under which the fragmented data at the healthcare institutions is stored, then we are led to the question about how such data will be entered.

EMR systems may evolve from one in which all entries are made by human users (be it the health institution, the clinician or the patient), into a system which also receives some direct input from sensory devices in the environment, and ones attached to patients using nanotechnologies and other relatively noninvasive methods. A large multi-country project called MobiHealth [9] has been funded by the European Commission to develop a system employing such devices.

Although sensory acquisition has been with us for decades (an early example being the Holter Monitor used to monitor irregular heart rhythms of known cardiac patients), the full potential of our ability to harness real-time acquisition of health data has really not yet been explored in the mainstream of medicine.

An example where an EMR system would benefit from data acquired in this way is supplied in [10]. This report describes a tiny wireless device which can be implanted in a tumor to tell doctors the precise location of the cancer and the exact amount of radiation it's receiving. A study of such data obtained from patient EMRs around the country, with information about the outcomes, would be of significant use in determining optimum therapy for such cases.

Clearly direct input from sensory devices provides us with a host of technical, social and legal challenges if it were to be adopted on a routine basis. The potential benefits are great however, especially in a world fraught with the scourge of an ever-increasing burden of cardiac disease and Diabetes Mellitus, to name just two of the diseases that could potentially be monitored in a connected world.

---

[12] USA: The Health Insurance Portability and Accountability Act of 1996.

7 The Impact of Bioinformatics and Genomics

Another future source of massive amounts of data to be collected and managed by the EMR will result from the appearance and availability of bioinformatic and genomic data.

Abnormalities related to over 1,600 genes have been linked to specific health conditions, and this number is rapidly growing with continued research [11] . About 2/3 of these genes are available for specific genetic tests ordered by physicians. Examples of such health conditions include:

(a) increased risks of multiple forms of cancer, with a consequent need for continual surveillance
(b) abnormally increased or decreased ability to metabolize certain drugs, with a consequent need for doses prescribed by physicians to be adjusted accordingly
(c) susceptibility to permanent hearing loss if certain drugs are taken
(d) susceptibility of infants to mental retardation on ingesting phenylalanine, an essential component of most sources of protein.

There is an obvious need for physicians to keep track of such factors, but the large number of known effects, and the rapidity with which others are being discovered, makes this extremely difficult. As [11] argues, EMR systems need to be altered to include a standard format for information obtained about a patient's genome. The entry of such information should elicit warnings about associated health conditions applicable to that specific patient. Furthermore, as new links between genes and health conditions are discovered, warnings should be sent out to the physician and/or the patient using a centralized computer system that identifies the patients concerned by accessing the genomic information in patient's records across the country [13]. Genes related to a disease often only increase the probability that the patient involved will suffer from it, but patients may misinterpret the advisory and think that it indicates that they actually already have the disease. Accordingly the data selected to be presented to patients should be accompanied where necessary with an interpretation of the possible impact and probabilities of progression, with references to the germane literature.

8 The Impact of the Personal Memex

A more speculative extension to the discussion about future sources of health data comes from Jim Gray's 1998 Turing Award Speech [12], in which he argued that, with Moore's Law, we will soon achieve the capability of creating what he calls a "Personal Memex". This is a system for recording everything one saw, read, or heard. Might there be benefits to linking the Personal Memexs of patients to an EMR system, such as for investigating the origin of health problems, and for extensions of, and additions to, the applications of sensory data input described above? What analysis and search tools would be needed to deal with such a large and complex data

---

[13] We fully acknowledge the huge cultural barriers which present themselves here. The idea of a "central computer system" which tracks everybody's genomic data raises major issues revolving around patient confidentiality and data security. Can they be overcome? This remains to be seen.

structure? One can only imagine the possibilities and the richness of new knowledge which could result[14].

9 Conclusion

We remain at present at the very infancy of understanding the true nature of the EMR. While today's efforts are largely focused on minimizing the fragmentation of medical information for direct patient care within one institution or healthcare organization, the potential sources of inputs into the EMR,, and the potential outputs of the EMR clearly goes far beyond the realm of the doctor's office or hospital bed.

One thing is clear, the full emergence of the EMR will impact our healthcare delivery system at many levels; the secondary and tertiary effects may be even more profound than the impact on direct patient care itself.

References[15]

1. Collen, M.: The History of Medical Information Systems in the United States. American Medical Informatics (1995)
2. Kohn, L.T., Corrigan, J.M., Donaldson, M.S. (eds.): To Err is Human: Building a Safer Health System. Institute of Medicine (2000) See http://www.iom.edu/CMS/8089/5575/4117.aspx
3. Electronic Health Information among Community Health Centers: Adoption and Barriers. Harvard Medical School/MGH, George Washington University and the Nation Association of Community Health Centers (2006)
4. See, http://www.gold.ahrq.gov/GrantDetails.cfm?GrantNumber=UC1%20HS16160
5. Health Trends in Hawaii. The Hawaii State Department of Health (2003)
6. Baldwin, G.: Emerging Technology: the patient-accessible EMR (2005) See, http://www.amkai.com/Emerging%20Technology.doc
7. See, http://www.myphr.com/resources
8. Goodman, G.: Wireless: Just what the Doctor Ordered. CIO Magazine (2003) See, http://www.cio.com/archive/080103/mobile.html
9. See, http://www.mobihealth.org/
10. Engineers creating small wireless device to improve cancer treatment. Purdue News Service (2006) See http://www.purdue.edu/UNS/html4ever/2006/060417.Ziaie.cancer.html
11. Mitchell, J.A.: The Impact of Genomics on E-Health. Stud Health Technol Inform. 106, 63–64 (2004)
12. Gray, J.: What Next? Microsoft Research Advanced Tech. Div., Tech. Report MS-TR-99-50 (1999)

---

[14] Even if the Personal Memex were never to come into ubiquitous use, it is possible that extensive diverse information about individuals will come to be collected, or linked together, in some standard format. In addition to EMRs, this could include such information as additional personal data, academic credentials, personal blogs, bank accounts, and perhaps credit reports, criminal histories, etc. Issues of security, confidentiality, privacy, and access rights will have to be addressed here not only with respect to EMRs, but also to these other categories of data.

[15] All the URLs listed here were last revisited on 2/14/2007.

Event-Related Brain Dynamics in Continuous Sustained-Attention Tasks

Ruey-Song Huang[1,2], Tzyy-Ping Jung[2], and Scott Makeig[2]

[1] Department of Cognitive Science
[2] Swartz Center for Computational Neuroscience, Institute for Neural Computation
University of California, San Diego
La Jolla, CA 92093, USA
{rshuang,jung,scott}@sccn.ucsd.edu

Abstract. Event-related brain dynamics of electroencephalographic (EEG) activity in a continuous compensatory tracking task (CTT) and in a continuous driving simulation were analyzed by independent component analysis (ICA) and time-frequency techniques. We showed that changes in the level of subject performance are accompanied by distinct changes in EEG spectrum of a class of bilateral posterior independent EEG components. During periods of high-error (drowsy) performance, tonic alpha band EEG power was significantly elevated, compared to that during periods of low-error (alert) performance. In addition, characteristic transient (phasic) alpha and other band increases and decreases followed critical task events, depending on current performance level. These performance-related and event-related spectral changes were consistently observed across subjects and sessions, and were remarkably similar across the two continuous sustained-attention tasks.

Keywords: EEG, ICA, brain dynamics, driving, drowsiness.

1 Introduction

In the real world, many tasks require sustained attention to maintain continuous performance. During the course of sustained-attention tasks, we usually receive continuous visual or auditory stimulus streams along with continuous performance feedback. Continuous efforts are required to resolve situations that last for less than a second to a few seconds. For instance, one of the goals of driving safely on a highway is to stay in the center of a cruising lane by continuously controlling the steering wheel. Small changes in road curvature or uneven pavement may make the vehicle drift off the lane center. Failure to respond to lane drifts could lead to catastrophic consequences.

Electroencephalographic (EEG) correlates of fluctuations in human performance and alertness have been demonstrated on time scales of one second to several minutes [1-8]. Event-related potentials (ERP) following sensory stimuli or events were often obtained by averaging time-domain EEG epochs precisely time-locked to stimulus onsets. In many ERP paradigms, participants respond to abrupt stimulus onset events

D.D. Schmorrow, L.M. Reeves (Eds.): Augmented Cognition, HCII 2007, LNAI 4565, pp. 65–74, 2007.

with single and discrete button presses. This might not be the case in real-world working environments that often involve more or less continuous efforts to maintain appropriate performance, instead of occasional impulsive and discretely cued behavioral choices (e.g., selective button presses). Furthermore, both ERP time courses and scalp distributions, among other ERP features, may change with onsets of drowsiness [9]. These limitations make ERP measures inappropriate or insufficient for assessing event-related brain dynamics during continuous sustained-attention tasks accompanied by fluctuating alertness levels.

In this study, we investigated event-related brain dynamics in response to random perturbations in two different continuous attention-sustained tasks. First, in an hour-long continuous compensatory tracking task (CTT), participants attempted to use a trackball to keep a randomly drifting disc in a bulls-eye on the center of screen. Second, during hour-long continuous driving simulation, participants tried to steer a drifting vehicle at the center of the left lane with arrow keys. Independent component analysis (ICA) [10-12] and event-related spectral perturbation (ERSP) [13] methods were applied to continuous EEG data collected in each of the 1-hour sessions. Event-related spectral changes were consistently observed across subjects and sessions in both continuous sustained-attention tasks.

2 Methods

2.1 Participants and Tasks

Non-sleep-deprived healthy adults with normal or corrected to normal vision were paid to participate in the experiment. All subjects gave informed consent before participating in a protocol approved by UCSD Human Research Protections Program. All subjects had lunch about two hours before arriving at the lab around 2:00 PM, and EEG recordings began near 3:00 PM. Subjects sat on a comfortable office chair with armrests and watched stimuli on a 19-inch screen in an EEG booth in which lighting was dim. Each subject took part in more than one hour-long session of sustained-attention tasks on different days.

The compensatory tracking task (CTT) required subjects (n=6) to attempt to use a trackball to keep a drifting ('wind-blown') disc as near as possible to a bulls-eye which was continuously visible in the center of screen (Fig. 1a), by making frequent (~3/s) movements of the trackball in the direction of intended movement, producing ('rocket-thrust' like) bursts of directional disc acceleration [14]. The coordinates and dynamics of the drifting disc, and the trackball velocity vector were recorded about 14 times per second via a synchronous pulse marker train that was recorded in parallel by the EEG acquisition system for subsequent analysis.

During the hour-long continuous driving simulation, every 3 to 7 seconds the car was linearly pulled towards the curb or into the opposite lane, with equal probability (Fig. 1b). Subjects (n=11) were instructed to compensate for the drift by holding down an arrow key, and to release the key when the car returned to the center of the cruising lane. Subjects were instructed not to make small corrections for precise alignment after they returned to the lane center.

In both tasks, subjects were instructed to maintain their best performance even if they began to feel drowsy. No intervention was made when subjects occasionally fell asleep and stopped responding.

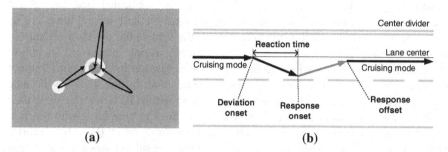

(a)   **(b)**

Fig. 1. Schematic plots of continuous sustained-attention tasks. (a) Compensatory tracking task. White ring: bulls-eye. Black curved arrows: trajectories of the drifting disc (white). (b) Driving simulation.

2.2 EEG Data Acquisition and Preprocessing

CTT. EEG activities were recorded from 70 scalp electrodes. Eye movements and blinks were recorded via two EOG electrodes placed below the right eye and at the left outer canthus, respectively. All electrodes used the right mastoid as reference. EEG and EOG activities were sampled at 250 Hz with an analog pass band of 0.01-100 Hz (SA Instrumentation, San Diego, CA).

Driving. 256-channel EEG/EOG/EKG signals were recorded at 256 Hz using a BioSemi system. The subject's behavior and driving trajectory were also recorded at 256 Hz, in sync with the EEG acquisition system.

All EEG data were digitally filtered with a linear 1-45 Hz FIR pass band filter before further analysis. Due to poor skin contacts and bad electrodes, several channels showed large fluctuations during the entire experiment. These channels were rejected from further data analysis.

2.3 Analysis of Behavioral Performance

CTT. The recorded time series of disc screen coordinates, $x(t)$ and $y(t)$, were converted into a disc error time series, $d(t)$, defined as the radial distance between the disc and the screen center. Local minima of disc error, $d(t)$, were identified as critical moments when the disc started to drift away from the bulls-eye (Fig. 1a). Each local minimum was defined as a time-locking event for a single trial in which participants had to attempt to use the trackball to return the disc back toward the central ring. Tracking performance was obtained by computing the root mean square (RMS) of $d(t)$ in a moving time window centered at each local minimum. RMS disc error in a (4-s) short moving window indexed the subject's current ('local') CTT performance, whereas RMS disc error in a long (20-s) window was computed to index longer term ('global') changes in CTT performance (Fig. 2a,b).

Driving. In a representative hour-long driving session, 666 drift events (trials) were recorded (Fig. 2c,d). The record of vehicle trajectory indicated that the subject became drowsy and hit the curb or drove into the opposite lane several times in this session. Similar to real-world driving experience, the vehicle did not always return to the same cruising position after each compensatory steering maneuver. Therefore, during each drift/response trial, driving error was measured by maximum absolute deviation from the previous cruising position rather than by the absolute distance from lane center. Behavioral responses and corresponding EEG epochs were then sorted by this error measure (Fig. 2d), which was linearly correlated with reaction time, the interval between deviation onset and response onset (Fig. 1b). Shorter reaction times or lower errors generally indicated that the subject was more alert, and vice versa.

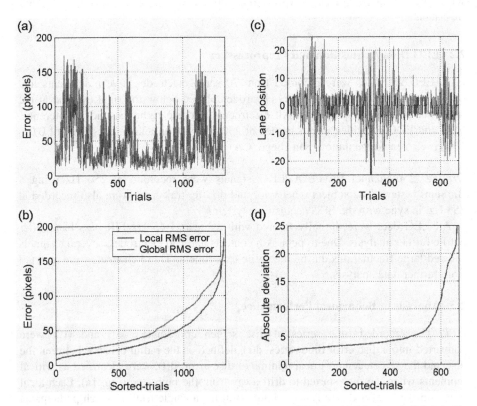

Fig. 2. Behavioral performance in hour-long sessions. (a) CTT. Local (blue) and global (red) RMS errors of trials in chronological order. (b) CTT. Trials sorted by local and global RMS errors. (c) Driving. Lane positions of trials in chronological order. (d) Driving. Trials sorted by absolute deviation.

2.4 Independent Component Analysis

Maximally independent EEG processes and their equivalent dipole source locations were obtained using the extended-infomax option of the *runica* algorithm and the DIPFIT tools in the EEGLAB toolbox (available for free download at http://sccn.ucsd.edu/eeglab) [15]. ICA finds an 'unmixing' matrix, W, which decomposes or linearly unmixes the multichannel EEG data, x, into a sum of maximally temporally independent and spatially fixed components u, where $u = Wx$. The rows of the output data matrix, u, are time courses of activations of the independent components (ICs). The ICA unmixing matrix was trained separately for each session and subject. Initial learning rate was 10^{-4}; training was stopped when learning rate fell below 10^{-7}. Some ICs were identified as accounting for blinks, other eye movements, or muscle artifacts [16]. Several non-artifact ICs showed event-related dynamics in various frequency bands that were time-locked to the lane drift or disc escape events. Below, we demonstrate time-frequency analysis of brain dynamics for a class of recovered ICs with equivalent dipole sources located bilaterally in lateral occipital cortex.

2.5 Time-Frequency Analysis

Epochs time-locked to drift events were extracted from the continuous IC time courses. In CTT sessions, each epoch contained data 1.5 s before and 3 s after each local minimum of disc error curve. In Driving task sessions, each epoch contained data 1 s before and 4 s after deviation onset (Fig. 1b). Epochs (trials) in each session were sorted by error, and then separated into five evenly spaced error-level groups. Here, we show results of time-frequency analysis on two groups of epochs, representing Alert (0-20%) and Drowsy (60-80%) performance in each session.

For each group of epochs, time series in each epoch k were transformed into time-frequency matrix $F_k(f,t)$ using a 1-s moving-window fast Fourier transforms (FFTs). Log power spectra were estimated at 100 linearly-spaced frequencies from 0.5 Hz to 50 Hz, and then were normalized by subtracting the log mean power spectrum in the baseline (pre-perturbation) periods for each group of epochs (Fig. 3). Event-related spectral perturbation (ERSP) images, were obtained by averaging n time-frequency matrices from the same group using:

$$ERSP(f,t) = \frac{1}{n}\sum_{k=1}^{n}\left|F_k(f,t)\right|^2 \qquad (1)$$

ERSP images were constructed to show only statistically significant ($p<0.01$) spectral perturbations (log power differences) from the mean power spectral baseline (Fig. 3). Significance of deviations from power spectral baseline was assessed using a surrogate data permutation method [15]. In the resulting ERSP images, non-significant time/frequency points were colored green (Figs. 4 and 5).

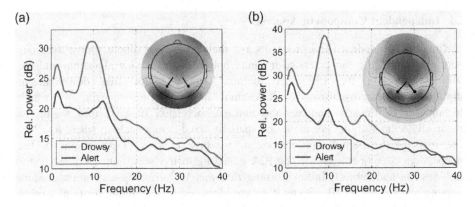

Fig. 3. Performance-related tonic increases in mean power spectra for independent components (ICs) with equivalent dipole sources located bilaterally in lateral occipital cortex, (a) from a CTT task session (70 channels), and (b) a Driving task session (256 channels). Insets: IC scalp maps and equivalent dipole source models.

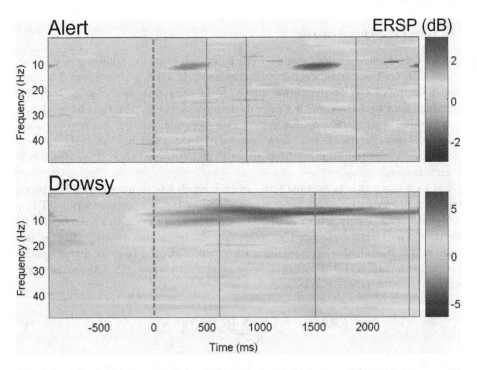

Fig. 4. Time-frequency images of event-related spectral perturbations (ERSPs) for the same IC in a CTT session (see Fig. 3). Dashed magenta line at time 0 marks a local error minimum in the disc trajectory. Solid magenta lines show median times of: 1) next subject response onset, 2) next local disc error maximum, 3) next disc error minimum.

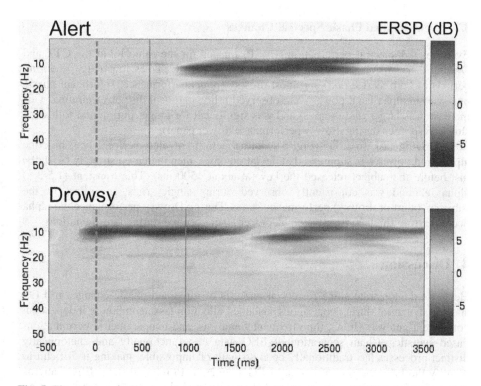

Fig. 5. Time-frequency images of event-related spectral perturbations (ERSPs) for the same IC in a Driving task session (see Fig. 3). Dash magenta lines: deviation onsets. Solid magenta lines: response onsets. Note that the initial alpha baseline power (not shown) was higher during Drowsy than during Alert performance (Fig. 3b).

3   Results

3.1   Performance-Related Tonic Spectral Changes

Fig. 3 shows scalp topographies and power spectral baselines for an IC appearing in separate decompositions of data recorded from the same subject during the two sustained-attention tasks. DIPFIT2 routines from EEGLAB were used to fit equivalent dipole source models to the IC scalp maps using a four-shell spherical head model [15, 17]. Results showed the equivalent dipole sources for this IC to be located in bilateral occipital cortex.

Wideband tonic increases were observed in the mean IC power spectra from low-error (Alert) to high-error (Drowsy) epochs, predominately in the alpha band (Fig. 3). Tonic brain activities in the occipital cortex have been shown to correlate with fluctuations of performance [3, 7]. Figure 3 shows that performance-related tonic spectral changes for equivalent ICs were very similar in two different sustained-attention tasks. ICs with quite similar scalp maps and tonic power spectral activities were consistently observed across sessions and subjects of both tasks (not shown because of space constraints).

3.2 Event-Related Phasic Spectral Changes

Event-related spectral perturbation (ERSP) images for the same IC in the CTT and Driving task sessions are shown in Figs. 4 and 5. In CTT sessions (Fig. 4) during periods of both alert (good) and most drowsy (poor) performance, significant phasic increases in alpha band power were observed following local disc error minima. This increase was larger (note scales) and was significant for longer during and following slower responses during drowsy performance (lower panel).

In Driving task sessions (Fig. 5), during periods of alert performance, baseline alpha band power was suppressed at deviation onset, then increased strongly (~10 dB) just before the subject released the key (at about 1500 ms). This transient (1.5-3 s) alpha rebound was consistently observed during single trials, regardless of the subjects' (alert or drowsy) performance status. During Drowsy performance, no alpha decrease from (higher) baseline alpha power level occurred during lane deviations.

4 Discussion

Here, we demonstrate some results of analysis of tonic and phasic changes in EEG spectral dynamics during continuous sustained-attention tasks combining independent component analysis (ICA), time-frequency analysis, and nonparametric permutation-based statistics. Clean separation of EEG data into functionally and anatomically distinct processes has traditionally been difficult or impossible, making it difficult to identify the brain origins of distinct EEG sources or to relate distinct EEG patterns originating in specific brain areas to behavior or pathology. In this study, we used ICA to blindly separate multi-channel data sets into statistically maximally independent components arising from distinct or overlapping brain and extra-brain networks. Time-frequency analysis could then be applied to the activations of the separated EEG source signals as opposed to the scalp-recorded mixtures of EEG activities, minimizing potential confounds arising from volume conduction and summation of source signals at the scalp sensors.

In two sustained-attention tasks, independent components (ICs) with equivalent dipole sources located in bilateral occipital cortex exhibited similar tonic and phasic performance-related power spectra changes. Tonic alpha-band power increased during periods of poor (high-error) compared to good (low-error) performance, while phasic alpha power increased following the drift events regardless of performance level.

The tonic increases in power spectra from alert to drowsy epochs were consistently observed across subjects and sessions, and were remarkably similar across two different sustained-attention tasks. The phasic power increases following lane-deviation events were very stable across subjects in the Driving experiments, possibly indexing subjects' visual relaxation of attention following each return to lane center. The phasic spectral perturbations were more variable for some subjects in the CTT experiments, possibly arising from our too uncritical selection of disc-escape moments to minor events to which subjects' brain activity might not have reacted strongly.

In real-world working environments, many tasks require sustained attention and responding to maintain continuous performance. It is critical for performers to detect significant events during continuous tasks, such as lane drifts during driving. In this study, we showed event-related phasic brain dynamic responses to events embedded in two tasks requiring continuous attention. These phasic event-related brain activities could be useful markers for measuring changes in the operator's awareness during tasks requiring continuous monitoring of information in their natural or machine environment.

Acknowledgments. This research was supported by gifts from The Swartz Foundation (Old Field, NY) and by grants from US National Aeronautics and Space Administration (NASA) and the United States Office of Naval Research. We thank Terrence J. Sejnowski for discussion and comments, and Julie Onton, Jennifer S. Kim, and Marisa Evans for help with experiment set-up.

References

1. Makeig, S., Inlow, M.: Lapses in alertness: coherence of fluctuations in performance and the EEG spectrum. Electroencephalogr. Clin. Neurophysiol. 86, 23–35 (1993)
2. Makeig, S., Jung, T.-P.: Changes in alertness are a principal component of variance in the EEG spectrum. NeuroReport 7, 213–216 (1995)
3. Makeig, S., Jung, T.-P.: Tonic, phasic and transient EEG correlates of auditory awareness in drowsiness. Cogn. Brain Res. 4, 15–25 (1996)
4. Jung, T.-P., Makeig, S., Stensmo, M., Sejnowski, T.J.: Estimating alertness from the EEG power spectrum. IEEE Trans. Biomed. Eng. 44(1), 60–69 (1997)
5. Jung, T.-P., Makeig, S., Sejnowski, T.J.: Awareness during drowsiness: dynamics and electrophysiological correlates. Canadian J. Exp. Psy. 54(4), 266–273 (2000)
6. Huang, R.-S., Tsai, L.L., Kuo, C.J.: Selection of valid and reliable EEG features for predicting auditory and visual alertness levels. In: Proc. Nat. Sci. Council, vol. 25, pp. 17–25 (2001)
7. Huang, R.-S., Jung, T.-P., Makeig, S.: Analyzing event-related brain dynamics in continuous compensatory tracking tasks. In: Proc. The 27th Annual International Conference of the IEEE Engineering in Medicine and Biology Society, Shanghai, China (2005)
8. Peiris, M.T., Jones, R.D., Davidson, P.R., Carroll, G.J., Bones, P.J.: Frequent lapses of responsiveness during an extended visuomotor tracking task in non-sleep-deprived subjects. J. Sleep Res. 15, 291–300 (2006)
9. Ogilvie, R.D.: The process of falling asleep. Sleep Med. Rev. 5(3), 247–270 (2001)
10. Bell, A.J., Sejnowski, T.J.: An information-maximisation approach to blind separation and blind deconvolution. Neural Comput. 7(6), 1004–1034 (1995)
11. Lee, T.W., Girolami, M., Sejnowski, T.J.: Independent component analysis using an extended infomax algorithm for mixed subgaussian and supergaussian sources. Neural Comput. 11(2), 417–441 (1999)
12. Jung, T.-P., Makeig, S., McKeown, M.J., Bell, A.J., Lee, T.-W., Sejnowski, T.J.: Imaging brain dynamics using independent component analysis. In: Proc. IEEE, vol. 89(7), pp. 1107–1122 (2001)
13. Makeig, S.: Auditory event-related dynamics of the EEG spectrum and effects of exposure to tones. Electroencephalogr. Clin. Neurophysiol. 86, 283–293 (1993)
14. Makeig, S., Jolley, M.: Comptrack: A compensatory tracking task for monitoring alertness (1995) ftp://ftp.snl.salk.edu/pub/scott/COMPTRACK.zip

15. Delorme, A., Makeig, S.: EEGLAB: an open source toolbox for analysis of single-trial EEG dynamics including independent component analysis. J. Neurosc. Meth. 134, 9–21 (2004)
16. Jung, T.-P., Humphries, C., Lee, T.-W., McKeown, M.J., Iragui, V., Makeig, S., Sejnowski, T.J.: Removing electroencephalographic artifacts by blind source separation. Psychophysiology 37, 163–178 (2000)
17. Oostenveld, R., Oostendorp, T.F.: Validating the boundary element method for forward and inverse EEG computations in the presence of a hole in the skull. Hum. Brain Mapp. 17, 179–192 (2002)

Information Filtering, Expertise and Cognitive Load

David N. Chin

University of Hawaii, Department of Information & Computer Sciences
1680 East West Rd, Honolulu, HI 96822, USA
chin@hawaii.edu

Abstract. Information filtering can be used to reduce cognitive load. However
the expertise level of the user will greatly affect the effectiveness of information
filtering. Any attempt to use neurophysiological measures of cognitive load for
information filtering should take these effects into account in the design of the
information filtering system. Combining information filtering, neurophysiological
measurements of cognitive load and user modeling of expertise can improve
performance. An integrated architecture for combining these techniques is
described along with its application to routing information within a crisis
management team.

Keywords: information filtering, cognitive load, expertise, stereotypes,
neurophysiological measures.

1 Introduction

Many computer applications have an excess of information that could be presented to
their users. Trying to make sense of too much information presented at once can lead
to cognitive overload for users. One technique for ameliorating such cognitive
overload is filtering the information that it presents to its users. Such information
filtering can be based on the requirements of the specific user task and/or based on
user preferences, either explicitly provided by the user or implicitly inferred by the
application and possibly stored in the application's user model. For example,
applications can filter Usenet news [9] and websites [11] based on inferred user
interests.

Even if applications filter information, there is still a question of how much
filtering to do. Too little information filtering can lead to missing important
information that is hidden by too much information and reduce user efficiency due to
cognitive overload. Too much filtering can lead to loss of important information that
isn't presented and can even reduce user performance due to inattention or boredom.
Different users vary in information processing capabilities and the same user can vary
in capability from moment to moment due to inebriation, tiredness, and/or
distractions. Ideally, the application should adapt its degree of filtering to the user's
actual cognitive load as roughly estimated with neurophysiological sensors [6, 7].

However, even a strong feedback loop that varies the degree of information
filtering to maintain a reasonable cognitive load must take into account the expertise

D.D. Schmorrow, L.M. Reeves (Eds.): Augmented Cognition, HCII 2007, LNAI 4565, pp. 75–83, 2007.
© Springer-Verlag Berlin Heidelberg 2007

of the user in processing information. For example, if the application wants to increase the cognitive load to prevent boredom, how much more information to present depends on the user's ability to process that information. That is, the expertise of the user in the information domain and the application should determine how much information to present. Expertise level can be inferred from user interactions with the application, represented as expertise stereotypes and used to adapt the application to the user's level of expertise such as in the domain of giving advice about how to use UNIX [2, 3].

Combining the three techniques of information filtering, neurophysiological estimation of cognitive load and user modeling of expertise can improve the performance of applications beyond the capability of any individual or pair of techniques.

2 Information Filtering

Information filtering can be viewed as the inverse of information retrieval [1], so many information retrieval techniques can be used to rate information relevance for filtering purposes. Techniques for personalized filtering include collaborative filtering [9], Bayesian classifiers [11], and others. However, in many applications the user is engaged in performing a specific task, so knowledge about the requirements of the task can be used to select information relevant for the current task. For example, Julier et al. filtered information presented in an augmented reality (AR) display based on factors such as task relevance and user location [8]. Julier et al.'s AR system used a detailed analysis of task structure for information filtering. Grootjen et al. have looked at task effort and their effects on operators [4]. However a much simpler analysis of user roles and the information requirements of common tasks performed by those roles would suffice for simple information filtering.

Also useful for information filtering is knowledge about the role of the user within a team. Information that might not be very relevant for a user's current task(s) may still be useful background information for that user's role. For example, a lieutenant who is in the midst of planning a perimeter defense would not need to know for the perimeter defense task that fuel reserves are running low, but would still benefit form the knowledge in future tasks. Likewise, a professor specializing in AI would not need to know about a breakthrough in chip design, but would still benefit from the knowledge in his/her role as a teacher of computer science.

A common problem in organizations is information routing: getting the right information to the right people in a timely fashion. Information routing can be viewed as the flip side of information filtering where information that is not routed to a user is in effect filtered out. For example, we (members of my lab and I) observed both the 2004 State of Delaware Division of Public Health "Operation Diamond Shield" and the 2004 State of Hawaii Department of Health "Bioterrorism Preparedness Exercise." Both exercises simulated a bioterrorism attack requiring activation of the Strategic National Stockpile (SNS). In both cases, the State health departments simulated loss of offices and their disaster response teams gathered in one location with portable office equipment to handle the simulated emergency.

Personnel were divided up into small teams to handle specific aspects of the disaster. We observed that a key problem in both exercises was information routing. During the exercises, people would often take down information and act upon it. However they would often forget to inform others, especially those in other teams, because they became caught up in handling their own responsibilities.

A computerized information routing system could easily be created to handle the needs of either health department. Such a system would require only a simple analysis of the roles and tasks of each member of the health teams combined with simple high-level ontology of information types. As information flowed into the disaster response team mostly by phone and sometimes by fax, email or web access, the receiving team member would typically jot down the information on a pad along with meta-data such as the source, date and time. Because each team member needed to immediately handle their own vital tasks, other people that might benefit from the received information would sometimes not be informed or informed late. By switching to an electronic pad such as a tablet PC and adding a checkbox for information type based on the ontology, an information routing system could easily forward the incoming information to the right people based on the information needs for their roles and tasks and/or based on their interests.

3 Neurophysiological Measurement of Cognitive Load

When too much information is presented at once to users, they experience information overload. On the other hand, too little information can lead to lower performance due to boredom or inattention. Ideally an application should adapt the information flow to maintain the user's cognitive load within some optimal range. The only way to do this is for the application to measure the user's actual cognitive load. Without measurements, it is very difficult to predict the cognitive load of information processing for a user. Not only do different users have different information processing capacities that vary with the type and difficulty of information, but also the same user can vary in capacity when tired, in pain, under the influence of psychoactive substances, or simply distracted by the environment or even his/her own thoughts.

One of the key research areas of Augmented Cognition [12] is the measurement of cognitive load. Although there is no single measurement technique that will work for all users across all tasks, certain techniques will work well for specific tasks. For example, the Warship Commander task in the DARPA Augmented Cognition Technical Integration Experiment [14] simulates a typical Navy air warfare task. Our Perceptual/Motor Load and Cognitive Difficulty measures were computed from eight pressure sensors on our Pressure Mouse [6, 7]. These measures correlated with two measures of task difficulty (number of airplane tracks and difficulty of plan tracks) at better than 95% consistently across experiment participants.

With the right neurophysiological measure for an appropriate task, an application can potentially adapt the information flow to a user. In the example application of routing information to disaster management team members, the application could vary the degree of information filtering to maintain the cognitive load of the user within a desired range (neither too much information at once, nor too little). As new information comes in, the application can consider the relevance of the information to the user's current task and role, the user's current cognitive load and the priority of the information (which can be determined by another check box when the information is first entered). Based on these factors, the application can decide whether the new information should be presented to the user immediately (thereby potentially increasing the user's cognitive load), delayed until the user is less loaded, or discarded as irrelevant to this user.

Another consideration is the interests of the user. Information that is not relevant to a particular user's tasks or role may still be of general interest to the user. Such lower priority information can be delayed until the user's measured cognitive load is low enough to warrant presentation of the interesting but irrelevant information.

4   User Model of Expertise

An important consideration for how much new information to present is an assessment of the difficulty of processing the new material for the specific user. That is, how much will the new information increase the cognitive load for this user? A new piece of information in the user's domain of expertise may only increase cognitive load slightly for the user. However another user without the domain expertise may find it very difficult to process the same information. Therefore a model of expertise that helps predict the difficulty of information processing is needed to properly decide how much information filtering should be done.

Our previous work in modeling expertise in UC (the UNIX Consultant system) used stereotypes for levels of expertise (novice to expert) in the UNIX domain [2, 3]. UC also had stereotype levels of difficulty for UNIX information (simple to complex). UC was able to infer the user's stereotype level from the user's interaction with the system. For example, if the user asked a question about something very simple like how to delete a file, then UC was able to rule out higher levels of expertise like intermediate or expert since it is almost a contradiction in terms to say that an expert or even an intermediate in the UNIX domain would not know how to delete a file in UNIX. Likewise, if a user demonstrates knowledge about something complex like file inodes (in UNIX, each file has a unique integer identifier called an inode), then UC could rule out lower levels of expertise like novice and beginner because such lower level users would not normally know such difficult UNIX concepts.

In the example application of routing information to disaster management team members, a user model of expertise similar to the stereotypes in UC could be created for each expertise area in disaster management. For example, one could have expertise stereotype levels for infectious diseases, hospital management, and crisis communication public relations.

Somewhat more problematic is determining the difficulty levels for incoming information. The problem is that the information taker may not be very knowledgeable in the domain, in which case the application cannot expect a non-expert to reliably judge the difficulty level of the incoming information. Fortunately, our observations of the actual information flow during both the Delaware and Hawaii SNS exercises showed that most of the time it was experts in the area that took down the information. This was partly due to the fact that about half of the time, it was the experts that were making phone calls or sending email or searching the web for information that they needed for their current task. The other half of the time, outsiders would call in or email information (called "injections" in the exercises) and if the wrong person answered the phone, the right person would usually be called over to handle it. So if this pattern is continued for an automated system, the great majority of the time the information entry will be by an expert in the domain who can easily judge the difficulty of processing the information.

In cases where the information taker is not an expert in the domain of the incoming information, the application could find a less cognitively loaded expert to quickly evaluate the difficulty of the information. Most likely, the evaluating expert would also find the information useful for his/her own purposes.

Another undetermined problem that will require investigation is whether expert judgments of difficulty really correlate well with the actual increase in cognitive load when an individual processes the information. Other potential problems include the degree of individual differences in processing efficiency. If such differences tend to stay fairly constant for any single individual, then it may be possible to correct for individual differences in processing efficiency by learning the correction factor for each individual.

5 An Integrated Architecture

To perform information filtering based on user expertise, cognitive load, roles and tasks, we propose a new integrated architecture. As shown in Fig. 1, key elements of the architecture include the Information Filterer, the Neurophysiological Sensor System, the User Model, the information ontology and a human Information Taker. The incoming information is processed first by the Information Taker who frequently will also be the one to enter the information into the application using a tablet PC or similar device. The Information Taker is asked to select the topic area of the incoming information from a high-level domain-specific ontology and rate the priority of the incoming information. If the Information Taker is an intermediate or expert in the information type, then he/she is also asked to rate the difficulty level of the incoming information. If the Information Taker does not have the expertise to rate the difficulty of the incoming information (based on the User Model's assessment of the Information Taker's expertise in the topic area of the incoming information), then another user with the right expertise is shown the incoming information and asked to rate its difficulty level. Which expert user to select and when to ask that user will depend on the measured cognitive loads of the available experts and the priority of the incoming information relative to the priority of their current tasks.

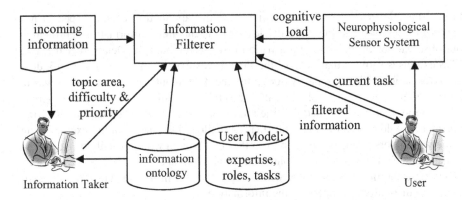

Fig. 1. An integrated architecture for information filtering based on neurophysiological sensors and a user model with expertise, role and task models

The Information Filterer decides which other users should be shown the incoming information based on the Information Taker's (or other expert's) assessment of the information's topic area, priority, and difficulty level. Note that the Information Filterer does not need to analyze the actual incoming information in any way and indeed the incoming information can remain in picture format exactly as scribbled on the tablet PC by the Information Taker. All required analysis is done by humans. If the incoming information is relevant to a user's tasks or role(s) or if it is of general interest to the user, then the incoming information becomes a candidate for display to the user. Otherwise, the information is filtered out for this particular user.

Determining when to actually show the candidate information to a user depends on the priority of the information (P), the user's current cognitive load (CL), the difficulty level of the information (D), the expertise level of the user in the topic area of the information (E), the user's current task and the relevance of the information to the user's current task (RT), the user's role(s) and the relevance of the information to the user's role (RR), and the user's interest in the topic area (I). First, the incremental cognitive load (ICL) of presenting the information is computed from D, E and CL. CL is required because ICL may not be linear with cognitive load. As a first approximation, $ICL \propto D / E$. However more research is needed to determine the exact nature of the relationship between ICL, D, E and CL.

Second, the relevance of the information to the user's current task, RT, is looked up in a table of task and information needs for the task. Relevance of the information to the user's role(s), RR, is likewise looked up in a table of roles and their information needs. The user's role is fixed at account setup and will change only as the user takes on new responsibilities or changes jobs. The user's current task is more problematic to determine. Automated plan recognition techniques such as used in the Microsoft Office Assistant [5] could infer the user's current task or the application could simply ask the user to select a task from a task hierarchy (users might be willing to do this if the information filtering works well enough to make it worth their while). Alternatively automated plan recognition could be combined with asking the user whenever the probability of the current task drops below a threshold.

Third, the relevance of the information to the user's role(s), RR, is looked up in a table of roles and information needs for those roles. Alternatively, the application could look up the role(s) in a table of roles and typical tasks for those roles, then determine the relevance of information to a role by checking whether the information is relevant for any of the tasks performed by that role. Fourth, the user's level of interest in the information, I, is computed using recommender techniques.

After computing ICL, RT, RR and I, the Information Filterer is ready to decide whether to display the information and when to display it. Table 1 summarizes the decisions. If RT is false, RR is false and I is low, then the information is filtered out and will never be displayed to this user unless the user selects it while browsing for information. This represents the case where the information is not needed for the user's current task nor for the user's role(s) nor is the user interested in the topic area of the information.

If RT is true and/or RR is true and CL + ICL <= the desired maximum cognitive load (MaxCL), then the candidate information is displayed to the user immediately. This represents the case where the information is needed by the user to do his/her current task and the user has the cognitive capacity to handle the information immediately.

If RT is true and CL + ICL > MaxCL, then the information is displayed only if P is greater than the average priority of all currently displayed information. This represents the case where the user needs the information to do his/her current task and the new information is more important than the information the user is already considering. Otherwise the information is delayed until CL drops enough to allow display, which will likely be after the user has finished processing the already displayed information. Note that if ICL > MaxCL, then the information may never be displayed to this user (even if CL drops to 0). In such cases if the information is relevant to the user's task, then a warning should be generated to let the supervisor know that this user does not have the expertise to handle some information required for his/her assigned task and perhaps a task reassignment is in order.

Table 1. Decision table for displaying information by the Information Filterer. RT = Relevance to Task, RR = Relevance to Role, I = Interest level of information to the user, CL = current Cognitive Load, ICL = Incremental Cognitve Load predicted for the incoming information, P = information Priority.

RT	RR	I	Cognitive load	P	Display?
False	False	Low	any	any	No
True	any	any	CL + ICL <= MaxCL	any	Yes
True	any	any	CL + ICL > MaxCL	P > displayed average	Yes
True	any	any	CL + ICL > MaxCL	P <= displayed average	Delay
False	True	any	CL + ICL <= MaxCL	any	Yes
False	True	any	CL + ICL > MaxCL	any	Delay
False	False	High	CL < MinCL & CL +ICL <= MaxCL	any	Yes
False	False	High	CL >= MinCL | CL + ICL > MaxCL	any	Delay

If RT is false but RR is true and CL + ICL > MaxCL, then the information is delayed. This represents the case where the information is not needed for the user's current task but may be needed for future tasks, but the user does not have the cognitive capacity to process the information immediately. If both RT and RR are false, but I is high, then the information is displayed immediately only if CL < the desired minimum cognitive load (MinCL) and CL + ICL <= MaxCL. This represents the case where the information is not needed for the user's current or future tasks, but the user is interested in the general topic area and the user is currently under stimulated and the user would not be over stimulated by the new information. Otherwise the information is delayed. Note that if ICL > MaxCL, then the user does not have the expertise to process this information, but there is no cause for alarm because this information is irrelevant to this user's job.

6 Related Architectures

Other augmented cognition systems have performed some types of information filtering. This review focuses only on their information filtering aspects and not on their many other related capabilities. One closed-loop system, the Boeing team's UCAV (Uninhabited Combat Air Vehicle) simulator, used a fog layer to obscure unimportant map details and used chunking to group related information about UCAVs and their recommended targets [13]. Higher levels of filtering reduced the number of visible UCAV chunks. The Boeing augmented UCAV system's information filtering can be modeled in the integrated architecture by assigning priorities to UCAVs by proximity to target.

The Lockheed Martin Advanced Technology Laboratories' simulated Tactical Tomahawk Weapons Control System (TTWCS) varied the pace of information presentation based on measured cognitive load using an architecture called PACE [10, 15]. The PACE architecture's information filtering components includes cognitive load and priority adaptation, but assumes all information is relevant and does not take into account the user's expertise in computing the potential increase in cognitive load caused by the new information.

7 Conclusions

Although there are many research questions that still need to be answered before a system will be able to adapt information filtering to a user's role, tasks, expertise and cognitive load, this integrated architecture represents an ideal that we should strive to attain. Such a system could potentially improve performance by ensuring that users gets the information that they need for their tasks and for their roles at a pace that they can handle. Such a system would likely improve user satisfaction because users would face fewer frustrations from missing vital information, would feel overwhelmed less often, and would experience fewer bouts of boredom.

Acknowledgements. This research was sponsored in part by Quantum Leap Innovations, Inc. (subcontracted from the Office of Naval Research contract N00014-02-C-0320), DARPA under grant no. NBCH1020004 and the Office of Naval Research under grants no. N000149710578 and N000140310135.

References

1. Belkin, N.J., Croft, W.B.: Information filtering and information retrieval: two sides of the same coin? Communications of the ACM 35(12), 29–38 (1992)
2. Chin, D.N.: KNOME: Modeling What the User Knows in UC. In: Kobsa, A., Wahlster, W. (eds.) User Models in Dialog Systems, pp. 74–107 Springer, Berlin (1989)
3. Chin, D.N.: Planning Intelligent Responses in a Natural Language System. In: Hegner, S.J., McKevitt, P., Norvig, P., Wilensky, R. (eds.) Intelligent Help Systems for UNIX, pp. 283–331. Kluwer Academic Publishers, Dordrecht, Netherlands (2001)
4. Grootjen, M., Neerincx, M.A., van Weert, J.C.M.: Learning Models of Scientific Problem Solving. In: Proceedings of 2006 Augmented Cognition International, San Francisco (2006)
5. Horovitz, E., Breese, J., Heckerman, D., Hovel, D., Rommelse, K.: The Lumière Project: Bayesian User Modeling for Inferring the Goals and Needs of Software Users. In: Proceedings of the Fourteenth Conference on Uncertainty in Artificial Intelligence, Madison, WI, pp. 256–265. Morgan Kaufmann, San Francisco (1998)
6. Ikehara, C.S., Chin, D.N., Crosby, M.E.: A Model for Integrating an Adaptive Information Filter Utilizing Biosensor Data to Assess Cognitive Load. In: Proceedings of Ninth International Conference on User Modeling, pp. 208–212 (2003)
7. Ikehara, C.S., Chin, D.N., Crosby, M.E.: Modeling and Implementing an Adaptive Human-Computer Interface Using Passive Biosensors. In: Proceedings of the 37th Hawaii International Conference on System Science (HICSS-37) (January 2004)
8. Julier, S., Lanzagorta, M., Baillot, Y., Rosenblum, L., Feiner, S., Höllerer, T., Sestito, S.: Information filtering for mobile augmented reality. In: Proceedings Augmented Reality (ISAR 2000), pp. 3–11 (October 2000)
9. Konstan, J.A., Miller, B.N., Maltz, D., Herlocker, J.L., Gordon, L.R., Riedl, J.: GroupLens: applying collaborative filtering to Usenet news. Communications of the ACM 40(3), 77–87 (1997)
10. Morizio, N., Thomas, M., Tremoulet, P.: Performance Augmentation through Cognitive Enhancement (PACE). In: the Proceedings of the International Conference on Human Computer Interaction, Las Vegas, NV (2005)
11. Pazzani, M., Billsus, D.: Learning and Revising User Profiles: The Identification of Interesting Web Sites. Machine Learning 27(3), 313–331 (1997)
12. Schmorrow, D.S. (ed.): Foundations of Augmented Cognition. Lawrence Erlbaum Associates, Mahwah (2005)
13. Snow, M.P., Barker, R.A., O'Neill, K.R., Offer, B.W., Edwards, R.E.: Augmented Cognition in a Prototype Uninhabited Combat Air Vehicle Operator Console. In: Proceedings of 2006 Augmented Cognition International, San Francisco (2006)
14. St. John, M., Kobus, D.A., Morrison, J.G.: DARPA Augmented Cognition Technical Integration Experiment (TIE). Technical Report 1905.San Diego: Pacific Science and Engineering Group, Inc. (2003)
15. Tremoulet, P., Barton, J., Craven, P., Gifford, A., Morizio, N., Belov, N., Stibler, K., Harkness Regli, S., Thomas, M.: Augmented Cognition for Tactical Tomahawk Weapons Control System Operators. In: Proceedings of 2006 Augmented Cognition International, San Francisco (2006)

Using Eye Blinks as a Tool for Augmented Cognition

Ric Heishman and Zoran Duric

4400 University Drive
Fairfax, Virginia 22030
{rheishman,zduric}@cs.gmu.edu

Abstract. The human face comprises a complex system integrated from tissue, bone and electricity. Biometrics associated with this region provide useful information for a wide range of research disciplines. For those interested in augmented cognition, the metrics and behaviors inherent to eye blinks are particularly valuable in the interpretation and understanding of an individual's affective and cognitive states. Our work involves a novel integration of computer vision techniques for observing and interpreting the biometric information flow inherent in human eye blinks, and using these behavioral patterns to gain insight into the cognitive engagement and fatigue levels of individual subjects. Of particular interest are behavioral ambiguities – both across multiple subjects and in individual subjects across various scenarios – that present problems to both the observation and interpretation processes. Our work is pertinent to system development efforts across a wide range of applications, including driver fatigue, medical patient monitoring and critical system operator vigilance.

Keywords: Eye, blink, cognition, affective computing, motion.

1 Introduction

The human face comprises a complex system integrated from tissue, bone and electricity. Biometrics associated with this region provide useful information for a wide range of research disciplines. For those interested in the general field of augmented cognition, the metrics and behaviors surrounding eye blinks can be particularly valuable in the understanding and interpretation of an individual's affective and cognitive states. Our work involves a novel integration of computer vision techniques for observing and interpreting the biometric information flow inherent in human eye blinks, and using these behavioral patterns to gain insight into the cognitive engagement and fatigue levels of individual subjects. Metrics such as blink frequency and blink transition time or blink closure duration can serve to characterize particular states in individual subjects. Of particular interest are behavioral ambiguities – both across multiple subjects and in individual subjects across various scenarios – that present problems to both the observation and interpretation processes. These ambiguities, such as incomplete or erratic eye closure, asymmetrical blink behavior, and minimal motion during transition, are present in one or more forms in a significant percentage of groups of random individuals.

D.D. Schmorrow, L.M. Reeves (Eds.): Augmented Cognition, HCII 2007, LNAI 4565, pp. 84–93, 2007.
© Springer-Verlag Berlin Heidelberg 2007

2 Experimental Framework

Our basic experimental design methodology engages random subjects with specific cognitive activities under contrasting conditions of mental and physical fatigue. The subjects were digitally videotaped from a frontal parallel view while participating in each of four experimental sessions: FD – Fatigued/Disengaged, FE – Fatigued/Engaged, ND – Non-Fatigued/Disengaged, NE – Non-Fatigued/Engaged. The FE/FD (fatigued) sessions were held late in the evening after a normal work day and the NE/ND (non-fatigued) sessions were held early in the morning after a full night's rest (minimum of eight hours). In the FD/ND (disengaged) sessions, the subject maintained continuous eye contact with the computer screen and was instructed to clear their minds (defocus) or "daydream". The length of these sessions averaged 15-20 minutes each. The FE/NE (engaged) sessions involved the subjects exercising problem-solving skills on a specific graphical puzzle activity. The length of these sessions averaged 20-25 minutes each.

The data processing and analysis stage involves five phases. In the manual *initialization* phase, the user chooses open and closed eye sample frames and sets the Region-Of-Interest (ROI) for each eye in these frames. The system then processes an initial frameset (1000 video frames) to gather a working set of eye transition ROIs. The *reduction* phase reduces this working set to a small number (~50) and the *clustering* phase uses k-means clustering to create a minimal eye transition alphabet (~12). The *classification* phase processes the remaining frames using a combination of static histogram analysis and dynamic image flow analysis to generate the eye state matrix. Finally, the *determination* phase employs a deterministic finite state machine to process the eye state matrix and generate the final blink behavior data.

Preliminary testing involved seven random volunteer subjects. Structured testing was then performed using five additional random volunteer subjects. Collectively, these experiments provided approximately 1.5 million color video frames for processing and analysis. For additional detail on these processes and techniques, please refer to prior publications by the authors and others [1,2,4].

3 Ambiguous Blink Behaviors

Figure 1 depicts an example of optimal eye biometric monitoring conditions, where there is clear definition of the open and closed eye states, sufficient transition range, and symmetry between the left and right eye regions.

Fig. 1. Example of optimal eye biometric monitoring conditions

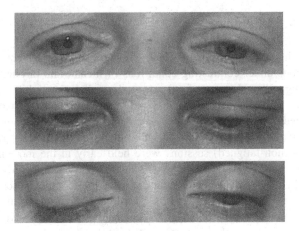

Fig. 2. Examples of ambiguous eye biometric monitoring conditions. Top – narrow eye openings and asymmetrical open states, Middle – incomplete closed state, Bottom – asymmetrical and incomplete closed state.

Figure 2 depicts three examples of ambiguous eye region behaviors. The *top* subject exhibits narrow eye openings and asymmetrical open states, which provide limited transition range and problematic correlation between the left and right eye regions. The *middle* subject exhibits an incomplete closed state, which provides a limited transition range. The *bottom* subject exhibits both an asymmetric and incomplete closed state, which causes problematic state correlation between the left and right eye regions.

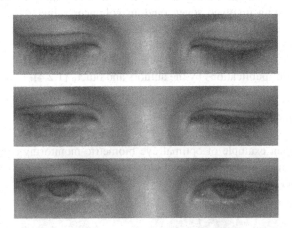

Fig. 3. Three different closed states for a single subject within a single HCI scenario

Figure 3 depicts three examples of differing blink behaviors exhibited by a single subject within a single HCI scenario testing session. This volatile behavior provides differing transition range metrics that cause problems with blink definition parameters. Our initial approach for eye ROI analysis involved the use of static frame-by-frame histogram analysis. However, given the frequency and breadth of the aforementioned blink behavior ambiguities, we shifted our subsequent analyses to a more dynamic approach using flow analysis across contiguous series of frames.

4 Comparison of Analysis Techniques

To compensate for the inadequacies inherent to static computer vision monitoring techniques, flow analysis can be used to enhance interpretation by compensating for processing anomalies that arise in problematic data streams. Flow analysis provides crisp parsing of the blink transition stages and is significantly more effective in delineation and classification when used in conjunction with or in lieu of static computer vision techniques such as histogram analysis using Euclidean Distances. Again, for detailed discussion of these techniques, refer to prior publications by the authors [2,4].

Table 1 provides a comparison of results from two of the processing extremes – subject CD (previously cited as an example of optimal eye biometric monitoring conditions (refer to Fig. 1) and subject SG (previously cited as an example of eye biometric pattern inconsistencies (refer to Fig. 3). The subject data was processed through three testing phases: *Manual* – manually counted while viewing video sequence at reduced speed, *Histogram* – (automatically processed using static

Table 1. Comparison between a subject exhibiting optimal eye biometric monitoring conditions (CD) and ambiguous eye biometric behavior (SG). Subject SG exhibited multiple completely-closed eye blink states (as depicted in Fig. 3).

	CD-FD			SG-ND		
	Manual	Histogram	Flow	Manual	Histogram	Flow
Blinks						
- total blinks in scenario	237	235	237	350	292	351
- blink frequency (seconds)	3.79	3.82	3.79	3.07	3.68	3.06
Steady-State (time between blinks)						
- min (seconds)	0.00	0.00	0.00	0.00	0.03	0.00
- max (seconds)	16.30	16.47	16.97	15.13	20.47	15.40
- mean (seconds)	3.39	3.47	3.43	2.76	3.15	2.66
- std dev (seconds)	2.57	2.65	2.97	2.55	2.55	2.28
Transition (blink duration – open/closed/open)						
- min (seconds)	0.30	0.07	0.10	0.10	0.10	0.10
- max (seconds)	0.77	4.23	0.53	0.43	0.43	0.63
- mean (seconds)	0.38	0.39	0.30	0.22	0.23	0.28
- std dev (seconds)	0.06	0.43	0.09	0.08	0.05	0.08

histogram analysis techniques, and *Flow* – hybrid process using both histogram and flow analysis techniques. Note that the *Manual* and *Flow* data are consistent across both subjects, with some differences due to inconsistencies inherent to manual objective dispositioning. Conversely, the *Histogram* results are consistent in the ideal subject but quite erratic in the problematic subject. Table 2 provides a sample data set of a single subject across all four HCI testing scenarios.

Table 2. Complete example data set for single subject using three techniques (M – manual, H – static histogram, F – dynamic hybrid histogram/flow) across all four HCI scenarios

Scenario	Method	Total Blinks	Blink Freq	Period (max)	Period (min)	Period (mean)	Period (sd)	Tran (max)	Tran (min)	Tran (mean)	Tran (sd)
FD	M	677	*	*	*	*	*	*	*	*	*
	H	638	1.97	8.57	0.00	1.66	1.30	5.00	0.10	0.36	0.35
	F	678	1.85	8.73	0.00	1.55	1.25	0.76	0.10	0.28	0.07
FE	M	511	*	*	*	*	*	*	*	*	*
	H	483	2.68	13.27	0.00	2.38	1.85	19.30	0.10	0.36	1.19
	F	510	2.54	8.27	0.00	2.28	1.61	0.60	0.10	0.24	0.05
ND	M	350	3.07	15.13	0.00	2.76	2.55	0.43	0.10	0.22	0.08
	H	292	3.68	20.47	0.03	3.48	3.15	0.43	0.10	0.23	0.05
	F	351	3.06	15.40	0.00	2.66	2.28	0.63	0.10	0.28	0.08
NE	M	267	*	*	*	*	*	*	*	*	*
	H	286	5.58	24.33	0.00	4.67	4.87	19.73	0.07	1.93	3.56
	F	266	6.00	31.60	0.07	5.71	5.04	0.06	0.10	0.26	0.06

5   Affective and Cognitive State Classification

Recent studies focused in areas relevant to eye blinks involving cognitive engagement and fatigue provide the following general assertions [3,6]:

- *blink rate* (BR) tends to increase as a function of cognitive workload, fatigue and time-on-task
- *blink closure duration* (BCD) tends to decrease as a function of cognitive work-load and increases as a function of fatigue

Fig. 4 provides the layout of our adaptation of Russell's conceptual framework – the Pleasure-Arousal psychological judgment space for affected feelings[5], which we refer to as the Fatigued, Engaged, Non-Fatigued, Disengaged (FEND) Condition Space. The horizontal plane represents the Fatigue state spectrum from Fatigued to Non-Fatigued. The vertical plane represents the Engagement state spectrum from Engaged to Disengaged. The quadrants formed by the integration of the two state dimensions provide the behavioral context for each of the four unique HCI scenarios. Each quadrant displays the corresponding Blink Rate (BR) and Blink Closure Duration (BCD) behaviors, based on historical empirical data from previous studies, for that particular state context.

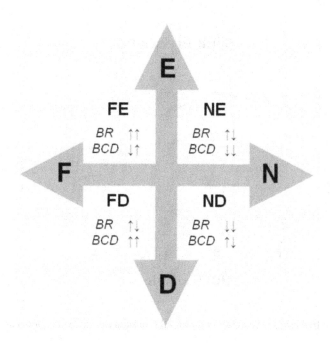

Fig. 4. Examples Fatigued, Engaged, Non-Fatigued, Disengaged (FEND) Condition Space – framework for the experimental domain

Given the aforementioned impact of fatigue and cognitive engagement on each scenario context, the following expectations regarding the Blink Rate (BR) and Blink Closure Duration (BCD) behaviors are implied. The magnitude of the impact of each state is assumed to be relatively equal for framework development purposes.

- *FE scenario* – elevated BR with moderate BCD
- *NE scenario* – moderate BR with suppressed BCD
- *ND scenario* – suppressed BR with moderate BCD
- *FD scenario* – moderate BR with elevated BCD

Figs. 5 & 6 provide the Blink frequency (blink rate – BR) and transition duration (blink closure duration – BCD) for all five subjects across the four HCI scenarios. In each plot, the dashed line represents the relative expected behavioral trend, as outlined in the FEND Condition Space (refer to Fig. 4). For blink frequency, the general expectation gleaned from cognitive psychology is that the highest blink rate should be exhibited by subjects in the FE state; the lowest blink rate should be exhibited by subjects in the ND state; and the subject's blink rates for the FD and NE states should fall somewhere between FE and ND. For transition duration, the general expectation is that the longest blink closure duration should be exhibited by subjects in the FD state; the lowest closure duration should be exhibited by subjects in the NE state; and the subject's blink closure duration for the FE and ND states should fall somewhere between FD and NE.

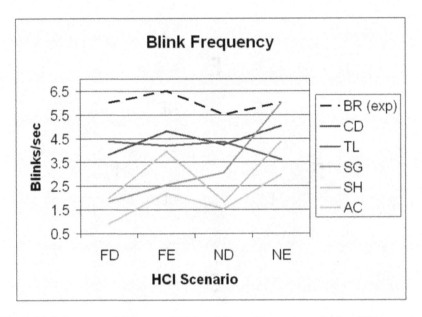

Fig. 5. Blink frequency (blink rate – BR) for all five subjects across the four HCI scenarios

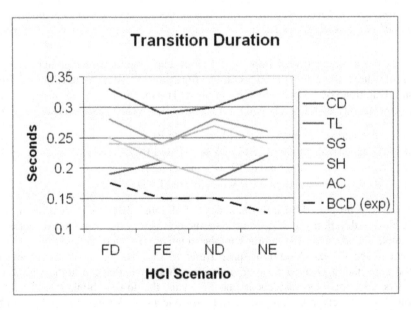

Fig. 6. Transition duration (blink closure duration – BCD) for all five subjects across the four HCI scenarios

This side-by-side comparison clearly illustrates one important fact – that there is no universal blink rate or blink closure duration that can be assumed for a generalized group of subjects. Another interesting thing to note here is that there was very little overlap in the results for each individual subject, thus each subject's behavioral range was unique on the relative magnitude scale. Finally, while the individual ranges of the transition durations projected by all subjects were relatively similar, some subjects expressed double (and in one case quadruple) the range of other subjects in the blink frequency data. We next present a more detailed examination of each individual subject.

Subject CD exhibits deviation from the expected behavior for blink rate. The NE and FD scenarios constitute the highest and lowest (respectively) blink rates while the FE and ND scenarios fall toward the middle of the range. The data does show elevated blink rates for the engaged versus disengaged sessions, however the fatigued versus non-fatigued sessions cover a similar, slightly translated trend. This subject's blink closure duration data tracks well with the expected trend, with the exception of the NE scenario – which is similar in value to the FD scenario. The summary for this subject is as follows:

- *FE scenario* – moderately elevated BR with moderate BCD
- *NE scenario* – elevated BR with elevated BCD
- *ND scenario* – moderately suppressed BR with moderate BCD
- *FD scenario* – suppressed BR with elevated BCD

Subject SG exhibits significant deviation from the expected behavior for blink rate in all scenarios. As with subject CD, the NE and FD scenarios constitute the highest and lowest (respectively) blink rates while the FE and ND scenarios fall toward the middle of the range. The data here show elevated blink rates for the non-fatigued versus fatigued sessions, however the engaged versus disengaged sessions provide little useful distinction. This subject's blink closure duration data is relatively flat, with minimal tracking with the expected trend. The summary for this subject is as follows:

- *FE scenario* – slightly suppressed BR with slightly suppressed BCD
- *NE scenario* – significantly elevated BR with moderate BCD
- *ND scenario* – slightly elevated BR with moderate BCD
- *FD scenario* – suppressed BR with moderate BCD

Subject TL exhibits nearly completely opposing trends to the expected behavior for blink rate in all scenarios. Additionally, there is significantly less variation in the data across scenarios compared to the other subjects. The only significant blink rate behavior is expressed in the NE scenario. As with the blink rate data, this subject's blink closure duration tracks nearly opposite to the expected trend. The data does reflect, however a distinction between the engaged versus disengaged sessions. The summary for this subject is as follows:

- *FE scenario* – slightly suppressed BR with slightly elevated BCD
- *NE scenario* – suppressed BR with elevated BCD
- *ND scenario* – slightly elevated BR with moderate BCD
- *FD scenario* – slightly elevated BR with slightly suppressed BCD

The subject SH blink rate data shows clear distinction between the engaged and disengaged sessions but no distinction between the fatigued and non-fatigued sessions. The blink closure duration data provides only slight distinction in the ND scenario. These biometric behaviors taken together provide the following general classification for this individual subject. As reflected in the classification rules, distinguishing between the FE and NE scenarios is problematic. The summary for this subject is as follows:

- *FE scenario* – significantly elevated BR with suppressed BCD ***
- *NE scenario* – significantly elevated BR with suppressed BCD ***
- *ND scenario* – significantly suppressed BR with slightly elevated BCD
- *FD scenario* – significantly suppressed BR with suppressed BCD

Subject AC exhibits deviation from the expected behavior similar to subject CD for blink rate, however with an exaggerated data spread. The NE and FD scenarios constitute the highest and lowest (respectively) blink rates while the FE and ND scenarios fall toward the middle of the range. The data does show elevated blink rates for the engaged versus disengaged sessions, however the fatigued versus non-fatigued sessions cover a similar, slightly translated trend. This subject's blink closure duration data generally tracks with the expected trend, except for the ND scenario, which is similar in value to the NE scenario. The summary for this subject is as follows:

- *FE scenario* – moderately elevated BR with moderate BCD
- *NE scenario* – significantly elevated BR with suppressed BCD
- *ND scenario* – moderately suppressed BR with suppressed BCD
- *FD scenario* – significantly suppressed BR with elevated BCD

Overall, none of the subjects tracked exactly with the expected behaviors, however, most provided adequate information for inferring a state from the blink rate and blink closure duration biometrics.

6 Conclusions

The experimental results of our study indicate that there are sufficient measurable behaviors inherent in the human eye blink for the reasonable determination of affective states (i.e., physical and/or mental fatigue) and cognitive states (i.e., task engagement) in individual subjects. However, this determination requires a priori knowledge of each individual gained through the learning process described above. Interestingly, six of the twelve subjects involved in our study exhibited one or more eye biometric ambiguities. These ambiguities can cause problems for static analysis techniques such as thresholding, but such anomalies can be interpreted effectively using techniques such as dynamic image flow analysis.

Finally, it has been suggested by some in the cognitive psychological community and others in HCI that blink frequency increases with cognitive workload and fatigue (or time-on-task) while blink closure duration decreases as a function of workload and increases as a function of fatigue. While we found this general assertion to largely hold true, in certain individuals the exact opposite was shown to be the reality. This understanding, coupled with other observations during the experimental phase, prevents us from generalizing the determination capability to a wider range of subjects.

References

1. Bhaskar, T.N., Keat, F.T., Ranganath, S., Venkatesh, Y.V.: Blink detection and eye tracking for eye localization. In: Proc. Conference on Convergent Technologies for Asia-Pacific Region, vol. 2, pp. 821–824 (2003)
2. Duric, Z., Li, F., Sun, Y., Wechsler, H.: Using normal flow for detection and tracking of limbs in color images. In: Proc. 15th International Conference on Pattern Recognition, vol. 4, pp. 40268–40271 (2002)
3. Fukuda, K., Stern, J.A., Brown, T.B., Russo, M.B.: Cognition, blinks, eye-movements, and pupillary movements during performance of a running memory task. Aviation, Space, and Environmental Medicine 76, C75–C85 (2005)
4. Heishman, R., Powers, W., Duric, Z.: Techniques for tracking and analyzing eye region biometrics in HCI Scenarios. In: Proceedings of the 19th British HCI Group Annual Conference, Edinburgh, Scotland, vol. 2, pp. 229–231 (2005)
5. Russell, J.A.: Reading emotions from and into faces: Resurrecting a dimensional-contextual perspective. In: Russell, J.A., Fernandez, J.M. (eds.) The Psychology of Facial Expression (chapter 13), pp. 295–320. Cambridge University Press, Paris (1997)
6. Stern, J.A.: The eye blink: Affective and cognitive influences. In: Forgays, D.G., Sosnowski, T., Wrzesniewski, K. (eds.) Anxiety: Recent Developments in Cognitive, Psychophysiological, and Health Research (chapter 8), pp. 109–128. Hemisphere Publishing, Washington (1992)

Assessing Information Presentation Preferences with Eye Movements

Laurel A. King[1] and Martha E. Crosby[2]

[1] Communication and Information Sciences, University of Hawaii at Manoa
`laurel.king@hawaii.edu`
[2] Information and Computer Sciences, 1680 East-West Road, POST 317, Honolulu, HI 96822

Abstract. This study investigates the relationship between participants' self-reported high verbal or high visual information preferences and their performance and eye movements during analytical reasoning problems. Twelve participants, six male and six female, were selected as being more visual than verbal or more verbal than visual in approach, based on the results of a questionnaire administered to 140 college students. Selected participants were tested for individual differences in spatial ability and working memory capacity. They completed a repeated measures experiment while their eye movements were tracked to examine any correlation with their stated preference for verbal or visual information presentation. Performance on analytical reasoning problems with and without an optional diagram is compared between groups and within-subjects. Due to the small number of participants, between-group differences, although indicated, were mostly statistically insignificant. Within-subject analysis is still being completed, but trends in diagram usage are examined.

Keywords: information presentation, eye tracking, analytical reasoning, problem representation.

1 Introduction

Various studies have found signs of cognitive style or learning preferences in some individuals for either a textual or text plus graphic representation of information[1, 2]. This is often referred to as a visual-verbal preference for information presentation and is dependent on the task and situation even for a given individual. Several tests have been used to measure any tendency for one or the other, but the construct is thought to be related to three factors: one's spatial visualization ability, visual-verbal learning preference and visual-verbal cognitive style [3]. The first factor refers to an ability one has developed to mentally manipulate and transform shapes. The second factor refers to one's preference for educational material to be presented textually or with graphics as well. The third factor refers to the tendency or belief that one's thoughts tend to be more visual or more verbal in nature, or that one has developed a habit of a visual or verbal approach to problem solving. At the same time, there has been conflicting usage of terminology, measurement, and significance of the construct.

D.D. Schmorrow, L.M. Reeves (Eds.): Augmented Cognition, HCII 2007, LNAI 4565, pp. 94–102, 2007.
© Springer-Verlag Berlin Heidelberg 2007

Studies have shown self-constructed representations for analytical reasoning falling into either diagrammatic or verbal categories [4, 5], and that some people may rely on mental imagery more to solve mechanical reasoning problems than others [6]. It is of interest in this study whether these groupings would correlate with other verbal-visual factors. Although correlating individual differences with behavior is difficult, it is necessary to try to determine whether visual-verbal factors influence problem representation preferences and whether visual strategy can be used to predict visual-verbal factors to be augmented.

Although the existence and possibility of visual imagery is a controversial topic in psychology [7-9], the current study is concerned more with the match between one's perception of oneself as a visualizer or verbalizer and one's actual perceptual practice than whether one is actually able to encode thoughts as images. There is also debate whether individual differences determine a significant level of variation between individuals or are reliable enough factors to be worthy of information system design research, because they can change with the task or context, even for a given individual [10].

However, as user modeling and augmentation improves, a better understanding of the verbal-visual construct, and what it means in terms of interface design and problem representation is warranted. There is indication that differences are very task dependent and studies have had conflicting results as to the importance of cognitive style because people are able to adapt to the information format as needed. Yet, there seems to have been little effort to find physiological evidence of visual-verbal individual differences that might provide behavioral support for any design implications. The work of Riding and Peterson are an exception to this [11, 12].The current study is an attempt to help clarify the perceptual aspects of the visual-verbal construct, if only in the narrow realm of solving relatively simple and determinate analytical reasoning problems on a computer screen.

2 Previous Studies

In this section a brief overview of some relevant eye tracking and visual representation research is provided.

2.1 Eye Tracking Studies

Eye tracking research has been instrumental in our understanding of visual perception processes. Although the technology for tracking eye movements is far from perfect, it is one physical measure that can help us understand what people look at in order to understand their environments. It is physically possible to track what a person is viewing within one degree of their pupil position, which represents the area that their foveal receptors can accurately perceive without eye movements. Peripheral vision outside the fovea is not usually clear enough for viewing details but is useful for drawing attention to a target. So, eye tracking allows us to know what a person is looking at within one degree of the eye position, and current accuracy is usually between one and two degrees where one degree is .4 inches or 40 pixels on a display placed 24 inches from the viewer [13]. The abrupt eye movements between one target and another are called saccades. Saccades can span from 1 to 40 degrees and are sudden movements during which the direction of the movement cannot be changed once started. They occur 100-300 milliseconds (1 ms. = 1/1000 sec.) after the target appears in peripheral vision. A saccade is usually followed by a fixation lasting between 200-600 milliseconds. During a fixation, small movements of less than a degree may occur to focus the area of interest on the fovea. Gazes are usually defined as collections of fixations and small saccades within an object or section of the viewing area [14]. The pupil size can also indicate things about the viewer and level of cognitive activity. Fixation duration is a measure of difficulty of information extraction and interpretation; while the number of fixations in a region indicates level of interest [15].

The literature on eye tracking in HCI is divided into three main groups: research to understand what the user is looking at on the screen, using eye tracking for interface evaluation, and most recently as an input device for attentive interfaces. This research falls into the first category, but the results could be important for the other two categories in the future. One general finding has been that eye movements in scene perception and search depend on the task. The author's previous studies have shown that it is possible to determine task and complexity from eye fixation data and train a neural network to recognize the task at very high levels of accuracy [16, 17].

Cognitive style as measured by the Meyers-Briggs Type Indicator's sensing/intuitive dimension was found to determine scanning patterns for both textual and graphic programming tasks, independent of the person's experience and comprehension level [18]. The sensing type has a preference for information "sensed" in the environment from concrete experience. The intuitive type prefers abstract possibilities, meanings and relationships. It is unclear how and if these types relate to a person's visual or verbal preferences, but the study shows a linkage between cognitive style and perceptual processing.

Much of the eye tracking research on diagrams for problem solving has focused on diagrams of mechanical devices. Of particular interest in these studies is a finding that subjects have a tendency to decompose the diagram into components that are believed to be mentally animated to help them determine causal relationships between different components [19]. Eye tracking showed that the relevant components are viewed during mental animation, and that working memory capacity limits constrain the ability to imagine component behavior. This is another indication of how working memory is important in problem solving.

Studies have shown that some people move their eyes in relation to their internal imagery even when looking at a blank screen and visualizing from memory after the image is removed. Eye movements matching the location of previously shown key components on the blank area of the screen were observed for 42% of participants in a problem solving task where the first problem was illustrated with a diagram and the second was not. It was hypothesized that those with eye movements in the blank area of the screen for the second problem were visualizing the diagram to solve the problem, even though the diagram was no longer present. The other 58% focused almost exclusively on the text of the question and problem on the second problem. This study did not test subjects for visual-verbal cognitive style or learning preferences, or memory capacity so it is impossible to know if it correlated with the imaging and non-imaging subjects [6].

2.2 Visual Representation

External representations facilitate problem solving by computational offloading among other functions [20-22]. Graphic representations accompanying text can improve retention of main facts by making concepts less abstract and emphasizing main points, e.g., [20, 21, 23-26]. Graphic representations are most useful in determinate problems because of increased notation and symbols for indeterminate problems [27]. Pictures and diagrams have been used to facilitate communication and understanding since the first cave drawings. Narayanan broadly defines diagrammatic communication as "an overarching theme that encompasses not only diagrammatic representation but also diagrammatic reasoning and diagrammatic interaction between humans and computers" in his review of taxonomy of diagrammatic communication [28]. Various aspects of diagrammatic communication are increasingly relevant with increasing information overload and the pressing need to communicate essential relationships and information from vast and complicated problems that we face as groups and individuals.

The best sources of information on how best to communicate information visually are found in Edward Tufte's aesthetically appealing and detailed work [29-31]. Although based more on his experience and aesthetic sense than empirical evidence, Tufte's main principal can be summarized that additional ink should always add meaning or it should not be used. In this study we are looking for differences in perceptual strategies in a problem-solving task and on the use of diagrams for communicating problems. Unfortunately, the literature is very sparse in this area and most deals with studies comparing different types of diagrams such as tables and bar charts.

Visual and verbal cognitive styles and learning preferences represent habits and approaches to thought and information processing [15, 32]. Visualizers prefer literal encoding (seeing, feeling physical features when relating information to prior knowledge), and use mental pictures when thinking. Verbalizers prefer linguistic encoding (reading how to do something), and use inner speech when thinking [15].

In a recent study on the effectiveness of visual interactive modeling on group decision making found that visualization improved efficiency and satisfaction, however, unexpectedly did not improve the quality of the decision made compared to a group not using the visualization technology [33]. Studies such as these may be explained if the decision maker's visual and verbal style is measured as well.

Another recent study on the effect of photos on newspaper processing found that verbalizers had better recall of both pictures and stories than visualizers, and that visualizers did not show more interest in stories with photos, and the best recall was by the high verbal/low visual type [34]. These results add to the evidence that visual-verbal style does affect learning, but leads one to the conclusion that reading a newspaper is a verbal task that visualizers may not excel at regardless of the use of photos to enhance interest. It would be interesting to know if diagrams would have had the same lack of enhancement in recall for those testing highly in visual style. The educational psychology literature has more work on the implications of cognitive style and other individual differences on curriculum, but much of the problem solving literature deals with teaching math and science using pictures, diagrams and animations as opposed to preferences for diagrams or text in analytical reasoning [1].

3 Methodology

To better understand the relationship between diagrammatic communication and problem representation in relation to the visual-verbal characteristics and preferences of the viewer, this study looks for eye movement and performance differences as evidence of preference differences in the use of diagrammatic and textual representations of problems. The visual-verbal factors were measured using established visual-verbal learning preferences and imagery questionnaires and psychological tests to measure spatial visualization ability and working memory capacity. Participants were observed and tested through an eye-tracking experiment to see if correlations between visual solution strategy and individual differences relating to verbal-visual preferences are detected and match the stated and expected preferences of the individual.

3.1 Research Design

This research is based on data from a repeated measures experiment where participants perform problem-solving tasks using analytical reasoning with and without ancillary graphic representations of some of the problem information. The performance on the tasks is based on the time to complete the problems and the number of correct answers. The performance with and without a graphic is being compared within subjects. The proportion of fixations and time spent on graphic elements, is compared both within subjects and between subject groups.

As a screening tool, participant pools were asked their preference for verbal or visual descriptions for learning and thinking using a verbal-visual preference questionnaire. The questionnaire is based on an adaptation of Richardson's Verbal-Visual Questionnaire [35], and Mayer's verbal, spatial, and visual-verbal learning style rating tests [3]. Mayer and Massa suggests that individual visual-verbal learning style rating correlates highly with other measures of visual-verbal cognitive style and learning preference [3]. The questionnaire was used to screen approximately 140 participants to find twelve that were measured as more verbal or more visual. This selection was done to accentuate any verbal and visual effect on eye movements.

In the experiment, the selected university students solved analytical reasoning problems to see how they view verbal and diagrammatic representations to solve a problem or accomplish a task. The participants were tested individually. First they were given a short test to measure their working memory span using a number span test and a timed paper folding test from the Kit of Factor Referenced Cognitive Tests [36] to measure their spatial ability. Then each participant performed a computerized experiment while connected to an ASL eye tracker. Their eye movements were tracked 60 times per second while they solved a series of problems using the textual and/or graphic information provided. Two sets of questions asked the participant to solve analytical reasoning problems. One set included an ancillary graphic representation with some of the information from the textual information. The other set of questions included only the textual information, and after finding the solution, they were asked to choose between Venn diagrams, a matrix, a network, and a hierarchy as the basic structure of the previous problem presented textually. Their performance was measured on the accuracy of their answers and the time taken to complete the problems.

Participants were given an opportunity to discuss the tasks and their experience after the experiment. The interaction between performance and type of representation is being analyzed in terms of other individual characteristics provided, such as spatial ability, visual-verbal preference profile, and memory capacity. All problems were designed to be solved while viewing a computer screen without additional notes or calculations, although for increased difficulty some require more working memory capacity than others.

3.2 Participants

Twelve participants were recruited from university students attending classes in language, information science, computer science, and business. A visual-verbal questionnaire was used to screen approximately 140 participants to find six extremely verbal and six extremely visual participants for the full experimental protocol. The participants were familiar with using a computer, mouse, and have some experience solving analytical reasoning problems such as those on standardized tests. The participants' data was grouped by spatial ability, working memory capacity, visual/verbal thinking, and visual/verbal learning preference to be compared for significant differences in performance and use of external representations.

3.3 Treatment

The eye movement data was collected while participants complete a computerized experiment. Section A contained a practice problem followed by five textual problems with graphic representations. Section B had a practice problem followed by five textual problems without graphics. This was followed by a question asking them to select the appropriate diagram for the problem.

The performance on the parallel problems in sections A and B are being compared for accuracy, and time to complete within subject. The performance is then analyzed in correlation to their measured or stated visual/verbal factors between subjects. The proportion of fixations on the graphic support in section A is also being analyzed for patterns relating to their visual/verbal factors.

The experiment takes about 45 minutes with breaks between the sections to allow the participant to relax. The questionnaires and psychological tests were done with paper and pencil and numbered to protect anonymity. Every attempt was made to make the participant feel relaxed and comfortable during the session.

4 Results

The data from this study is still being analyzed. The between group results show a trend for differences between the visual and verbal groups in duration of time spent on the text plus graphic section and the text only section. The differences in the means for the visual and verbal groups are not statistically significant for most variables.

Table 1. The means for the different measures for the visual and verbal groups

	Type	N	Mean	Std. Deviation	Std. Error Mean
Spatial test (max 10)	visual	6	5.7917	2.16458	0.88369
	verbal	6	6.9583	1.56857	0.64037
Memory (max 53)	visual	6	45.50	5.244	2.141
	verbal	6	46.00	5.329	2.176
Sect A w/ diagram correct (5)	visual	6	4.50	0.837	0.342
	verbal	6	4.17	0.983	0.401
Sect B w/o diagram correct (5)	visual	6	3.17	0.408	0.167
	verbal	6	3.83	0.983	0.401
Sect C correct (5)	visual	6	4.00	1.095	0.447
	verbal	6	4.17	1.169	0.477
Total Correct (15)	visual	6	11.67	1.033	0.422
	verbal	6	12.17	1.941	0.792

However, it is interesting to note that despite the lower average spatial visualization score, the visual group scored higher on the problems with diagrams. This is being investigated within subject to see if the trend is based on a particular strategy.

The duration of time spent on each problem is similarly interesting yet there is no clear statistical result in the between group comparisons. There seems to be a trend for the visual participants to spend more time on the diagram, and the verbal participants to spend more time on the text, but this analysis is incomplete. These results will be presented and clarified at the time of the conference.

5 Conclusion

Through this study we hope to gain a better understanding of how and when external representations are effective for analytical problem solving and for whom. The results and analysis should add to our knowledge of representations used in diagrammatic communication as well. It has been shown that illustrations can both distract and enlighten the viewer during learning. The same should be true for diagrammatic communication and it is hoped that eye tracking will lead us to a better understanding of the user of diagrams for representing analytical reasoning problems. If information presentation preferences are relevant to systems design and diagrammatic communication, it should be evident in the eye movements and performance of the participants doing analytical reasoning problems.

References

1. Sternberg, R.J., Zhang, L. (eds.): Perspectives on thinking, learning, and cognitive styles. Erlbaum, Mahwah (2001)
2. Jonassen, D., Grabowski, B.L.: Handbook of individual differences, learning, and instruction. Erlbaum, Hillsdale (1993)

3. Mayer, R.E., Massa, L.J.: Three Facets of Visual and Verbal Learners: Cognitive Ability, Cognitive Style, and Learning Preference. Journal of Educational Psychology 95, 833–846 (2003)
4. Cox, R.: Representation construction, externalized cognition and individual differences. Learning and Instruction 9, 343–363 (1999)
5. Cox, R., Brna, P.: Supporting the use of external representations in problem solving: The need for flexible learning environments. Journal of Artificial Intelligence in Education 6, 239–302 (1995)
6. Yoon, D., Narayanan, N.H.: Mental imagery in problem solving: an eye tracking study. In: Proceedings of the Third ACM Symposium on Eye Tracking Research & Applications, ACM Press, New York (2004)
7. Pylyshyn, Z.W.: What the mind's eye tells the mind's brain: a critique of mental imagery. Psychological Bulletin 80, 1–24 (1973)
8. Kosslyn, S.M., Pinker, S., Smith, G.E., Schwartz, S.P.: On the demystification of mental imagery. Behavioral and Brain Sciences 2, 535–581 (1979)
9. Anderson, J.R.: Arguments concerning representations for mental imagery. Psychological Review 85, 249–277 (1978)
10. Huber, G.P.: Cognitive Style as a Basis for MIS and DSS Designs: Much Ado About Nothing. Management Science 29, 511,567 (1983)
11. Peterson, E.R., Deary, I.J., Austin, E.J.: A new measure of Verbal–Imagery Cognitive Style: VICS. Personality and Individual Differences 38 (2005)
12. Riding, R.J.: Cognitive Styles Analysis. Learning and Training Technology, Birmingham (1991)
13. Jacob, R.J.K.: Eye Tracking in Advanced Interface Design. In: Barfield, W., Furness, T.A. (eds.) Virtual Environments and Advanced Interface Design, pp. 258–288. Oxford University Press, New York (1995)
14. Just, M.A., Carpenter, P.A.: Eye fixations and cognitive processes. Cognitive Psychology 8, 441–480 (1976)
15. Richardson, A.: Mental imagery and memory: Coding ability or coding preference? Journal of Mental Imagery 2 (1978)
16. King, L.: Predicting User Task with a Neural Network. In: HCI International, vol. 1, pp. 332–336. Lawrence Erlbaum Associates, Mahwah, NJ, New Orleans, LA (2001)
17. King, L.: The Relationship between Scene and Eye Movements. In: Hawaii International Conference on System Sciences. IEEE, Hawaii (2002)
18. Crosby, M.E., Stelovsky, J.: Using enhanced eye monitoring equipment to relate subject differences and presentation material. In: Groner, R., d' Ydewalle, R., Parham, R. (eds.) From eye to mind: information acquisition in perception, search and reading, Elsevier, North-Holland (1990)
19. Hegarty, M.: Mental animation: inferring motion from static diagrams of mechanical systems. Journal of Experimental Psychology: Learning, Memory and Cognition 18, 1084–1102 (1992)
20. Scaife, M., Rogers, Y.: External cognition: how do graphical representations work? International Journal of Human-Computer Studies 45, 185–213 (1996)
21. Larkin, J.H., Simon, H.A.: Why a diagram is (sometimes) worth ten thousand words. Cognitive Science 11, 65–99 (1987)
22. Cheng, P.C.-H.: Functional Roles for the Cognitive Analysis of Diagrams in Problem Solving. In: Cottrell, G.W. (ed.) Proceeding of the Eighteenth Annual Conference of the Cognitive Science Society, pp. 207–212. Lawrence Erlbaum and Associates, Hillsdale (1996)

23. Mayer, R.E.: Thinking, problem solving, cognition. W.H. Freeman and Company, New York (1983)
24. Koedinger, K.R., Anderson, J.R.: Abstract planning and perceptual chunks: elements of expertise in geometry. Cognitive Science 14, 511–550 (1990)
25. Mayer, R.E., Gallini, J.K.: When Is an Illustration Worth Ten Thousand Words? Journal of Educational Psychology 82, 715–726 (1990)
26. Carney, R.N., Levin, J.R.: Pictorial illustrations still improve students learning from text. Educational Psychology Review 14, 5–26 (2002)
27. Stenning, K., Oberlander, J.: A cognitive theory of graphical and linguistic reasoning: logic and implementation. Cognitive Science 19 (1995)
28. Narayanan, N.H.: Technical Report CSE97-06: Diagrammatic Communication: A Taxonomic Overview. Auburn University (1997)
29. Tufte, E.R.: Visual and Statistical Thinking: Displays of Evidence for Making Decisions. Graphics Press LLC, Cheshire (1997)
30. Tufte, E.R.: Envisioning information. Graphics Press LLC, Cheshire (1990)
31. Tufte, E.R.: The Visual Display of Quantitative Information. Graphics Press LLC, Cheshire (1983)
32. Paivio, A.: Imagery and verbal processes. Holt, Rinehart and Winston, Inc., New York (1971)
33. Jain, H.K., Ramamurthy, K., Sundaram, S.: Effectiveness of Visual Interactive Modeling in the Context of Multiple-Criteria Group Decisions. IEEE Transactions on Systems Man. and Cybernetics Part. A:Systems and Humans 36, 298–318 (2006)
34. Mendelson, A.L., Thorson, E.: How verbalizers and visualizers process the newspaper environment. Journal of Communication 54, 474–491 (2004)
35. Richardson, A.: Verbalizer-visualizer: a cognitive style dimension. Journal of Mental Imagery 1, 109–126 (1977)
36. Ekstrom, R.B., French, J.W., Harman, H.H.: Manual for kit of factor-referenced cognitive tests. Educational Testing Service, Princeton, NJ (1976)

Inclusive Design for Brain Body Interfaces

Paul Gnanayutham[1] and Jennifer George[2]

[1] Department of Computing, University of Portsmouth, Buckingham Building, Lion Terrace,
Portsmouth, PO1 3HE, United Kingdom
[2] SAE Institute, United House, North Road, London, N7 9DP, United Kingdom
paul.gnanayutham@port.ac.uk, jennifer.george@sae.edu

Abstract. In comparison to all types of injury, those to the brain are among the most likely to result in death or permanent disability. A certain percentage of these brain-injured people cannot communicate, recreate, or control their environment due to severe motor impairment. This group of individuals with severe head injury has received little from assistive technology. Brain computer interfaces have opened up a spectrum of assistive technologies, which are particularly appropriate for people with traumatic brain-injury, especially those who suffer from "locked-in" syndrome. Previous research in this area developed brain body interfaces so that this group of brain-injured people can communicate, recreate and launch applications communicate using computers despite the severity of their brain injury, except for visually impaired and comatose participants. This paper reports on an exploratory investigation carried out with visually impaired using facial muscles or electromyography (EMG) to communicate using brain body interfaces.

Keywords: Brain-Body Interface, Inclusive design, Neuro-rehabilitation, Assistive Technology and visual impairment, EEG, EMG and EOG.

1   Introduction

As medical technology not only extends our natural life span but also leads to increased survival from illness and accidents, the number of people with disabilities is constantly increasing. World Health Organization [1] estimates that there are more than 600 million people who are disabled as a consequence of mental, physical or sensory impairment thus creating one of the world's largest minorities. It has been estimated that 80 to 120 million European citizens have some form of disability, exceeding the population of almost every European state [2] In comparison to different types of injury, those to the brain are among the most likely to result in death or permanent disability. In the European Union, brain injury accounts for one million hospital admissions per year. A certain percentage of these brain-injured people cannot communicate, recreate, or control their environment due to severe motor impairment. This group of severely head injured people is cared for by nursing homes that cater for their wellbeing in every possible way. Their loved ones also play a major role in the wellbeing of this group of people.

D.D. Schmorrow, L.M. Reeves (Eds.): Augmented Cognition, HCII 2007, LNAI 4565, pp. 103–112, 2007.
© Springer-Verlag Berlin Heidelberg 2007

1.1 Brain Injury

There are two stages in traumatic brain injury, the primary and the secondary. The secondary brain injury occurs as a response to the primary injury. In other words, primary brain injury is caused initially by trauma amyotrophic lateral sclerosis, brain stem stroke etc., but includes the complications, which can follow, such as damage caused by lack of oxygen, and rising pressure and swelling in the brain. A brain injury can be seen as a chain of events beginning with the first injury which occurs in seconds after the accident and being made worse by a second injury which happens in minutes and hours after this, depending on when skilled medical intervention occurs. There are three types of primary brain injury - closed, open and crush. Closed head injuries are the most common type, and are so called because no break of the skin or open wound is visible. Open head injuries are not so common. In this type of injury the skull is opened and the brain exposed and damaged. In crush injuries the head might be caught between two hard objects. This is the least common type of injury, and often damages the base of the skull and nerves of the brain stem rather than the brain itself. Individuals with brain injury require frequent assessments and diagnostic tests [3]. Most hospitals use the Glasgow Coma Scale for predicting early outcome from a head injury, for example, whether the person will survive or Rancho Levels of Cognitive Functioning for predicting later outcomes of head injuries [4].

1.2 Brain Body Interface Devices

The brain is the centre of the central nervous system in humans as well as the primary control centre for the peripheral nervous system (Fig.1.). The building blocks of the brain are special cells called neurons. The human brain has approximately hundred billion neurons. Neurons are the brain cells responsible for storing and transmitting information from a brain cell. The adult brain weighs three pounds and is suspended in cerebrospinal fluid. This fluid protects the brain from shock. The brain is also protected by a set of bones called the cranium or a skull.

The three main components of the brain are the cerebellum, cerebrum and brainstem. The cerebellum is located between the brainstem and the cerebrum. The cerebellum controls facial muscle co-ordination and damage to this area affects the ability to control facial muscles thus affecting signals (eye movements and muscle movements) needed by Brain-Body Interfaces. The cranial nerves that carry the signals to control facial movements also originate in the brainstem, hence the brainstem is of interest when using Brain-Body Interfaces.

Assistive devices are essential for enhancing quality of life for individuals with severe disabilities such as quadriplegia, amyotrophic lateral sclerosis (ALS), commonly referred to as Lou Gehrig's disease or brainstem strokes or traumatic brain injuries (TBIs). Research has been carried out on the brain's electrical activities since 1925 [5]. Brain-computer interfaces (BCIs), also called brain-body interfaces or brain-machine interfaces provide new augmentative communications channels for those with severe motor impairments. In 1995 there were no more than six active brain computer interface research groups, in 2000 there were more than twenty and now more than thirty laboratories are actively researching in BCI [6]. A BCI is a communication system that does not depend on the brain's normal output pathways

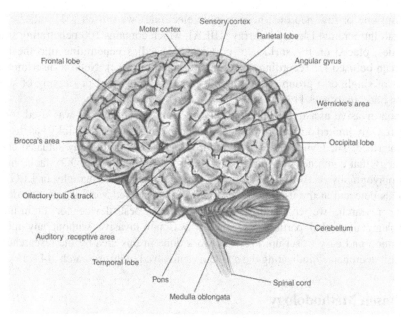

Fig. 1. Brain Map (Courtesy of www.headinjury.com)

such as speech or gestures but by using electrophysiological signals from the brain as defined by Wolpaw [7]. There are two types of brain body interfaces namely invasive (signals obtained by surgically inserting probes inside the brain) and non-invasive (electrodes placed externally on part of the body).

Brain activity produces electrical signals that can be read by electrodes placed on the skull, forehead or other part of the body (the skull and forehead are predominantly used because of the richness of bio-potentials in these areas). Algorithms then translate these bio-potentials into instructions to direct the computer, so people with brain injury have a channel to communicate without using the normal channels.

Non-invasive technology involves the collection of control signals for the brain computer interface without the use of any surgical techniques, with electrodes placed on their face, skull or other parts of their body. The non-invasive devices show that, signals obtained are first amplified, filtered and thereafter converted from analogue to digital signal. Various electrode positions are chosen by the developers, who choose electrode caps, electrode headbands with different positions and number of electrodes or the international 10-20 system [8]. Authorities dispute the number of electrodes needed for collection of usable bio-potentials [9]. There is only one agreed standard for the positions and number of electrodes that is the International 10-20 system of electrodes [10].

Invasive electrodes can give better noise to signal ratio and obtain signals from a single or small number of neurons. Signals collected from the brain require expensive and dangerous measures such as surgery. Neurons are the brain cells responsible for storing and transmitting information from a brain cell. Any mental experience even if unconscious has a signal associated with it. There are two types of electrodes used for invasive brain body interfaces. If signals needed to be obtained with the least noise and from one or few neurons, neurotrophic electrodes were used [11], other choice was Utah Intracranial Electrode Array (UIEA), which contains 100 penetrating silicon electrodes, placed on the surface of cortex with needles penetrating into the brain, which can be used for recording and simulating neurons [12]. Neuron discrimination (choice of single or a group of neurons) does not play any part processing of signals in brain body interfaces [13].

A non-invasive assistive technology device named Cyberlink™ was used for this research. Only limited amount of research has been done using Cyberlink™ as the brain body interface. The Cyberlink™ used in our research, is a brain-body actuated control technology that combines eye-movement (Electrooculargraphy or EOG), facial muscle (Electromyography or EMG) and brain wave (Electroencephalalography or EEG) bio-potentials detected at the user's forehead. Having considered various assistive devices for our research, we chose the Cyberlink as the best device for brain-injured quadriplegic nonverbal participants, since it was non-invasive without any medical intervention and easy to set-up. Previous work done in this area by the researcher has been well documented indicating the challenges involved in this research [14 – 19].

2   Chosen Methodology

Having considered the research methodologies on offer the appropriate one for this investigation was chosen, where the final artefact was evaluated by a small number of severely brain-injured participants [20]. A medical practitioner chose suitable brain-injured participants for the research analysing their responses and medication. Comatose and medication that restricted response were used as the criteria for exclusion from this research.

The approach chosen is shown in diagrammatic form in figure 2. The diagram shows the three phases of the research and the iterative processes that were used to develop the paradigms. The iterative processes that were employed in the design and development of the novel interaction paradigms are shown on the left of the diagram and the other issues that influenced the processes are shown on the right side of the diagram. Iteration driven by phenomenological formative and summative evaluations [21], gives the opportunity for building artefacts that can evolve into refined, tried and tested end products when developing artefacts [22]. The final feedback from each phase is shown in the text boxes in figure 2. One method of conducting scientific research in a new area of study with a new tool is to use the tool with a group of participants and to collect data from the performance of tasks with the tool. The data then display trends that allow other questions to be formed. These questions can be used to form a hypothesis that may be evaluated in further experiments. This method is known as Naturalistic Inquiry [23]. Williams states "naturalistic inquiry is disciplined inquiry conducted in natural settings (in the field of interest, not in laboratories), using natural methods (observation, interviewing, thinking, reading, writing)". Naturalistic inquires were used in this research for investigating topics of interest. Formative research methods and empirical summative methods were used to evaluate the paradigms being investigated in this research [24]. Developed prototypes

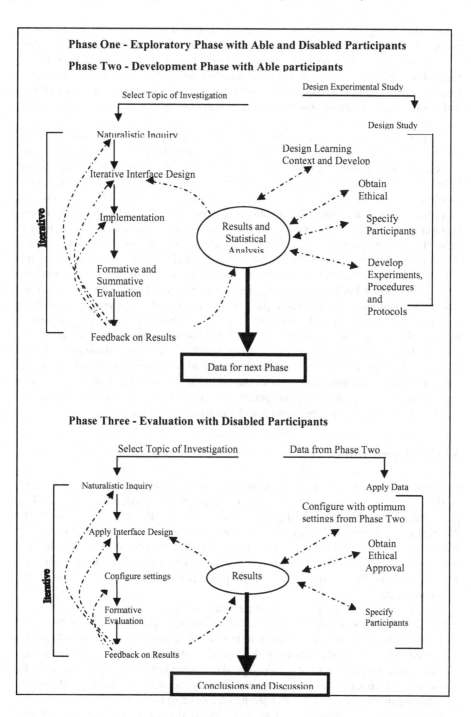

Fig. 2. Chosen Research Methodology

were tested using able users as test subjects before being evaluated with disabled users. Iteration allowed better feedback for faster interface development. Many versions of the interface program were developed to get the final artefact. Formative method or formative evaluation can be conducted during the planning and delivery of research. This method is based on scientific knowledge based on application of logic and reasoning. It produces information that is used to improve a program while it is in progress.

First phase of the research aimed to replicate Doherty's work with his tunnel interface [19]. Once replicated, a small change, adding discrete acceleration to cursor movement, was made to the interface that greatly improved performance overall. However, this change was not enough to make the most of the wide variations in capability in the user population. This meant that the users could not be grouped according to their disability classification but every user had to have an individually personalised interface [19]. The second phase incorporated discrete acceleration into a more flexible and personalised interface (Fig. 2). It also introduced a control system, which controlled the movements of the cursor by dividing the computer screen into configurable tiles and delaying the cursor at each tile. This new paradigm also brought the cursor back to a starting point after an elapsed period of time, avoiding any user frustration. Able-bodied participants evaluated this paradigm to obtain optimum settings that can be used in phase three thus avoiding any unnecessary training. Re-configuration facility was available for users by running the target test again and replacing the previous personalised interface. The third phase evaluated the novel interface paradigm developed in phase two incorporating the optimum settings. This novel interface paradigm was evaluated with the disabled participants. This proved to be usable by a larger percentage of brain-injured population than in previous Doherty's studies, and over a wider range of functionality.

3 Developed Interface

Prototypes were used for this study from previous research. Fig. 2 shows an example of this interface. The interface was tested with the able participants then disabled participants, using the individual abilities and bio-potentials that could be used. If a disabled user moves a cursor in any direction consistently we were able to create an individual interface and communicate effectively. The initial tests with the disabled participants were to find out how much EEG, EOG or EMG that can be harnessed. The severity of the brain injury of the participants gave only EEG signal for communicating.

In order to support discrete acceleration, the computer screen is divided into tiles, which support discrete jumps from one tile to the next predicted tile on the user's route. However, the lack of regularity in user's cursor paths in study one ruled out a wholly adaptive algorithm, with the following algorithm being implemented instead:

The configuration took care of all timings, there were individual times allocated for every task, which mean the interface automatically recovered to the original position (i.e. starting point in the middle) this taking care of error recovery.

The above is still however a universal design that only takes account of user differences at run-time. Irregularities in user input rule out jumping directly to the

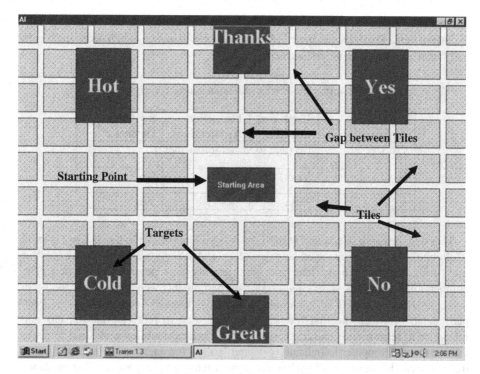

Fig. 3. Interface Used for this research

nearest predicted target. Instead, a step by step approach is taken that leaves the user in control at each point. A wholly automated approach would introduce high error recovery costs given the limited capabilities of the traumatic brain-injured. Thus, the interface has further features that allow the cursor's path to be controlled by settings for a specific user. The personalised settings include time spent on the starting area to relax the user before navigating to a target, time spent on each tile to control the bio-potential in such a way controlled navigation can take place, size of tile to suit each user etc.

4 Experiments and Results

The approach chosen was iteration driven by phenomenological formative and summative evaluations, which gives the opportunity for building artefacts that can evolve into refined, tried and tested end products when developing artefacts. Formative approaches are based on the worldview belief that reality based on perceptions is different for each person. Formative research has to be systematic and subjective, indicating the experience of individual users. Formative and summative methods compliment each other since they generate different types of data that can be used when developing interfaces. Results obtained in summative methods should be tested using statistical methods, statistical significance, hypothesis validation, null hypothesis etc. Previous research [18] showed how five out of ten were unable to participate due to the visual impairment.

Table 1. Previous results with brain injured participants

Participant	Used text to audio	Launched Applications	Switched Devices
1,2,3, 6, 7	No (due to visual impairment)		
5, 10	Yes	No	No
4, 8, 9	Yes	Yes	Yes

This new research conducted at the Low Vision Unit of the National Eye Hospital (Colombo) for participants aged between seven and seventy were able to say 'yes' or 'no' using the brain body interface with seventy five percent consistency. The numbers of participants were eight and seven participants were able to use the brain body interface. Overall a maximum of twenty minutes was spent with each participant, of which the first few minutes were used to relax the participants and relieve or at least reduce muscle tension. Then forehead muscles were used to move the cursor of a computer to indicate 'yes' and 'no', to the questions being asked using the interface shown in Fig. 2. Although certain tensed participants needed guidance and help seven out of eight participants could control the curser to say yes and no by frowning and relaxing (using electromyography).

5   Conclusions and Future

A flexible interface was developed to suit each person, with targets positioned by either using the target test program or manually placing them where participants wish. As a result, it has been possible to extend effective interaction for some users to tasks beyond simple communication. This was achieved with less need for adjusting the Cyberlink™ settings before use. Brain-body interfaces for rehabilitation are still in their infancy, but we believe that our work could be the basis for their more widespread use in extensively extending the activities of severely impaired individuals. It is possible to see this as the main current viable application of brain-body interfaces, since anyone who can use a more reliable and efficient alternative input device should do so.

Vision impaired participants and comatose participants were the two groups of non-verbal quadriplegic brain-injured people who could not be included in the previous study. But exploratory study showed how the vision impaired could also now be included in using brain body interfaces to communicate in the future.

At present the researchers are working in three areas. Exploratory work is being been done for blind participants navigate computer screen using musical guidance. Research is also being carried out on rehabilitation robotics for the brain injured.

Acknowledgments. Dr. Chris Bloor, Professor Gilbert Cockton, Dr. Ivan Jordanov, Dr. Eamon Doherty and to the following institutes Vimhans Delhi, Mother Theresa's Mission of Charity Delhi, Holy Cross Hospital Surrey, Castel Froma, Leamington spa and Low Vision Unit of the National Eye Hospital Colombo.

References

1. World Health Organization, Disability, Including Prevention, Management and rehabilitation, Report by the Secretariat document A58/17, World Health Organization Publications (April 2005)
2. Council of Europe, Towards full social inclusion of persons with disabilities, Report Social, Health and Family Affairs Committee, Doc. 9632, Communication Unit of the Assembly (December 2002)
3. Sears, A., Young, M.: Physical Disabilities and Computing Technologies: An Analysis of Impairments. In: Jacko, J.A., Sears, A. (eds.) The Human-Computer Interaction Handbook, pp. 482–503. Lawrence Erlbaum Associates, Mahwah (2003)
4. Roy, E.A.: The anatomy of a head injury (2004), accessed 1st May 2005. http://www.ahs. uwaterloo.ca/~cahr/headfall.html
5. Kozelka, J., Pedley, T.: Beta and MU Rhythms. Journal of Clinical Neurophysiology, vol. 7(2), pp. 191–207. Raven Press Ltd. (1990)
6. Vaughan et al.: Brain-Computer Interface Technology: A Review of the Second International Meeting. IEEE Transactions on Neural Systems and Rehabilitation Engineering 11(2), 94–109 (2003)
7. Wolpaw, J., Birbaumer, N., Heetderks, W.J., McFarland, D.J., Peckham, P.H., Schalk, G., Donchin, E., Quatrano, L.A., Robinson, C.J.: IEEE Transactions on Rehabilitation Engineering. In: Wolpaw, J., Vaughan, T. (eds.) Brain-Computer Interface technology: A review of the First International Meeting, vol. 8(2), pp. 164–173 (2000)
8. Pregenzer, M., Pfurtscheller, G., Flotzinger, D.: Selection of electrode positions for an EEG-based Brain Computer Interface (BCI). Biomedizinische Technik 39, 264–269 (1994)
9. Berg, C., Junker, A., Rothman, A., Leininger, R.: The Cyberlink Interface: Development of A Hands-Free Continuous/Discrete Multi-Channel Computer Input Device, Small Business Innovation Research Program (SBIR) Phase II Final Report, Brain Actuated Technologies, Ohio, USA (1998)
10. Jasper, H.: The Ten-Twenty Electrode System of the International Federation in Electroencephalography and Clinical Neurophysiology. Electroencephalographic Clinical Neurophysiology 10, 371–375 (1958)
11. Siuru, B.: A brain /Computer Interface. Electronics Now. 70(3), 55–56 (1999)
12. Spiers, A., Warwick, K., Mark Gasson, M.: Assessment of Invasive Neural Implant Technology. In: HCI International 2005 (CD-ROM), Lawrence Erlbaum Associates, Las Vegas (2005)
13. Sanchez, J.C., Principe, J.C., Carne, P.R.: Is Neuron Discrimination Preprocessing Necessary for Linear and Nonlinear Brain Machine Interface Models? In: HCI International 2005 (CD-ROM), Lawrence Erlbaum Associates, Las Vegas (2005)
14. Gnanayutham, P.: Assistive Technologies for Traumatic Brain injury. ACM SIGACCESS Newsletter (80), 18–21 (2004)
15. Gnanayutham, P.: The State of Brain Body Interface Devices, UsabilityNews (October 2006) http://www.usabilitynews.com/

16. Gnanayutham, P., Bloor, C., Cockton, G.: Robotics for the brain injured: An interface for the brain injured person to operate a robotic arm. In: Antoniou, G., Deremer, D. (eds.) ICCIT'2001, pp. 93–98. New York (October 2001)
17. Gnanayutham, P., Bloor, C., Cockton, G.: AI to enhance a brain computer interface. In: Stephanidis, C. (ed.) HCI International 2003, pp. 1397–1401. Lawrence Erlbaum Associates, Mahwah, Crete (2003)
18. Gnanayutham, P., Bloor, C., Cockton, G.: Discrete Acceleration and Personalised, Tiling as Brain Body Interface Paradigms for Neurorehabilitation. In: CHI 2005, pp. 261–270. ACM Press, Portland, Oregon (2005)
19. Gnanayutham, P.: Personalised Tiling Paradigm for Motor Impaired Users. In: HCI International 2005 (CD-ROM), Lawrence Erlbaum Associates, Las Vegas (2005)
20. Preece, J., Rogers, Y., Sharp, H.: Interaction Design. Wiley, USA (2002)
21. Munhall, P.L.: Philosophical ponderings on qualitative research methods in nursing. Nursing Science Quarterly 2(1), 20–28 (1989)
22. Abowd, G., Bowen, J., Dix, A., Harrison, M., Took, R.: User Interface Languages: a survey of existing methods, Oxford University Computing Laboratory, Programming Research Group, UK (October 1989)
23. Williams, D.D.: When is Naturalistic Evaluation Appropriate? In: Williams, D, D. (ed.) Naturalistic Evaluation. New Directions for Program Evaluation, vol. 30, San Francisco: Jossey-Bass (1986)
24. Nogueira, J.L., Garcia, A.C.B.: Understanding the Tradeoffs of Interface Evaluation Methods. In: Jacko, J., Stephanidis, C. (eds.) HCI International 2003, pp. 676–680, Crete (2003)

A Human Computer Interface Using SSVEP-Based BCI Technology

Chuan Jia, Honglai Xu, Bo Hong, Xiaorong Gao,
Zhiguang Zhang, and Shangkai Gao

Dept. of Biomedical Engineering, School of Medicine
Tsinghua University, Beijing 100084, China
hongbo@tsinghua.edu.cn

Abstract. To address the issue of system simplicity and subject applicability, a brain controlled HCI system derived from steady state visual evoked potential (SSVEP) based brain computer interface (BCI) is proposed in this paper. Aiming at an external input device for personal computer, key issues of hardware and software design for better performance and user-friendly interface are introduced systematically. With proper parameter customization for each individual, an average information transfer rate of 46bits/min was achieved in the operation of dialing a phone number. With encouraging online performance and advantages of system simplicity, the proposed HCI using SSVEP-based BCI technology is promising for a substitute of standard computer input device for both health and disabled computer users.

Keywords: brain-computer interface (BCI); steady state visual evoked potential (SSVEP); input device.

1 Introduction

Much effort has been made to develop various forms of augmented device for those computer users with motor impairments. Besides traditional technologies, such as voice recognition, eye-tracker and breath controller [1], brain-computer interfaces (BCI) has been adopted as a new media to facilitate the human computer interaction in recent years. BCI translates the human intents encoded in the brain signal into control commands of computer or devices. Because of its non-invasive operation and easy system implementation, electroencephalogram (EEG) recorded on the surface of human head are widely used for BCI clinical trials [2].

Currently there are several types of EEG signal, such as motor related μ rhythm, visual evoked potential, slow cortical potential, P300, can be modulated by user's intent and/or attention and act as neural media in the brain controlled HCI system [2]. However, with its limitation of poor subject applicability (only intensively trained user can operate the system easily), low information transfer rate (usually lower than 25bits/min) and high system complexity (typically with tens of EEG electrodes), the current brain controlled HCI systems are far from user friendly.

D.D. Schmorrow, L.M. Reeves (Eds.): Augmented Cognition, HCII 2007, LNAI 4565, pp. 113–119, 2007.
© Springer-Verlag Berlin Heidelberg 2007

Based on our prototype BCI system [3][4][5], a novel design and implementation of the brain controlled HCI is introduced in this paper. Aiming at a brain controlled input device for personal computer, key issues of hardware and software optimization for better performance and user-friendly interface are addressed systematically.

2 System Design and Implementation

2.1 System Configuration

Our HCI system is composed of visual stimulation and feedback unit (VSFU), EEG Data Acquisition Unit (EDAU) and personal computer (Fig.1a). In the VSFU, compact LED modules flicking at predefined frequency bands were employed as visual stimulator. For a typical setting, 12 LEDs in a 4 by 3 array formed an external number pad with numbers 0-9, 'Backspace' and 'Enter' key (Fig.1b). When the user focused his/her visual attention on the flickering LED labeled with the number that he/she wanted to input, the EDAU and software running on PC identified the desired number by analyzing the EEG signal recorded from the user's head surface. By this means, the computer user was able to input number 0-9 and other characters with proper design of the input method. In the mode of mouse cursor control, 4 of the keys were assigned as UP, DOWN, LEFT and RIGHT movement of the cursor. Real-time feedback of input characters was provided by means of visual display and voice prompts.

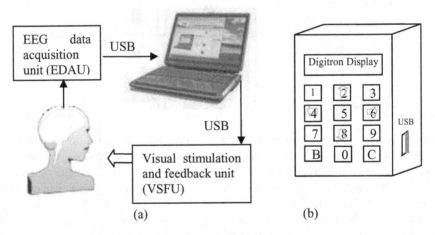

(a)   (b)

Fig. 1. Brain controlled HCI system using SSVEP. (a) System configuration and main components; (b) External number pad for visual stimulation and feedback.

2.2 Hardware Implementation

Aiming at a PC peripheral device with standard interface, the hardware of our brain controlled HCI system was designed and implemented as a compact box containing both EEG data acquisition unit and visual stimulation and feedback unit. Two USB ports are used for real-time data streaming from EDAU and online control of VSFU respectively.

EEG Data Acquisition Unit. In the EDAU, a pair of bipolar Ag/AgCl electrode was placed over the user's occipital region. A tennis headband was modified to harness the electrodes on the head surface.The EEG signal was amplified by a customized amplifier and digitized at a sampling rate of 256Hz. After a 50Hz notch filtering to remove the power line interference, the digital EEG data were streamed to PC memory buffer through USB port.

Visual Stimulation and Feedback Unit. As shown in Fig.2, for the precision of frequency control, the periodical flickering of each LED was controlled by a separate lighting module, which downloads the frequency setting from the PC through master MCU.

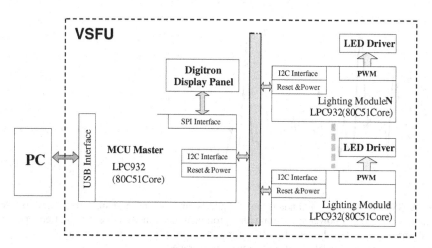

Fig. 2. Schematic diagram of visual stimulation and feedback unit

In one of the application, our brain controlled HCI system was used for dialing a phone number. In that case, a local telephone line was connected to the RJ11 port of internal modem of the personal computer.

2.3 Software and Algorithm

The main software running on the PC consists of key parts of the EEG translation algorithm, including signal enhancing, feature extraction and pattern classification. The following algorithms were implemented in Microsoft Visual C/C++ and compiled into a stand alone program. The real time EEG data steaming was achieved by using a customized dynamic link library (DLL).

In the paradigm of SSVEP, the target LED evokes a peak in the amplitude spectrum at the flickering frequency. After a band filtering of 4-35Hz, fast Fourier transform (FFT) was applied on the ongoing EEG data segments to obtain the running power spectrum. If a peak value was detected over the frequency band (4-35Hz), the frequency corresponding to the peak was selected as the candidate of target frequency. To avoid a high false positive rate, a crucial step was to make sure that the amplitude of candidate frequency was higher enough than the mean power of the whole band. Herein, the ratio between the peak power and the mean power was defined as:

$$Q = P_{peak}/P_{mean}. \tag{1}$$

Basically, if the power ratio Q was high than the predefined threshold T (T>2), the peak power was considered as significant. For each individual, the threshold T was estimated beforehand in the parameter customization phase. The optimal selection of the threshold made a tradeoff between the speed and accuracy of the HCI operating. Detail explanation of this power spectrum threshold method can be found in our previous study[4][5].

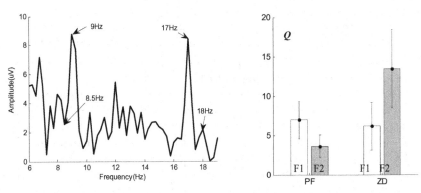

Fig. 3. SSVEP response at fundamental frequency and second harmonic frequency. (a) An instance of user ZD's power spectrum with a prominent peak in second harmonic frequency F2 (b) Comparison of Q value at F1 and F2 for subject PF and ZD, in which the Q value at 27 frequencies between 6-19Hz (0.5Hz spacing) was averaged.

During the algorithm testing and verifying, we notice that the fundamental target frequency F1 of some users does not give a prominent response, while the second harmonic frequency F2 (F2=2F1) displays more significant peak power. As shown in Fig.3a, for the user ZD and the target frequency 8.5Hz, the power of fundamental frequency is lower than the neighboring peak frequency 9Hz, which misled the algorithm. It can be easily found that, if the power at second harmonic frequency (17Hz) were taken into account, the situation would changed a lot. The further comparison of Q value between fundamental frequency and second harmonic frequency gives us a clear idea as shown in Fig.3b. For the user PF, the fundamental frequency F1 is a better feature to detect the target frequency, while the user ZD prefers the second harmonic F2. For this reason, we further improved the algorithm by incorporating the power value at the second harmonic frequency and the P_{peak} in Eq.1 was substituted by the linear combination of power amplitude at F1 and F2.

$$P_{peak} = \alpha P_{F1} + (1-\alpha)P_{F2} \tag{2}$$

The weight coefficient α was optimally predefined in the parameter customization phase. Basically, for users like ZD, weight coefficient α should be set lower than that of users like PF.

2.4 Parameter Customization

To address the issue of individual diversity and to improve the subject applicability, a procedure of parameter customization was conducted before the HCI operating. Our previous study suggests that the crucial system parameters include EEG electrode location, visual stimulus frequency band, and threshold (T) for target frequency determination [5]. To maintain the simplicity of operation and efficiency of parameter selection, a standard procedure was designed to help the system customization, which consists of the following steps:

Step1 - Frequency Scan. 27 frequencies in the range of 6-19Hz (0.5Hz spacing) were randomly divided into 3 groups and the 9 frequencies in each group were randomly assigned to number 1-9 on the aforementioned LED number pad. Then the frequency scan was conducted by presenting the number 1-9 on the digitron display one by one and each for 7 seconds. During this time period, the user was asked to gaze at the LED number pad corresponding to the presented number. This kind of scan was repeated for 3 groups containing all 27 frequencies. There was 2 seconds of resting period between each numbers and 1 minutes of resting between groups. It took about 8 minutes for a complete frequency scan. The 7-second SSVEP response during each frequency stimulus was saved for the following offline analysis. In the procedure of frequency scan, the bipolar EEG electrodes were placed at Oz (center of the occipital region) and one of its surrounding sites (3cm apart on the left or right side). According to our previous study[6], this electrode configuration was the typical one for most of the users.

Step2 - Simulation of Online Operating. The saved EEG segments were analyzed using FFT to find the optimal frequency band with relatively high Q values. The suitable value of the threshold T and the weight coefficients α were estimated in a simulation of online HCI operating, in which the saved EEG data were fed into the algorithm in a stream.

Step3 -Electrode Position Optimization. For some of the subjects, when the above two steps do not provide a reasonable performance, the advanced method using independent component analysis was employed to find the optimal position of EEG electrodes. The best electrode pair for bipolar recording with highest signal-to-noise ratio was selected by mapping the EEG signal and noise amplitude over all possible electrodes[6].

3 Result

Ten subjects participated in the online experiment of dialing a telephone number and all of them succeeded in the operation. As shown in Fig.4, the brain controlled BCI box acts as an external input device of a laptop computer. With only two EEG electrodes attached on the surface of the head, the HCI user could obtain an easy control of number inputting through directing his/her gaze on the external flickering number pad.

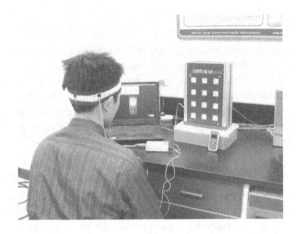

Fig. 4. The brain controlled HCI box in the operation of dialing a cell phone number

Table 1. Online operation performance of 5 subjects with parameter optimization

Subject	Time/selection (seconds)	Accuracy (%)	ITR (bits/min)
ZD	2.7	93	66.7
SY	3.5	100	61.5
PF	4.6	100	46.8
XH	5.0	88	31.9
JC	6.8	93	26.5
Average	4.52	94.8	46.68

With optimized system parameters for 5 participants, an average information transfer rate (ITR) of 46.68bits/min and an average accuracy of 94.8% were achieved. The best performance was the 93% accuracy at an ITR of 66.7bits/min (Table 1). In another testing of operating Microsoft Internet Explorer, 8 of the participants were able to implement the task of opening a target web link.

4 Conclusion

To address the issue of system simplicity and subject applicability, a SSVEP-based brain controlled HCI system was proposed in this paper. Comparing with other brain controlled HCI systems, it bears the following major characteristics: 1) non-invasive harnessing; 2) PC compatible operating; 3) few EEG electrodes without using EEG cap; 4) little training and setting; 5) high information transfer rate; 6) low cost of the system hardware.

With encouraging online performance and advantages of system simplicity, the proposed HCI using SSVEP-based BCI technology is promising not only for the prosthetics of the disabled people, but also for a substitute of standard computer input device in the case of inconvenient use of one or both hands of the health people[5][7], such as the situation of using a cell phone or other handheld devices.

Acknowledgments. This work was supported by the Science and Technology Ministry of China under Grant 2006BAI03A17 and the National Science Foundation of China under Grant 30630022.

References

1. Jacko, J.A., Sears, A.: The Human Computer Interaction Handbook: Fundamentals, Evolving Technologies, and Emerging Applications, pp. 246–343. Lawrence Erlbaum Associates, London (2003)
2. Lebedev, M.A., Nicolelis, M.A.L.: Brain–machine interfaces: past, present and future. Trends in Neurosciences 29(9), 536–546 (2006)
3. Cheng, M., Gao, X., Gao, S., Xu, D.: Design and implementation of a brain–computer interface with high transfer rates. IEEE Trans. Biomed. Eng. 49(10), 1181–1186 (2002)
4. Gao, X., Xu, D., Cheng, M., Gao, S.: A BCI-based environmental controller for the motion-disabled. IEEE Trans. Neural. Sys. Reh. Eng. 11(2), 137–140 (2003)
5. Wang, Y., Wang, R., Gao, X., Hong, B., Gao, S.: A Practical VEP-Based Brain–Computer Interface. IEEE Trans. Neural. Sys. Reh. Eng. 14(2), 234–239 (2006)
6. Wang, Y., Zhang, Z., Gao, X., Gao, S.: Lead selection for SSVEP-based brain–computer interface. In: Proc. Annual International Conference of IEEE EMBS, pp. 4507–4509 (2004)
7. Trejo, L.J., Rosipal, R., Matthews, B.: Brain–Computer Interfaces for 1-D and 2-D Cursor Control: Designs Using Volitional Control of the EEG Spectrum or Steady-State Visual Evoked Potentials. IEEE Trans. Neural. Sys. Reh. Eng. 14(2), 225–229 (2006)

Enhanced P300-Based Cursor Movement Control

Zhongwei Ma, Xiaorong Gao, and Shangkai Gao

Dept. of Biomedical Engineering, School of Medicine, Tsinghua University, Beijing
100084, China
gsk-dea@mail.tsinghua.edu.cn

Abstract. In order to build a high-performance brain-computer interface (BCI) for cursor movement control, a P300-based BCI system using a five-select oddball paradigm was designed and implemented. We found that high intensity visual stimuli (HIVS) can improve the performance of BCI. 9 subjects participated in the test of the proposed BCI system. Each subject completed 40 epochs with HIVS and low intensity visual stimuli (LIVS) respectively. The preprocessed data were classified by support vector machines (SVM). The averaged waveforms both from HIVS and LIVS proved that this new paradigm can elicit evident P300 potentials. Furthermore, the results indicated the information transfer rate (ITR) of HIVS could reach 5.4 bit/min, which was higher than 4.6 bit/min of LIVS.

Keywords: brain-computer interface (BCI), P300, support vector machine (SVM), information transfer rate (ITR), stimulus intensity, electrophysiological (EEG).

1 Introduction

To help paralyzed persons regain the ability of environment control is an important goal of the field of Augmented Cognition (AugCog). Many groups are eager to find a new channel, which does not depends on human peripheral muscle or nerve system, to translate information and commands between human and external world, namely called Brain-Computer Interface (BCI)[1].

Among the applications of BCI, cursor movement control is studied frequently. Several electrophysiological (EEG) signals can be used for cursor movement control BCI, such as steady-state visual evoked potential (SSVEP)[2], P300 potentials[3], mu rhythm[4, 5]. Because of the short latency and no long-lasting operant training, P300 potentials were applied widely[6]. Farwell and Donchin first applied P300 to brain-computer interface in 1988, a 6*6 matrix of characters was presented to realize a P300 speller[7]. Several methods can be utilized to distinguish P300 potential from background noise, such as independent component analysis (ICA)[8, 9], wavelet transform[10], step discriminant analysis (SWDA)[11] and support vector machine (SVM)[9, 12]. SVM is a supervised learning method used for classification and regression, and has been successfully applied in BCI [13]. In this paper, we utilized SVM to identified P300 potentials.

D.D. Schmorrow, L.M. Reeves (Eds.): Augmented Cognition, HCII 2007, LNAI 4565, pp. 120–126, 2007.

To develop a simple and practical BCI for cursor movement control, a P300-based BCI system with a five-choice (stand for UP, DOWN, LEFT, RIGHT and OK in virtual mouse) oddball paradigm was designed and implemented in our work. Our study demonstrated that high intensity visual stimulus (HIVS) could enchant the performance of this kind of BCI.

2   Experiment Methods

2.1   Subjects

Nine subjects (five males and four females) aged between twenty one and twenty eight participated in the test of the proposed BCI system, all of them are right-handed, had normal or corrected-to-normal vision.

2.2   Paradigm

Subjects were seated in a comfortable chair, 100 cm from a 15-inch TFT monitor on which the stimulus interface was displayed. The circumstance brightness was $120cd/m^2$, the maximal illumination of TFT monitor was 150Lx. Five small crosses that help subjects locate the target were shown on the screen in a cross-order form (see Fig.1(a)).

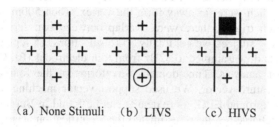

(a) None Stimuli   (b) LIVS   (c) HIVS

Fig. 1. The stimulus interface

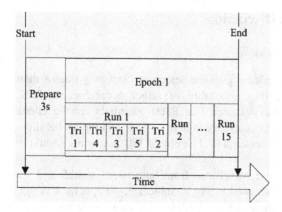

Fig. 2. The proceeding of an epoch

During the experiment, a mark that stood for target was put onto one of the five small crosses in random order for a period of 100ms. Between two successive appearances of the marks, there was a 75ms of rest time. So, the time duration of each trial was 175ms, namely 5.7 trails appeared in a second. The mark appeared on each of the five small crosses once in a run, and each epoch consists of 15 runs. The total duration of an epoch was 13.125s. An interval of 3s was inserted into two serial epochs to make subjects take a short rest and prepare for next epoch. Fig.2 gives the exact details of an epoch.

Every subject completed 40 epochs with low intensity visual stimulus (LIVS) and HIVS respectively. In LIVS experiment block, the mark was a white hollow circle in order to reduce the stimulus at visual cortex (see Fig.1(b)). In HIVS experiment block, the mark was a full rectangle, which would arouse high visual stimulus at visual cortex (see Fig.1(c)).

2.3 Data Recording

32-channel data was recorded with a BioSemi Active Two system at 256 Hz, but only six channels (Fz, Cz, Pz, Oz, T7 and T8) were used for further analysis. We placed the ground electrode at the top of the head as the system default.

2.4 Analysis Methods

After band-pass filtering between 1 and 16Hz, data was referred to the mean of T7 and T8, both of which were far away form the vertex. Then 500ms length data was extracted after each trigger, there were overlap between two serial data segments obviously. For every subject, we got totally 75 (5 selections, 15 repetitions) segments in each epoch. Data downsampled to 32Hz from four electrodes (Fz, Cz, Pz, Oz) were chosen for further analysis. Time-domain waveforms of the four electrodes were cascaded as the feature vector. We used support vector machine to identify P300 potential from background EEG, more details can be found in Burges's paper[14]. In order to obtain a reliable result, we estimated the identification accuracy by a 10-fold cross-validation.

3   Result and Discussion

3.1 P300 Waveform

The paradigm included 5 possible selections, but only one of them was attended by subjects at once, the probability of target occurrence is 20%. Sellers and his coworkers have demonstrated that P300 potentials can be elicited even when the probability of target occurrence is high as 33% and the probability manipulation does not compromise accuracy[15]. Thereby, P300 potentials should be aroused by this new paradigm.

Averaged response waveforms from both target stimuli and non-target Stimuli at electrode Cz were showed in Fig.3 (subject 3, 40 epochs, LIVS). We could become conscious of that there was an evident peak around 300ms from target stimulus and none significant feature around 300ms from non-target stimulus. The waveform from target stimuli was similar with the reports in the literature. We believed that P300 potentials were elicited by this new paradigm.

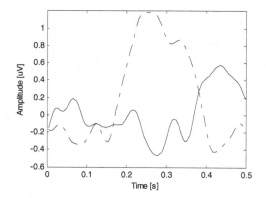

Fig. 3. Averaged response waveforms from both target stimuli (dotted line) and non-target Stimuli (solid line) at electrode Cz

3.2 Difference in HIVS and LIVS

Polich et al. have demonstrated that the increase in stimulus intensity will bring on increases in P300 amplitude and decreases in peak latency[16]. Two kinds of stimulus intensity were applied in this paper, the averaged response waveforms in both HIVS and LIVS were illustrated in Fig.4 (All subjects).

The waveforms from target stimuli both for HIVS and LIVS at electrode Pz were very similar. The effects of stimulus rhythm of 5.7Hz could be found. The amplitude of P300 potential was higher in HIVS than the one in LIVS, which agreed with the former report. But there were no significant difference between the latencies of P300 potential for HIVS and LIVS.

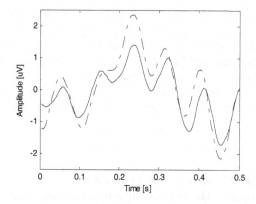

Fig. 4. Averaged response from target stimuli both for HIVS (dotted line) and LIVS (solid line) at electrode Pz

3.3 Identification Accuracy

For each subject, the identification accuracy versus the number of repetition trials was calculated. The averaged varying curve of all subjects was presented in Fig.5.

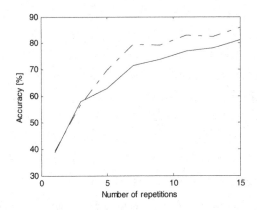

Fig. 5. The identification accuracies of HIVS (dotted line) and LIVS (solid line)

Along with the increase of the number of trial repetitions, the identification accuracies increased monotonously in both HIVS and LIVS. Nevertheless, the identification accuracy in HIVS was higher around 5% than the one in LIVS when the number of trial repetitions exceeded 3.

3.4 Information Translate Rate

One of the measurements to evaluate the performance of a BCI is the information translate rate (ITR)[9]. Three factors influence the ITR: the number of possible selections, the identification accuracy and the duration of each selection. The bit rate B should be calculated before the ITR R is acquired. The bit rate is defined as follows:

$$B = \text{Log}_2 N + p\text{Log}_2 P + (1 - P)\text{Log}_2[(1 - P)/(N - 1)] \tag{1}$$

N is the number of possible selections and P is the identification accuracy. The bit rate is information translated per epoch, we can convert the bit rate into ITR by $R = BM$, M is number of epoch per minute.

The results of offline analysis indicated that the information transfer rate of this BCI in high intensity reached 5.4 bit/min, apposed to 4.6 bit/min in low intensity.

4 Conclusion

A novel enhanced P300-based cursor movement control was designed and implemented in this paper. The new paradigm was demonstrated to evoke robust P300 potentials from all subjects; also the ITR in HIVS was higher than the one in LIVS.

Acknowledgements. This work was supported by National Natural Science Foundation of China (NSFC) 60318001 and Tsinghua-Yuyuan Medicine Research fund to the third author.

References

1. Wolpaw, J.R., Birbaumer, N., McFarland, D.J., Pfurtscheller, G., Vaughan, T.M.: Brain-computer interfaces for communication and control. Clinical Neurophysiology 113(6), 767–791 (2002)
2. Cheng, M., Gao, X.R., Gao, S.G., Xu, D.F.: Design and implementation of a brain-computer interface with high transfer rates. IEEE Transactions on Biomedical Engineering 49(10), 1181–1186 (2002)
3. Piccione, F., Giorgi, F., Tonin, P., Priftis, K., Giove, S., Silvoni, S., Palmas, G., Beverina, F.: P300-based brain computer interface: Reliability and performance in healthy and paralysed participants. Clinical Neurophysiology 117(3), 531–537 (2006)
4. Wolpaw, J.R., Flotzinger, D., Pfurtscheller, G., McFarland, D.J.: Timing of EEG-based cursor control. Journal of Clinical Neurophysiology 14(6), 529–538 (1997)
5. Fabiani, G.E., McFarland, D.J., Wolpaw, J.R., Pfurtscheller, G.: Conversion of EEG activity into cursor movement by a brain-computer interface (BCI). IEEE Transactions on Neural Systems and Rehabilitation Engineering 12(3), 331–338 (2004)
6. Birbaumer, N.: Breaking the silence: Brain-computer interfaces (BCI) for communication and motor control. Psychophysiology 43(6), 517–532 (2006)
7. Wolpaw, J.R., Loeb, G.E., Allison, B.Z., Donchin, E., do Nascimento, O.F., Heetderks, W.J., Nijboer, F., Shain, W.G., Turner, J.N.: BCI Meeting 2005 - Workshop on signals and recording methods. IEEE Transactions on Neural Systems and Rehabilitation Engineering 14(2), 138–141 (2006)
8. Xu, N., Gao, X.R., Hong, B., Miao, X.B., Gao, S.K., Yang, F.S.: BCI competition 2003 - Data set IIb: Enhancing P300 wave detection using ICA-based subspace projections for BCI applications. IEEE Transactions on Biomedical Engineering 51(6), 1067–1072 (2004)
9. Serby, H., Yom-Tov, E., Inbar, G.F.: An improved P300-based brain-computer interface. IEEE Transactions on Neural Systems and Rehabilitation Engineering 13(1), 89–98 (2005)
10. Bostanov, V.: BCI competition 2003 - Data sets Ib and IIb: Feature extraction from event-related brain potentials with the continuous wavelet transform and the t-value scalogram. IEEE Transactions on Biomedical Engineering 51(6), 1057–1061 (2004)
11. Donchin, E., Spencer, K.M., Wijesinghe, R.: The mental prosthesis: Assessing the speed of a P300-based brain-computer interface. IEEE Transactions on Rehabilitation Engineering 8(2), 174–179 (2000)
12. Kaper, M., Meinicke, P., Grossekathoefer, U., Lingner, T., Ritter, H.: BCI competition 2003 - Data set IIb: Support vector machines for the P300 speller paradigm. IEEE Transactions on Biomedical Engineering 51(6), 1073–1076 (2004)
13. Blankertz, B., Dornhege, G., Lemm, S., Krauledat, M., Curio, G., Muller, K.R.: The Berlin brain-computer interface: Machine learning based detection of user specific brain states. Journal of Universal Computer Science 12(6), 581–607 (2006)
14. Burges, C.J.C.: A tutorial on Support Vector Machines for pattern recognition. Data Mining and Knowledge Discovery 2(2), 121–167 (1998)

15. Sellers, E.W., Krusienski, D.J., McFarland, D.J., Vaughan, T.M., Wolpaw, J.R.: A P300 event-related potential brain-computer interface (BCI): The effects of matrix size and inter stimulus interval on performance. Biological Psychology 73(3), 242–252 (2006)
16. Covington, J.W., Polich, J.: P300, stimulus intensity, and modality. Evoked Potentials-Electroencephalography and Clinical Neurophysiology 100(6), 579–584 (1996)

Low Power Technology for Wearable Cognition Systems

David C. Yates, Alexander Casson, and Esther Rodriguez-Villegas

Circuits and Systems, Dept. Electrical and Electronic Engineering,
Imperial College London, UK, SW7 2AZ
{david.yates,alexander.casson06,e.rodriguez}@imperial.ac.uk

Abstract. This paper analyses a key tradeoff behind miniature devices intended to monitor cognition-related parameters. These devices are supposed to be worn by people that would otherwise be carrying on a normal life and this factor imposes important constraints in the design. They have to be wireless, wearable, discrete, low maintenance and reliable. In order to reduce power intelligence will be built into the sensors aiming to reduce the data transmission to only that information that it is strictly necessary. This intelligence will be in the form of an algorithm which will be required to be implemented in electronic circuits as part of the system. The complexity of the algorithm affects the complexity of the electronics and hence the power consumption. This, in turn affects the size of the battery and the overall size of the device. For the sensor to be low maintenance the device must operate for extended periods from the battery, adding more constraints to the power consumption of the electronic circuits. The battery must be kept small so that the overall size of the device is small and lightweight enough to be worn on the body and the more discrete the device the higher consumer compliance. A tradeoff has to be met between the algorithm complexity, the power consumption of the electronics required to realize the latter, the power consumption required to transmit data and the battery size and lifetime.

Keywords: Ambulatory EEG, low-power, wearable, wireless, cognition.

1 Introduction

Augmented cognition aims to improve human performance by modifying an operator's interaction with a machine depending on their mental state. Central to this vision is the development of wearable psychophysiological sensors, capable of both monitoring and transmitting data to be used in a closed-loop system. User acceptability requires that the presence of such technologies causes minimum inconvenience. This places stringent limits on both the size and weight of these devices and makes wireless operation highly desirable [1]. It is envisioned that a variety of sensor technologies would be combined in order to recognise a more complete set of cognitive states [2]. A short battery lifetime for the nodes of a dense network of wireless body sensors is impractical for the user, yet the battery capacity is

D.D. Schmorrow, L.M. Reeves (Eds.): Augmented Cognition, HCII 2007, LNAI 4565, pp. 127–136, 2007.

limited by the size restrictions. Particularly challenging are mobile environments in which size and weight limitations are more acute [2]. Moreover, there are important augmented cognition scenarios, such as the dismounted soldier, where the user may be expected to operate for extended periods of time with an extremely limited supply of power [3]. Energy efficient circuits and systems will thus be required to maximise the ratio of battery lifetime to battery size.

Electroencephalography (EEG) is a key enabling technology for augmented cognition [1]. It has been successfully employed to measure a number of cognitive states including workload [1], alertness [4], working memory [5], and selective attention [6]. Ambulatory EEG (AEEG) is currently widely used in the context of healthcare [7]. The patient is either monitored in-house or at home but very rarely in a more challenging environment. In order to apply this technology to the field of augmented cognition the EEG headset must be made less bulky, lighter, wireless, lower power and the electrodes must be easy to position. This paper focuses on the first four of these requirements by identifying and analyzing a key trade-off in the design of AEEG headsets. This trade-off enables us to maximize the battery lifetime to battery size ratio.

2   System Power Consumption

Table 1 details three groups of batteries, classified according to the total energy available, and which have been named AA, the large coin cell (LCC) and the small coin cell (SCC). The table includes off-the-shelf examples of each group and primary and secondary cells are denoted by (P) and (S) respectively. To give a brief indication of the energy available for each group, operation for one working week (5 days) would require a power consumption of 29 mW for the AA battery, 3 mW for the LCC and 250 μW for the SCC.

Table 1. Specifications for batteries of various sizes

Group	Energy / mWh	Examples				
		Make	Type	Voltage	Capacity /mAh	Size /mm (diam.×height)
AA	3500	Sanyo HR-3U-4BP	NiMH (S)	1.2 V	2500	15 × 51
AA	3500	Duracell Ultra MX1500	Alkaline MnO_2 (P)	1.5 V	2500	15 × 51
LCC	400	VARTA	NiMH (S)	1.2 V	250	25.1 × 6.7
LCC	400	Panasonic	$LiMnO_2$ (P)	3 V	165	20 × 2.5
SCC	30	RS RX364-2C5	AgO_2 (P)	1.5 V	23	6.8 × 2.15
SCC	30	Power Paper STD-1	$ZnMnO_2$ (P)	1.5 V	15	39 × 0.6

A number of groups have designed wireless headsets based on off-the-shelf components. One representative prototype, developed by IMEC [8] achieves 3 day operation from 4 AA batteries. It is likely that successful AEEG wireless headsets suitable for augmented cognition would have to operate for longer off a smaller power supply.

The electronics in a wireless AEEG headset consists of at least an amplifier, an ADC and a radio transmitter. Recently ultra low power amplifiers for EEG systems have been reported which achieve the required performance whilst dissipating only around 1 μW [9, 10]. The noise performance of these circuits, designed for monitoring neurological illnesses, is based on a bandwidth of 30 Hz, whereas monitoring cognitive states often requires a slightly larger bandwidth of 44 Hz [11]. To achieve a similar noise performance with a larger bandwidth requires a higher power consumption. Hence, this analysis assumes that a suitable amplifier will consume 2 μW. A sub-microwatt ADC suitable for the application is presented in [12]. Based on a number of publications [1, 5, 11] this work conservatively assumes that 9 EEG/EOG channels will be required. Considering that each channel will need one amplifier and one ADC, the total power consumed by these two circuit blocks will be no more than about 30μW.

Table 2 shows the power consumption and data rates of various `state-of-the-art' low power transceivers. Where the required data rate is significantly less than the achievable data rate the transmitter can be operated at a low duty cycle, considerably reducing the average power dissipation. The energy used per bit transmitted, also given in table 2, is therefore a useful metric. Two energy per bit values are used in the remainder of this paper. Based on the performance of the nRF2401 [13] and the BRF6150 [14], 50 nJ/b is taken as a conservative value, definitely achievable in most environments for short range communications, whereas 5 nJ/b is taken as a more speculative but still realistic figure, based on the reported performance of UWB devices such as the XS110 [15] or on cutting edge narrowband device such as Zarlink's ZL70100 [16].

Table 2. Low power off-the-shelf transceivers

	nRF2401 [13]	BRF6150 [14]	XS110 [15]	ZL70100 [16]
Type	GFSK	Bluetooth	UWB	MICS
Data rate (b/s)	1 M	1 M	110 M	800 k
TX power (mW)	21	75	750	5
Energy/bit (nJ/b)	21	75	6.8	6.25

Based on 9 channels, a sampling rate of 256 Hz and a resolution of 16 bits, the required data rate of the AEEG systems is approximately 37 kb/s. This can be reduced to only 23 kb/s by removing the large DC offset at the scalp-electrode interface, which is almost 1000 times the signal amplitude [17]. This corresponds to a transmitter power consumption of 1.15 mW in the conservative case and 115 μW in the speculative case. It can thus be clearly seen that the transmitter will dominate the system power consumption in both cases, and this is neglecting the power needed to control the transmitter or store the data to be transmitted.

3 Data Compression

In order to reduce the power consumption of the system it is necessary to dissipate less power in the transceiver. One way to achieve this is to reduce the amount of data to be transmitted. Duty-cycling the transmitter according to the ratio of the required data rate to the maximum   possible data rate results in the following average transmitter power consumption, $P_{TX,u}$:

$$P_{TX,u} = \frac{b_{r,u}}{b_{r,\max}} \cdot P_{TX,\max} \quad . \tag{1}$$

where $b_{r,u}$ is the required data rate before compression, $b_{r,max}$ is the maximum possible data rate and $P_{TX,\ max}$ is the transmitter power consumption at that maximum data rate. Using the same argument, compressing the data to give a data rate of $b_{r,c}$ will result in an average transmitter power dissipation, $P_{TX,c}$, which is given by:

$$P_{TX,c} = \frac{b_{r,c}}{b_{r,u}} \cdot P_{TX,u} \quad . \tag{2}$$

The compression technique will consume a certain amount of power, P_{comp}, which includes any extra short term data storage and duty cycle control of the transceiver. The total system power consumption, P_{sys}, is thus given by:

$$P_{sys} = P_{amp} + P_{ADC} + P_{comp} + C \cdot P_{TX,u} \quad . \tag{3}$$

where P_{amp} are P_{ADC} are the power consumption of the amplifiers and ADC(s) respectively; C is the compression ratio, which is equal to $b_{r,c}/b_{r,u}$. If $P_{comp} + C \cdot P_{TX,u} < P_{TX,u}$ then the total system power is reduced. Reducing C will generally require an increase in P_{comp}. The remainder of this paper analyses this key design trade-off by detailing the combinations of C and P_{comp} which will improve the lifetime to battery size ratio.

4 Improving Battery Lifetime

For a battery powered system with battery capacity, C_{cell} and voltage, V_{cell}, designed to operate for a lifetime, t_l the total system power, P_{sys}, is given by:

$$P_{sys} = \frac{C_{cell} \cdot V_{cell}}{t_l} \quad . \tag{4}$$

Figures 1 and 2 show the system designer which combinations of P_{comp} and C will be required to achieve a certain lifetime for a given amount of available energy. Both graphs assume a total amplifier and ADC power consumption of 30 μW and that the

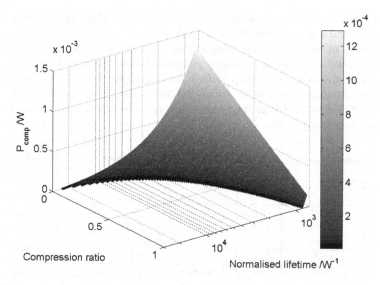

Fig. 1. Maximum power for compression against compression ratio and normalised lifetime for a transmitter which consumes 50 nJ/b

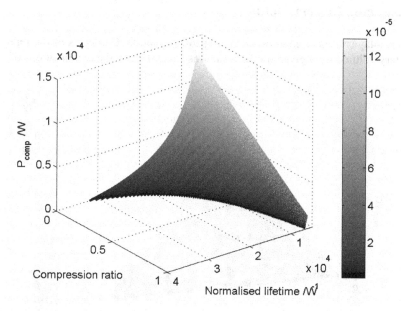

Fig. 2. Maximum power for compression against compression ratio and normalised lifetime for a transmitter which consumes 5 nJ/b

uncompressed data rate is 23 kb/s. The lifetime is normalised with respect to the available energy of the battery given by $C_{cell} \cdot V_{cell}$. Table 3 shows the lifetime for the different battery groups of table 1 with and without compression. The table gives specific values of a realistic compression ratio and P_{comp} combination which would result in a useful but reasonable increase in lifetime. $t_{l,c}$ and $t_{l,u}$ represent the battery lifetime with and without compression respectively.

The figures of table 3 are promising in that even for the conservative estimate of transmitter power, if compression ratios of around 0.25 can be achieved for no more than 200 μW then the SCC battery class could operate for 3 days, and the LCC battery class could operate for 2 weeks, the latter being much longer than current medical AEEG devices, where the headset is wired to a belt or an over-the-shoulder battery and data storage pack.

Table 3. Comparison of battery lifetime with and without data compression

TX Energy/bit	Group	$t_{l,u}$	$t_{l,c}$	C	P_{comp} /mW
50 nJ/b	SCC	25 hrs	72 hrs	0.2	0.16
50 nJ/b	LCC	2 weeks	1 month	0.3	0.17
50 nJ/b	AA	17 weeks	6 months	0.4	0.3
5 nJ/b	SCC	8 days	2 weeks	0.3	0.025
5 nJ/b	LCC	3.8 months	6 months	0.4	0.015
5 nJ/b	AA	33 months	5 years	0.2	0.027

5 Reducing Battery Volume

The advantages of data compression can also be quantified in terms of the reduction in battery volume for a given lifetime. Figures 3 and 4 show the combinations of P_{comp}

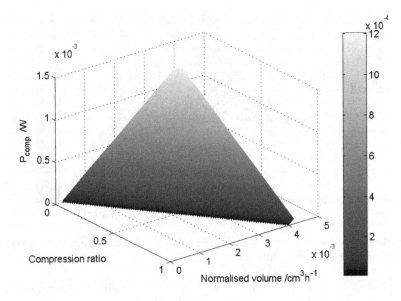

Fig. 3. Maximum power for compression against compression ratio and battery volume normalised to lifetime for a battery with energy density equal to 1100 J/cc, and a transmitter which consumes 50 nJ/b

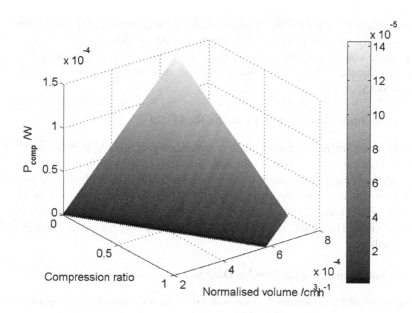

Fig. 4. Maximum power for compression against compression ratio and battery volume normalised to lifetime for a battery with energy density equal to 1100 J/cc, and a transmitter which consumes 5 nJ/b

and C required for a particular battery volume based on the energy density of a lithium secondary cell, which is 1100 J/cc [18]. Battery volume has been normalised to lifetime measured in hours. It can be seen from figure 4 that to achieve a volume to lifetime ratio of less than 0.004 cm^3/h, data compression is needed for a transmitter which consumes 50 nJ/b. For the 5 nJ/b transmitter no compression is needed until the desired volume to lifetime ratio drops below about 0.0006 cm^3/h.

6   Data Reduction Mechanisms

Three principle methods of data reduction are discussed here, with some results summarised in table 4.

6.1   Reduce the Quality of the Recording

Modern AEEG systems record digitally allowing the sampling resolution and rate to be varied. Reducing these will reduce the data to be transmitted, but also reduce the recording quality. Clearly minimum values will be required to accurately represent the EEG signal. [19] notes that most EEG signals studied are in the range 0.5–60Hz, although there is also some higher frequency content. A minimum sampling frequency of 120Hz is thus required. Most EEG systems use between eight and 16 sampling bits, and using the lower end of this range would produce the least amount of data. The data could also be reduced by simply monitoring fewer channels; recording only two EEG channels is enough to monitor alertness [4] and three EEG channels are enough to determine cognitive workload [1]. These methods, however, reduce the quality of the EEG recording and the quality of the cognitive state assessment [5] .

6.2 Use Compression Algorithms on the Raw Data

There has been interest in recent years in using compression algorithms on raw EEG streams. This has shown good results with a compression ratio of approximately 0.5 being achievable using a lossless compression techniques [20], which can reduced to a compression ratio of approximately 0.15 when lossy compression is deemed acceptable [21]. These levels are impressive and the schemes should certainly be used where possible. The major barrier to their use is their implementation in suitably low power hardware.

6.3 Do Not Transmit a Continuous Data Set

Transmission of the complete data set is not necessary if some form of cognitive state assessment can be performed locally. There are essentially three methods which could be used individually or in some combination to reduce the transmitted data.

1   Implement an algorithm which detects any significant changes of state, without determining that change of state. The relevant data could then be transmitted for more detailed analysis at a node with more data processing capability.
2   Detect the cognitive state locally and simply transmit the new cognitive state each time it changes.
3   It may be the case that particular cognitive state can only be determined in conjunction with other sensors, in which case no local decision about the change of state can be made. In such a case the cognitive state could be monitored only when some action needs to be taken (for instance the communication of some new information to a dismounted soldier).

The first of the three methods has been researched in detail by the authors to aid in the diagnosis and treatment of people suffering from epilepsy. In this case data that is potentially important is recorded for closer analysis by the neurologist. Epileptic EEG traces can be broken down into two phases: ictal (seizure activity) and interictal (spikes and spike-and-waves) [22]. Interictal activity usually contains isolated events along with *normal* background signals. By recording only the ictal and interesting interictal activity it is estimated that a compression ratio of 0.1 can be achieved [23]. For comparison, table 4 illustrates preliminary results for a wavelet transform based interictal detection algorithm developed from [24] and [25] (labelled 'example CWT method' in table 4) and analysed with new data as part of this work. Similar algorithms can be used to detect cognitive states [26].

Figures 1, 2, 3 and 4 indicate that the challenge for the designer is to implement such algorithms at sub-milliwatt power levels.

Table 4. Performance comparison of data reduction schemes

Method	Notes	Lossy	C
Reduced quality	3 channels, 8 bits, 120 Hz	Yes	0.12
Lossless compression	See [20]	No	0.4
Lossy compression	See [21]	Yes	0.1-0.2
Discontinuous (Gotman)	See [23]	Yes	0.05-0.1
Example CWT method	140 ms window	Yes	0.06
Example CWT method	5 s window	Yes	0.5

7 Conclusion

Graphs have been presented which aid the designer in determining when it is advantageous to employ data compression. These graphs show the improvement in lifetime or battery volume possible for varying compression ratios, and give the corresponding power available to perform this compression. It is shown that data compression ratios of between 0.2 and 0.4 using only a few hundred microwatts can significantly improve the lifetime for a given battery size in the case of a 50 nJ/b transmitter. Such compression would make it feasible to operate a wireless headset from a small coin cell for about 3 days and from a large coin cell for up to 1 month. For the 5 nJ/b transmitter compression algorithms could consume no more than a few tens of microwatts to significantly increase the ratio of lifetime to battery size.

References

1. Berka, C., et al.: Real Time Analysis of EEG Indexes of Alertness, Cognition, and Memory Acquired With a Wireless EEG Headset. International Journal of Human-Computer Interaction 17(2), 151–170 (2004)
2. St. John, M., et al.: Overview of DARPA Augmented Cognition Technical Integration Experiment. International Journal of Human-Computer Interaction 17(2), 131–149 (2004)
3. Energy Efficient Technologies for the Dismounted Soldier. Committee on Electric Power for the Dismounted Soldier. National Academy Press, Washington D.C. (1997)
4. Lin, C.-T., Wu, R.-C., Liang, S.-F., Chao, W.-H., Chen, Y.-J., Jung, T.-P.: EEG-Based Drowsiness Estimation for Safety Driving Using Independent Component Analysis. IEEE Transactions on Circuits and Systems—I: Regular Papers 52(12), 2726–2738 (2005)
5. Berka, C., et al.: EEG Indices Distinguish Spatial and Verbal Working Memory Processing: Implications for Real-Time Monitoring in a Closed-Loop Tactical Tomahawk Weapons Simulation. Foundations of Augmented Cognition. In: Schmorrow, D.D. (ed.) Proceedings of the International Conference on Human Computer Interaction, vol. 11, Las Vegas, Nevada (July 2005)
6. Hillyard, S.A., Hink, R.F., Schwent, V.L., Picton, T.W.: Electrical Signs of Selective Attention in the Human Brain. Science, New Series 182(4108), 177–180 (1973)
7. Waterhouse, E.: New horizons in ambulatory electroencephalography. IEEE Engineering in Medicine and Biology Magazine, 74-80 (May/June 2003)
8. Ambulatory, E.E.G.: R & D Fact sheet, IMEC 2004, [online]. Available at http://www.imec.be/human/

9. Harrison, R.R., Charles, C.: A low-power low-noise CMOS amplifier for neural recording applications. IEEE Journal of Solid-State Circuits 38(6), 958–965 (2003)
10. Yates, D.C., Villegas-Rodriguez, E.: An ultra low power low noise chopper amplifier for wireless EEG. Invited Paper. In: 49th IEEE Midwest Symposium on Circuits and Systems, Suan Juan, Puerto Rico (August 6-9, 2006)
11. Erdogmus, D., Adami, A., Pavel, M., Lan, T., Mathan, S., Whitlow, S., Dorneich, M.: Cognitive State Estimation Based on EEG for Augmented Cognition. In: Proc. 2nd International IEEE EMBS Conference on Neural Engineering, Arlington, Virginia, v – viii (March 16-19, 2005)
12. Sauerbrey, J., Schmidt-Landsiedel, D., Thewes, R.: A 0.5 V 1 mW Successive Approximation ADC. IEEE Journal of Solid-State Circuits 38(7), 1261–1265 (2003)
13. Product specification: Single-chip 2.4 GHz Transceiver, Nordic Semiconductor (2004), [online]. Available: http://www.nordicsemi.no
14. Bluetooth solutions from Texas Instruments. Product bulletin, Texas Instruments (2004) [online]. Available: http://focus.ti.com/
15. XS110 UWB solution for media-rich wireless applications. Freescale Semiconductor (2004) [online]. Available: http://www.freescale.com/
16. Zarlink ZL70100 Datasheet (May 2005). [Online]. Available at: http://www.zarlink.com/
17. Cooper, R., Osselton, J.W., Shaw, J.C.: EEG Technology, 2nd edn. Butterworth & Co, London (1974)
18. Roundy, S., Steingart, D., Frechette, L., Wright, P., Rabaey, J.: Power Sources for Wireless Sensor Networks. In: Karl, H., Wolisz, A., Willig, A. (eds.) Wireless Sensor Networks. LNCS, vol. 2920, pp. 1–17. Springer, Heidelberg (2004)
19. Binnie, C.D., Rowan, A.J., Gutter, T.: A manual of electroencephalographic technologyz. Cambridge University Press, Cambridge (1982)
20. Antoniol, G., Tonella, P.: EEG data compression techniques. IEEE Transactions on Biomedical Engineering 44(2), 105–114 (1997)
21. Cardenas-Barrera, J., Lorenzo-Ginori, J., Rodriguez-Valdivia, E.: A wavelet-packets based algorithm for EEG signal compression. Medical Informatics and the Internet in Medicine 29(1), 15–27 (2004)
22. Smith, P.E.M., Wallace, S.J.: Clinicians guide to epilepsy. London: Arnold (2001)
23. Gotman, J.: Automatic detection of seizures and spikes. J Clinical Neurophysiology 16(2), 130–140 (1999)
24. Coninx, N.: Automated detection of epileptic events in the interictal EEG using the wavelet transform. Bachelors thesis, Universiteit Maastricht (2005)
25. Patel, S.: Intelligent low power circuit for electroencephalography. Master's thesis, Imperial College London (2006)
26. Parikh, P., Micheli-Tzanakou, E.: Detecting drowsiness while driving using wavelet transform. Bioengineering Conference. In: Proceedings of the IEEE 30th Annual Northeast, pp. 79–80 (April 17-18, 2004)

Novel Hybrid Bioelectrodes for Ambulatory Zero-Prep EEG Measurements Using Multi-channel Wireless EEG System

Robert Matthews, Neil J. McDonald, Harini Anumula, Jamison Woodward,
Peter J. Turner, Martin A. Steindorf, Kaichun Chang, and Joseph M. Pendleton

Quantum Applied Science and Research, 5764 Pacific Center Blvd., #107,
San Diego, CA, USA, 92121
{robm,neil,harini,jamison,peter,msteindorf,kai,joe}
@quasarusa.com

Abstract. This paper describes a wireless multi-channel system for zero-prep electroencephalogram (EEG) measurements in operational settings. The EEG sensors are based upon a novel hybrid (capacitive/resistive) bioelectrode technology that requires no modification to the skin's outer layer. High impedance techniques developed for QUASAR's capacitive electrocardiogram (ECG) sensors minimize the sensor's susceptibility to common-mode (CM) interference, and permit EEG measurements with electrode-subject impedances as large as 107 Ω. Results for a side-by-side comparison between the hybrid sensors and conventional wet electrodes for EEG measurements are presented. A high level of correlation between the two electrode technologies (>99% for subjects seated) was observed. The electronics package for the EEG system is based upon a miniature, ultra-low power microprocessor-controlled data acquisition system and a miniaturized wireless transceiver that can operate in excess of 72 hours from two AAA batteries.

Keywords: EEG, biosensors, high impedance, wireless.

1 Introduction

This paper discusses a novel hybrid (capacitive/resistive) EEG biosensor that can make measurements of through-hair EEG with zero preparation of the scalp. This sensor technology is used as part of an unobtrusive wireless EEG system for ambulatory EEG. In order to be truly unobtrusive, the system (including the sensors) should be donned or doffed quickly by the wearer, be easy to use, worn comfortably for extended periods and require no skin preparation for the sensors to operate with sufficient fidelity.

The EEG is most frequently used in clinical settings for monitoring and diagnosis of epilepsy and subjects with sleep disorders. However, measurements of the EEG have applications in operational settings, in which knowledge of an individual's cognitive state can be used to predict impending cognitive failure and trigger

D.D. Schmorrow, L.M. Reeves (Eds.): Augmented Cognition, HCII 2007, LNAI 4565, pp. 137–146, 2007.

appropriate countermeasures [1]. The ability to separate cognitive states, such as cognitive fatigue or overload, has been demonstrated for several applications under the Defense Advanced Research Projects Agency's (DARPA) Augmented Cognition (AugCog) program [2]. Military applications for this technology, such as command and control, communication, and security, have civilian counterparts such as developing countermeasures for pilot or driver fatigue [3]. Future research will lead to a new generation of computer interfaces that can act as brain-computer interfaces for the severely disabled [4].

The implementation of EEG-based systems in operational settings for determining cognitive state is limited, however, by the lack of an EEG sensor technology with high user compliance. Conventional 'wet' electrode technology presently requires preparation of the skin or the application of conductive electrolytes at the skin-sensor interface, which can be time consuming and unpleasant for the subject. Preparation of the electrode site involves abrading the scalp, with consequent discomfort for the subject and an associated risk of infection if the electrodes are not sterilized between subjects [5]. Similarly, a conductive gel leaves a residue on the scalp, and furthermore may leak, resulting in an electrical short between two electrodes in close proximity.

Quantum Applied Science and Research (QUASAR) has recently developed novel capacitive biosensors that meet the AugCog requirements for operational recordings of electrocardiograph (ECG), electrooculograph (EOG), and electromyograph (EMG) signals [6]. The QUASAR sensors couple to the electric fields of the body capacitively, requiring no skin contact and no skin preparation. Further development of QUASAR's capacitive bioelectrode technology was funded through Aberdeen Test Center as part of an effort to develop a biomonitoring sensor suite for Test & Evaluation (T&E) applications. Measuring EEG using the capacitive bioelectrodes became problematic when operating through hair. The sensors' high impedance made them susceptible to triboelectric charge generation due to rubbing between the sensor and hair.

The novel hybrid electrode described in this paper is the result of a research program funded by Aberdeen Test Center to develop a through-hair EEG sensor that is capable of making high fidelity EEG measurements with zero preparation of the scalp. This effort will culminate in a biomonitoring system, measuring EEG, EOG, ECG and EMG signals for T&E monitoring of human-computer interactions.

The miniature data acquisition system and wireless transceiver is discussed with regard to recording fidelity and noise characteristics.

2 Experimental

The measurements described herein were made using the novel hybrid EEG sensor technology developed at QUASAR. We report on simultaneous tests of QUASAR biosensors side-by-side with conventional 'wet' electrodes in laboratory tasks designed to produce variations in EEG rhythms such as theta and alpha bands or spectral patterns. Our focus was on limited tests to permit qualitative and semi-quantitative comparisons with wet electrodes. A total of 5 subjects (divided into two groups) were included in this study, and as such, the present sample sizes do not permit statistical comparisons.

2.1 QUASAR Hybrid EEG Electrodes

The hybrid biosensor (Fig. 1a) uses a combination of high impedance resistive and capacitive contact to the scalp, thereby enabling through-hair measurements of EEG without any skin preparation. The hybrid biosensor contacts the skin with a set of 'fingers,' each of which is small enough to reach through hair without trapping hair beneath the finger (thereby preventing electrical contact to the scalp). The sensors were held in place using the cap in Fig. 1b.

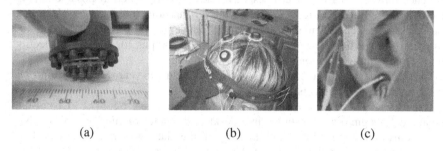

(a)   (b)   (c)

Fig. 1. (a) QUASAR hybrid biosensor. (b) Harness for holding QUASAR biosensors on scalp. (c) Common-mode follower (CMF) placed on earlobe of subject.

In contrast to conventional EEG electrode technology, which relies on a low impedance contact to the scalp (typically less than 5 kΩ in clinical applications), the contact impedance between the scalp and each electrode finger can be as high as $10^7\,\Omega$ in the bandwidth of interest. Therefore the amplifier electronics are shielded and placed as close as possible to the electrode in order to limit interference caused by the pickup of external signals, and innovative processing electronics are used to reduce pickup of and susceptibility to common-mode signals on the body [6].

The sensor is used in combination with QUASAR's proprietary common-mode follower (CMF) technology (situated on the subject's earlobe in Fig. 1c). The CMF is a separate biosensor that is used to reduce the sensitivity of the hybrid biosensor to common mode signals on the body. It operates by measuring the potential of the body relative to the ground of the amplifier system. The ultra-high input impedance of the CMF (~$10^{12}\,\Omega$) ensures that the output of the CMF tracks the body-ground potential with a high degree of accuracy.

The output of the CMF is then used as a reference for EEG measurements by the hybrid sensors. In this way, the common-mode signal appearing on the body is dynamically removed from the EEG measurement. This typically achieves a common-mode rejection ratio (CMRR) of 50 to 70 dB.

2.2 Data Acquisition

During these experiments, six channels of EEG were recorded simultaneously: three QUASAR hybrid biosensors and three conventional wet electrodes. The hybrid electrodes were positioned at the nominal Cz, Fz and F$_3$ positions [7], and the wet electrodes were positioned 2 cm to the right and posterior to the hybrid electrodes

(Subjects 1 and 2), or 2 cm anterior to the hybrid electrodes (Subjects 3-5). Preparation of the scalp for the wet electrodes included abrasion with Nu-Prep, followed by cleaning with alcohol and then application of Grass EC2 electrode paste. No preparation of the scalp was performed at the QUASAR electrode sites.

Independent grounds were used for the wet and hybrid electrodes. The electrical ground for the hybrid electrodes was a high impedance ground via a fabric strip in contact with the subject's forehead. The site was not prepared. The high impedance ground was connected to the ground of the data acquisition system. The ground reference for the wet EEG electrodes was a standard pre-gelled disposable Ag-AgCl electrode placed upon a prepared site on the left mastoid (Subjects 1 and 2), or the mid-posterior aspect of the subject's right pinna, as in Fig. 1c (Subjects 1-3). Differential amplifiers were used to generate the output for each wet electrode, thereby maintaining isolation between the two grounds.

The CMF for the hybrid electrodes was placed below the ear (Subjects 1 and 2), or on the right earlobe (Subjects 3-5).

The data acquisition system was a National Instruments NI-4472 PCI (24-bit, 8 channel delta-sigma) card installed in a desktop computer running a LabView-based data acquisition application. Anti-aliasing of the data was not necessary before digitization because of the details of the sigma-delta data acquisition. Signals were sampled at 12 kHz, then digitally filtered with a 300 Hz (-3dB) low-pass anti-alias filter before the samples were decimated to a sample rate of 1200 Hz. Each signal was corrected for the intrinsic gain of the sensors and ancillary electronics (gain=20 for all EEG channels). Signals were displayed in real time for monitoring purposes and saved on the hard disk drive.

For the purposes of analysis, the time series data were digitally filtered using a 8th order Butterworth bandpass filter between 1 and 40 Hz (with an additional notch filter at 60 Hz). Power Spectral Density functions (PSDs) were computed using Welch's method from the digitally filtered EEG with window length = 2 s, overlap = 1 s and FFT length = 2400 (sample frequency 1200 Hz).

2.3 Tasks

Task 1 - Eyes Open/Closed (Desynchronization of EEG alpha rhythm). Recording of EEG with a subject at rest with eyes open or closed is part of a standard clinical EEG test. A prominent feature of the eyes-closed EEG is a pronounced alpha rhythm, which disappears (or desynchronizes) when the eyes are opened [8]. To measure this effect, we recorded EEG with the subject's eyes open while the subject was still for a period of 30 seconds. This was repeated with the subject's eyes closed. This was repeated at the conclusion of the tests for Subjects 1 and 2.

Task 2 - Memory/Cognition Measurements (Modulation of EEG alpha and theta rhythms). Memory load and mental arithmetic are frequently used to control mental workload and produce distinct effects on EEG spectra, including modulation of theta (4-7 Hz) and alpha (8-12 Hz) bands [8], [9], [10]. Such effects are key features used by real-time algorithms to monitor human cognition during decision-making and control tasks [11], [12].

This task was conducted with the subjects seated and then walking in place. While seated, Subjects 1 and 2 were asked to count down from 1000 in steps of 2 for a period of 120 seconds (easy task), and then count down from 1000 in steps of 7 for a period of 120 seconds (hard task). The easy and hard tasks were then repeated while the subject walked in place.

While seated, Subjects 3-5 responded to a sequence of alphabetic characters displayed on a screen with either a 'y' or 'n', depending upon whether the current character was the same as the previous character, for a period of 300 seconds (N0, easy task), and then responded to a sequence of alphabetic characters displayed on a screen with a 'y' or 'n', depending upon whether the current character was the same as that prior to the previous character, for a period of 300 seconds (N2, hard task). The easy and hard tasks were then repeated while the subject walked in place.

3 Results

3.1 Sample Recordings and Inter-sensor Correlations

A segment of a time-series recording comparing the signals obtained for Subject 3 from the Cz electrodes during the eyes closed session is shown in Fig. 2. Also included on the plot is the Pearson correlation over 0.25 second segments. Although only a single 4-s segment is shown, the recording quality was consistent for all subjects without obvious changes in signal quality or noise levels. Very significant correlations, in excess of 90%, are evident throughout the record.

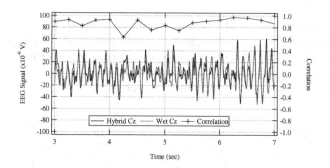

Fig. 2. Comparison of wet and hybrid Cz signals for Subject 3 during eyes closed session. The correlation data are calculated using 0.25 second segments.

However, regions of low EEG signal level reduce the Pearson correlation coefficients for the QUASAR-wet electrode pairs at Cz, Fz, and F_3 in 1-second segments of the sensor time series, averaged over the entire 30 second record, to 0.7423, 0.7691, and 0.7106, respectively. The average correlation coefficients were not observed to vary significantly as the segment length was varied between 0.25 seconds and 1 second.

A segment of a time-series recording comparing the signals obtained for Subject 2 from the Fz electrodes during the hard counting task (walking in place) is shown in

Fig. 3. The benefit of the CMF is illustrated in these data because although triboelectric charge generation while walking increases the CM signals appearing on the body, very significant correlations, in excess of 80%, are evident throughout the record.

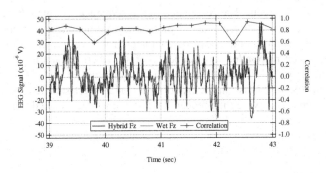

Fig. 3. Comparison of wet and hybrid Fz signals for Subject 2 performing the hard counting task while walking in place. The correlation data are calculated using 0.25 second segments.

The average Pearson correlation coefficients for the QUASAR-wet electrode pairs at Cz, Fz, and F_3 in 1-second segments over the entire 120 second time-series were 0.8226, 0.8409, and 0.8350, respectively.

3.2 Eyes-Open/Eyes-Closed EEG Task

The power spectral density (PSD) functions of the EEG signals for QUASAR and wet sensors were highly similar across eyes-open and eyes-closed tasks. Desynchronization of the alpha rhythm was observed in both electrode technologies for all five subjects when their eyes were open. For Subject 3 (Fig. 4), the beta rhythm (15-25 Hz) also desynchronized when the eyes were open.

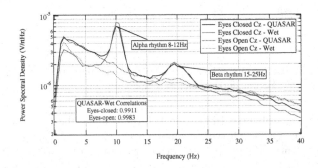

Fig. 4. Power spectral density functions of 30-s EEG recordings for Subject 3 at Cz during the eyes-open session and the following eyes-closed session

In the eyes-open/eyes-closed session for Subject 3, the inter-sensor Pearson product-moment correlation coefficients of the PSDs for QUASAR-wet sensor pairs at Cz, Fz, and F_3, calculated for all frequency bins below 40 Hz, were 0.9911, 0.9898, and 0.9825, respectively. In the eyes-open session, the corresponding correlation coefficients for QUASAR-wet sensor pairs at Cz, Fz, and F_3 were 0.9983, 0.9975, and 0.9976, respectively. Correlation coefficients in excess of 0.957 were observed across all 5 subjects for QUASAR-wet sensor pairs at Cz, Fz, and F_3 for EEG data sets recorded during this task.

3.3 Memory/Cognition Task

The PSD functions of the EEG signals for QUASAR and wet sensors were highly similar for all subjects across the two levels of the memory/cognition tasks. The inter-sensor Pearson correlation coefficients of the PSDs for QUASAR-wet sensor pairs at Cz, Fz, and F_3, calculated for all frequency bins below 40 Hz were in excess of 0.935 for all subjects in each cognition task, with the exclusion of Subject 3 while walking. The residual CM signal on Subject 3 resulted in a 2 Hz peak in the PSD, corresponding to the impact frequency while walking. However, the correlation coefficients for QUASAR-wet pairings for the bipolar derivations Cz-Fz, Cz-F_3 and Fz-F_3 for Subject 3 (walking) possess correlation coefficients greater than 0.96.

Other authors have reported synchronization of theta band power and desynchronization of alpha band power as the difficulty of cognition task increases [8], [9]. We observed modulation of alpha band and theta band power in data for individual subjects, though not consistently across all 5 subjects. For example, the data for Subjects 1, 3 and 4 show evidence of a decrease in alpha band power during the hard counting and N2 task while seated, but no effect is evident in the theta band for either electrode technology. Alternatively, Subject 2 possesses a decrease in theta band power, but no change in alpha band power, while seated during the hard counting task. No modulation of the theta and alpha and band powers is evident in the data for Subject 5. Similarly, neither is any modulation of the theta and alpha band powers evident for any subject for either sensor technology.

4 Deployable Neurocognitive Monitoring System

A truly deployable mobile neurocognitive monitoring system must possess several key features. The electrodes for the system must be noninvasive and require no modification of the outer layer of the skin to obtain EEG recordings with sufficient fidelity to classify cognitive states. Furthermore, in order to be deployed in operational settings, the electrodes must operate for periods longer than 8 hours with no maintenance and no discomfort for the user. The harness holding the sensors must also be comfortable and, not least when considering user compliance, have a stylish appearance. The electronics to digitize and record the signals need to be small and lightweight, have a sleek appearance, and operate for a minimum of 24 hours using small batteries that are easy to obtain.

4.1 Data Acquisition/Wireless Electronics for EEG System

The electronics package for the EEG system is based upon a miniature, ultra-low power microprocessor-controlled data acquisition system (DAQ) and a miniaturized wireless transceiver (Fig. 5). Presently, power consumption of the system is dominated in approximately equal parts by the DAQ and the transceiver. In order to conserve power, the microprocessor operates in a low-power "sleep" mode when not acquiring data and the wireless transceiver transmits information in a data "burst" mode. Wireless data rates up to 2.5 ksamples per second have been achieved using the present system operating in a low power mode. Current estimates show that the run time for the system is in excess of 72 hours from two AAA batteries.

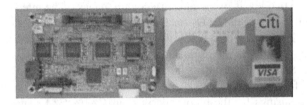 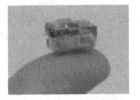

Fig. 5. (left) Prototype data acquisition board with credit card for scale. (right) Prototype miniature wireless transmitter.

In order to facilitate the calculation of high CMRR difference signals in software, the input filters on each analog channel have been matched to better than -72 dB below 50 Hz. Additionally, the timing error between ADC channels is less than 1 μs (i.e., a phase error less than -80 dB below 100 Hz).

Data acquisition is performed using 16-bit sigma-delta ADCs. The input noise of the DAQ channels has been measured to be 400nV/√Hz for a sampling frequency of 4 kHz. Aliasing of out-of-bandwidth signals is less than -80 dB below 50 Hz.

4.2 Sensor Harness

One of the principal benefits of the QUASAR hybrid sensor is the ease with which the sensors may be applied. The user can simply pull the sensors on using a simple combing motion to work them through the hair. Ideally, the harness will serve several functions, primarily as a set of headphones or glasses and secondly, but equally important, to hold the sensors to the head in a comfortable manner (Fig. 6). Note that in the glasses configuration, extra sensors can be included for measurements of the EOG.

The sensor harness will also need to hold the electronics package which will provide power to the sensors, digitize the signals and either write the data to flash memory or wirelessly transmit it to a base station. The base station can be a central computer, or a PDA carried by the user, allowing full deployment of the system in the field.

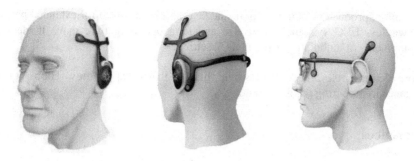

Fig. 6. Two concepts for a sensor harness suitable for operation in a C2 environment

5 Discussion

Although the present experiments were limited to five subjects, the quality and consistency of the recordings and the effects we measured show that the QUASAR hybrid biosensors function as well as conventional 'wet' sensors. Our results provide clear and convincing evidence of EEG signals which correlate extremely well with simultaneously recorded wet electrodes. Correlations of alpha activity in the time domain were typically in excess of 0.8-0.9, but correlation coefficients averaged over an entire data set were found to be considerably lower. This is due to the effect of regions of low EEG signal level and the presence of skin noise reducing the signal-to-noise ratio (SNR) of the EEG signal. Regions of low SNR have a correspondingly small correlation coefficient.

In the spectral domain, the PSD functions of QUASAR and wet EEG recordings within the EEG band of 0-40 Hz were remarkably high, typically above 0.99. The frequency domain correlations appear to be immune to SNR considerations because of the stability of the skin noise, which possesses a predominantly $1/f$ characteristic. Only one subject recorded correlations below 0.9 for EEG measured while walking in place due to interference from common-mode signals.

Besides showing that the signals of interest are correlated across sensor types, both sensor technologies demonstrate sensitivity to the effects typically used for human-computer interaction – namely modulation of EEG rhythms, such as alpha and theta. These effects were seen in both sensor technologies when present in a particular subject, but the results were not observed consistently across all 5 subjects in the memory/cognition task. It is likely that the small sample size and limited acquisition time are responsible.

Performance tests for the EEG system have demonstrated that the system possesses specifications suitable for multi-channel EEG acquisition. The common-mode follower technology enables measurements of EEG using contact impedances several orders of magnitude greater than that considered acceptable for conventional electrodes. The pickup of common-mode interfering signals will be further reduced by the wireless nature of the system because the coupling of the system's ground to earth ground is considerably reduced.

The technology described in this paper directly addresses user compliance issues. The biosensors can be donned or doffed quickly by the wearer, require no skin preparation, produce no skin irritation, and be comfortably worn for extended periods. The wireless EEG system's small size and long operating time make it ideal for measurements of ambulatory EEG in a C2 setting.

Acknowledgments. The authors would like to thank Dr. Andrew Hibbs for his assistance in preparing the document.

References

1. Matthews, R., McDonald, N.J., Trejo, L.J.: Psycho-Physiological Sensor Techniques: An Overview. In: 11th International Conference on Human Computer Interaction (HCII), pp. 22–27. Las Vegas, NV (July 2005)
2. St. John, M., Kobus, D.A., Morrison, J.G., Schmorrow, D.: Overview of the DARPA Augmented Cognition Technical Integration Experiment. International Journal of Human-Computer Interaction. 17, 131–149 (2004)
3. Sullivan IV, J.J.: Fighting Fatigue. Public Roads 67, 18–23 (2003)
4. Wolpaw, J.R., McFarland, D.J.: An EEG-based brain-computer interface for cursor control. Electroenceph. Clin. Neruphysiol. 78, 252–259 (1991)
5. Ferree, T.C., Luu, P., Russell, G.S., Tucker, D.M.: Scalp electrode impedance, infection risk, and EEG data quality. Clinical Neurophysiology 112, 536–544 (2001)
6. Matthews, R., McDonald, N.J., Fridman, I., Hervieux, P., Nielsen, T.: The invisible electrode - zero prep time, ultra low capacitive sensing. In: 11th International Conference on Human Computer Interaction (HCII), pp. 22–27. Las Vegas, NV (July 2005)
7. Jasper, H.H.: The ten-twenty electrode system of the international federation. Electroencephalogr. Clin. Neurophysiol. 10, 371–375 (1958)
8. Klimesch, W.: EEG alpha and theta oscillations reflect cognitive and memory performance: a review and analysis. Brain Research Reviews 29, 169–195 (1958)
9. Gevins, A., Smith, M.E., Leong, H., McEvoy, L., Whitfield, S., Du, R., Rush, G.: Monitoring working memory load during computer-based tasks with EEG pattern recognition. Human Factors 40, 79–91 (1998)
10. Wallerius, J., Trejo, L.J., Matthews, R., Rosipal, R., Caldwell, J.A.: Robust feature extraction and classification of EEG spectra for real-time classification of cognitive state. In: 11th International Conference on Human Computer Interaction (HCII), pp. 22–27. Las Vegas, NV (July 2005)
11. Trejo, L.J., Matthews, B., Rosipal, R.: Brain-computer interfaces for 1-D and 2-D cursor control: designs using volitional control of the EEG spectrum or steady-state visual evoked potentials. IEEE Trans. Neural Syst. Rehabil. Eng. 14, 225–229 (2006)
12. Wilson, G.F., Russell, C.A.: Real-time assessment of mental workload using psychophysiological measures and artificial neural networks. Human Factors 45, 635–643 (2003)

Measuring Cognitive Task Load on a Naval Ship: Implications of a Real World Environment

Marc Grootjen[1,2], Mark A. Neerincx[2,3], Jochum C.M. van Weert[3], and Khiet P. Truong[3]

[1] Defense Materiel Organization, Directorate Materiel Royal Netherlands Navy, P.O. Box 20702, 2500 ES The Hague, The Netherlands
[2] Technical University of Delft, P.O. Box 5031, 2628 CD Delft, The Netherlands
[3] TNO Human Factors, Kampweg 5, P.O. Box 23, 3769 ZG Soesterberg, The Netherlands
Marc@Grootjen.nl, {mark.neerincx, khiet.truong}@tno.nl, jochum@gmail.com

Abstract. Application of more and more automation in process control shifts the operator's task from manual to supervisory control. Increasing system autonomy, complexity and information fluctuations make it extremely difficult to develop static support concepts that cover all critical situations after implementing the system. Therefore, support systems in dynamic domains should be dynamic as the domain itself. This paper elaborates on the state information needed from the operator to generate effective mitigation strategies. We describe implications of a real world experiment onboard three frigates of the Royal Netherlands Navy. Although new techniques allow us to measure, combine and gain insight in physiological, subjective and task information, many practical issues need to be solved.

1 Introduction

Designing highly complex interactive man-machine systems in process control has been subject of many studies. Due to ongoing automation, major changes in information technology have taken place, causing a radical change in the position of the operator from monitoring and control to supervision. Grootjen et al. [1] defined six main problem areas: (1) Increasing complexity; (2) Changing of information type and volume; (3) Increasing system autonomy causing 'out of the loop' operator problems; (4) Task integration from different domains; (5) Decreasing personnel and training budgets; (6) Increasing legislative constraints.

Human-centered design methods are often proposed to establish for the human a central and distinct position from other aspects of the system [2,3]. In the design of a new system, different configurations are tested and evaluated. Finally, the most efficient configuration which fits on a generic set of constraints will be implemented. However, a different configuration could be more efficient for a specific situation or subset of constraints, although it would be less efficient generally. Even if we follow a human-centered design method, the six defined problem areas make it extremely difficult to develop static support concepts that cover all critical situations after implementing the system. Therefore, support systems in dynamic domains should be

D.D. Schmorrow, L.M. Reeves (Eds.): Augmented Cognition, HCII 2007, LNAI 4565, pp. 147–156, 2007.
© Springer-Verlag Berlin Heidelberg 2007

dynamic as the domain itself. For example Niwa and Hollnagel [4] use dynamic mapping of alarm support of to enhance operator performance in nuclear power plants. Another example is the alarm handling support system of Dutch navy ships, which has different levels of automation [5].

A way of optimizing human-machine interaction by dynamic or adaptive automation is the use of augmented cognition. Augmented cognition symbiotically integrates man and machine in a closed-loop system. The machine's task is to detect both operator cognitive state and the operational context and to then dynamically adapt in real time in response, with the goal being to improve total man machine performance [6]. Taking the limitations of human information processing as a starting point, measurements of the cognitive state of the operator are used to trigger mitigation strategies to bypass or overcome the bottleneck e.g. [7-9]. Next to cognitive state measurements, a wide variety of data is proposed [10,11]. Our approach is multimodal sensing for complementary and more robust measurements. In Grootjen et al. [1] we describe a high level framework for HMC consistsing of four models (operator, task, system and context model), and an allocator which generates a work plan (i.e. mitigation strategy). This paper gives an overview which permanent and dynamic operator characteristics should be sensed and recorded in the operator model, classified in five categories (Section 2). Section 3 describes an experiment on board of three frigates of the Royal Netherlands Navy and shows which state-of-the-art sensing and fusing tools were applied. Section 4 presents implications and future directions, Section 5 the conclusion.

2 Operator Model

An essential source of information for effective and efficient mitigation is the operator model. The operator model contains a large variety of information (see [1] for a literature overview), we propose classification in five categories (Fig. 1).

1. Permanent characteristics. This category contains fixed personal characteristics, which can be used to uniquely identify an operator. Characteristics like age and gender can affect a person's cognitive abilities and can be used in classification of operator groups.
2. Dynamic characteristics. This category contains characteristics that can change gradually over time. Like with some permanent characteristics, this information can be used for classification of operator groups.
3. Baseline state. This category contains baseline values of the operator's state.
4. Momentary state. This category contains real-time operator state measurements and task information (i.e. on which task the operator is working). Note that this information is also used to update the baseline state information.
5. Critical load areas: This category describes critical load areas using the CTL model of Neerincx [3].

The allocator uses information from the operator model to determine critical load areas, which are stored in the operator model itself. Furthermore, the actual real-time CTL is also calculated by the allocator. Comparing actual CTL and critical areas enables determination of a work plan.

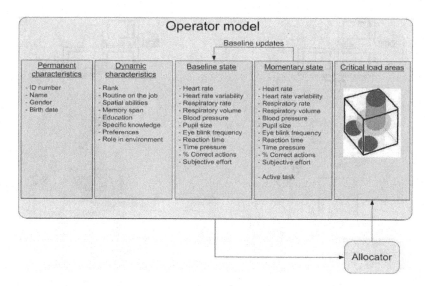

Fig. 1. Classification of operator information in five categories

3   Real World Experiment

The Royal Netherlands Navy started in 1991 with the development of a new type of frigate: the Air Defense and Control Frigate (ADCF). In 2001 the first of four ADCFs was commissioned. For monitoring and control of all platform, energy and propulsion systems the ship has been equipped with an IMCS (Integrated Monitoring and Control System). During multiple sailing sessions on board of the ADCFs, the ship control centre (SCC) was evaluated using machinery breakdown drills. An important part of this evaluation was the collection of a wide variety of data for development of the operator model. Section 3.1 will focus on the method used to collect this data, the complete experimental setup used for the total SCC evaluation is out of the scope of this paper. Section 3.2 describes the organization of data afterwards.

3.1   Method

Three ADCFs participated in the experiment, each contained four active teams responsible for around the clock SCC operation. All teams consisted of four persons, a manager (sergeant), an operator (corporal), and two engine room operators (sailors). The participants had to deal correctly with the emergencies that appeared. In our experiment we focused only on the manager and the operator (12 of each in total, all males). The manager and operator used an IMCS console consisting of three screens, a keyboard and trackball for system operation. For communication purposes they had a voice terminal, several telephones and a separate push-to-talk engine room communication system. Fig. 2 shows the experimental setup.

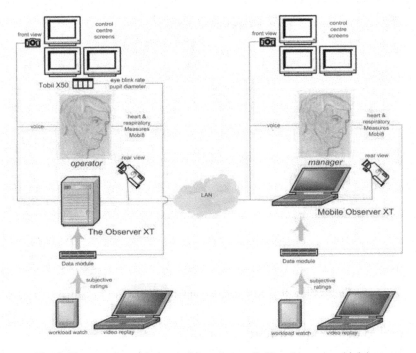

Fig. 2. The experimental setup of the operator (left) and manager (right)

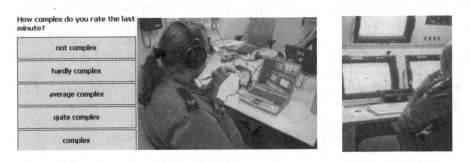

Fig. 3. Operator scoring complexity and effort during video replay of the just performed scenario (left and middle). Measuring pupil dilation (right).

For the operator and for the manager we installed a small spy camera (1/3" Sony super HAD color CCD) between the SCC screens to record a front view. On the ceiling we installed two digital cameras for the rear view. After each scenario, the participants had to do an individual video evaluation of the tasks just performed, using a laptop and handheld device. Each minute they were asked to rate task complexity and subjective effort on a five point scale (Fig. 3, based on the workload watch of Boer [12]. For heart and respiratory measures a Mobi8 recording device was used [13]. During the experiment we had one eye tracker available [14], which was used for the operator (Fig. 4, right). High quality voice recordings were made using 2 wireless headsets (Img Stageline HSE-210/SK), a receiver (Img Stageline TXS-890/TXS-890HSE) and amplifier (InterM PP-9214/R150Plus). Two Observer XT systems [15] were used to record all video and audio data. The external data module of the Observer XT system was used to import and synchronize data afterwards (Section 4). Individual systems were connected by a Netgear Fast Ethernet Switch FS608 v2.

The scenarios took place during the day or night, depending on the availability of the ship and working schedules of the participating SCC teams. The total time needed for one team was about 4 hours.

3.2 Organizing Data

After a challenging period of collecting data at sea, the next exercise was organizing the data and prepare it for interpretation. To do this, we used the Observer XT of Noldus. This section will give an overview of the steps followed in organizing the data for the *operator*. Data for the manager was organized in a similar way, except for the eye tracker data. Fig. 4 shows part of the data in a screen dump of the Observer software.

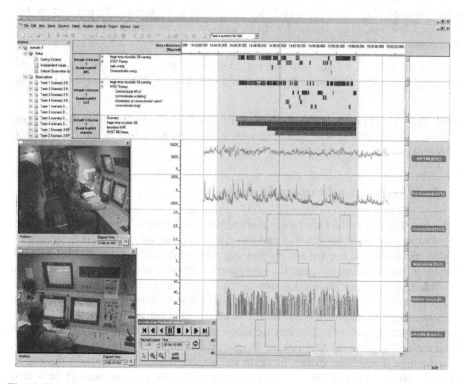

Fig. 4. The Observer XT (Noldus, 2006 192 /id). From top to bottom: three rows of task data, heart rate, respiratory rate, complexity, effort, voice stress and performance.

Video and audio. With the Observer we recorded rear and front images of the operator. The rear recordings included low quality audio, the front high quality. Using this high quality audio we measured four raw speech features that are likely to correlate with stress (F0, SLOPE, COG and HI). See Section 5 for a short description. All features were extracted with Praat, a tool for speech analysis [16]. Furthermore, the front images were analyzed using Vicar Vision's FaceReader software [17]. To get the best results, we configured the FaceReader to do two frame-by-frame analyses. The first time we configured the FaceReader as if the spycam was positioned under the IMCS screen. The second time we took the default position. See Section 5 for a short description. Each analysis gives 7 output variables: happy, sad, angry, disgusted, surprised, scared and neutral.

Physiological Mobi data. We measured the expansion of the abdomen and the thorax due to breathing, the electrocardiogram and a sync signal. This data was downloaded from the flash card and analyzed with external software. Six variables were imported into the Observer: instantaneous respiratory rate (Hz), instantaneous heart rate (bpm), heart rate variability (0.04-0.15 Hz and 0.15-0.4 Hz), the sync signal and an artifact signal.

Subjective data. There are 3 subjective variables: complexity, effort and expert performance rating. All three variables were scored every minute. To import this data into the Observer, the variables had to be converted from single values every minute to a continuous block signal.

Tobii data. The eye tracker data was recorded on a separate computer. This data was exported with using Clearview [14], analyzed with MatLab [18] and imported into the Observer.

Task data. To obtain task data, videos were analyzed by experts using the observer software. Behavioral scoring schemes were composed according to the CTL method of Neerincx [3].

4   Implications and Future Directions

Observer XT. During and after the experiment the Observer XT was intensively used. We linked two Observer systems and the eye tracker so we could start recording all audio, video and the eye tracker by pressing one button. This saved us a lot of work synchronizing data streams after the experiment. Imported data using the external data module had to be synchronized manually. Having all data on the same timeline gives great insight, for example one can easily detect that missing eye tracker data often occurs simultaneously with high subjective effort. Clicking on an interesting part of a variable directly shows accompanying video images. However, such a big amount of data requires datamining techniques. We planned to import all data into the Observer, synchronize it and then export in again in one datasheet. Unfortunately the export option was not working in this specific way, and will be implemented in a next version of the software. Future research will hopefully reveal the real meaning of this data.

Voice analysis. Many studies have tried to determine a general acoustic profile of stressed speech. In order to find a general acoustic stress profile, Scherer et al. [19] suggest different types of stress should be defined (e.g., emotional stress and cognitive stress). Although some acoustic features seem to correlate with stressed speech, a general "acoustic stress profile" has yet to be found. Most of the studies report higher values for speech rate, mean F0, mean intensity/energy, and the energy in the higher frequency regions of the spectrum in speech under stress [19,20]. We have measured four raw speech features that are likely to correlate with stress. First, we measure F0 which is expected to increase in speech under stress. The other three measures are based on the observation that the proportion of energy in the higher frequency regions increases in stressed speech. This can be measured in several ways: 1) by measuring the slope of the long-term averaged spectrum (SLOPE), 2) by measuring the centre of gravity (COG) and 3) by measuring the Hammarberg Index (HI) which is defined as the maximum energy below 2000 Hz minus the maximum energy between 2000 - 5000 Hz (HI). Thus, it is expected that F0, SLOPE and COG increase, while HI decreases in stressed speech. We experienced some difficulties during feature extraction that were due to the real world nature of the data: e.g., background noise like alarm signals, clipping of the signal by the ship's communication system and crosstalk.

Facial emotion. Automatic facial expression analysis usually consists of 3 tasks: 1) detection of the face, 2) feature detection and extraction and 3) classification of emotions. The best known method for facial data extraction is the facial action coding system (FACS, see [21]). The FACS system describes facial movements in terms of Action Units (AU). The system consists of a taxonomy of 44 AUs with which facial expressions can be described, and has attracted many researchers from the field of computer vision to develop automatic facial expression analyzers based on AUs. The automatic facial expression analyzer we have used, is based on Active Appearance Models and can classify emotions in six basic universal emotion categories. The FaceReader can only give output when the image quality is at an acceptable level, which is difficult given the real world conditions under which the data was recorded. Bad illumination, different poses of the head and background noises are some of the difficulties that the recognition software has to deal with. Fig. 5 shows classification of one image using the model where the camera is positioned under the screen. In contrast with this result, image quality is too poor for classification if we use the default model. Also due to background clutter, image quality can decrease making a classification impossible [22]. For future research we would recommend to reduce background clutter as much as possible, for example with a curtain. Furthermore, increase the amount of light in the face with a evenly distribution and zoom in as much as possible.

We did not yet analyze the seven output variables of the FaceReader for a stress related component due to export problems. As was stated earlier this Section, future research should reveal correlations.

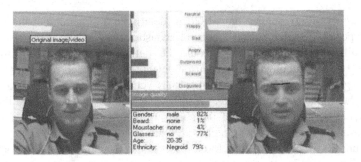

Fig. 5. Classification by the FaceReader [17] with a "below screen model". Using a default model for the camera position decreases image quality and makes classification impossible.

Heart and respiratory rate. During the experiment, the operator and manager wore the Mobi8. This is a small and light 8 channel physiological recording system. Data can be recorded on a flash card, or can be directly transferred using Bluetooth to a computer. Our initial plan was to use Bluetooth and link the system to the Observer so data would be automatically synchronized. Due to unknown problems with Bluetooth connection, we chose for recording with the more reliable flash card. At the start of every scenario the participants gave a synchronization pulse by pressing a button on the device, which could later be used when importing the data into the Observer. In future experiments we strongly recommend to use an automatic synchronizing feature.

Eye tracker. In the SCC, the participants had three screens available. Because the screen on top wasn't used very often, the eye tracker was configured for the two lower screens. Unfortunately, the operator moved around a lot. Communication devices, talking to colleagues or simply moving from the screen to relax or to the screen to read something, caused missing data. Because of the missing data, we were not able to subtract eye blinks from the pupil dilation information. In future real world experiments we would recommend a mobile, wearable eye tracking system. A multiple camera system could also work.

Follow up. We are planning the next experiment for spring 2007. For this experiment, experiences of real world experiments like this one and Grootjen et al. [23] and more controlled experiments [24,25] will be combined into an augmented cognition Closed Loop Integrated Prototype (CLIP). Although a lot preparation has already been done, some challenges are:

The allocator. The allocator should construct critical (and optimal) CTL areas, be able to generate a real time CTL operator signal and generate mitigation strategies. After analyzing data described in Section 3, we will select measurements and develop a method to fuse this data into one or two variables. With SOWAT [1] we will create CTL areas. Using information from other models (e.g. task model) should prevent us from an oscillating system [26].

Trust, situational awareness (SA) and locus of control. Being able to know when to mitigate is just one side of the story. Harkness-Regli et al. [27] state: "Adjusting non-optimal cognitive states can be at least as difficult as recognizing them." Our experiment will include a full usability evaluation. To improve trust and SA, we will evaluate usage of visual load feedback and a special SA display. We expect to increase trust and SA by giving the operator insight in the adaptive process. Furthermore, we will compare a situation in which the user is in charge of mitigation with one where the system is in charge.

5 Conclusion

Application of more and more automation, increasing system autonomy, complexity and information fluctuations make it extremely difficult to develop static support concepts that cover all critical situations after implementing the system. Augmented cognition offers a possible solution: symbiotic integration of man and machine in a closed-loop system. Although theoretical frameworks and methods are being developed [1,28,29] and controlled experiments have proven to increase performance [8], experience with real world environments is crucial in the development of new augmented cognition systems. This paper showed the implications of a real world environment during measurement and processing of data. Although new techniques allow us to measure, combine and gain insight in physiological, subjective and task information, many practical issues need to be solved.

References

1. Grootjen, M., Neerincx, M.A., Weert, J.C.M.v.: Task Based Interpretation of Operator State Information for adaptive support, Foundations of Augmented Cognition, 2nd edn. pp. 236–242 (2006)
2. Stanton, N.A., Baber, C.: The ergonomics of command and control. Ergonomics 49(12-13), 1131–1138 (2006)
3. Neerincx, M.A.: Cognitive task load design: model, methods and examples. In: Hollnagel, E. (ed.) Handbook of Cognitive Task Design, pp. 283–305. Lawrence Erlbaum Associates, Mahwah (2003)
4. Niwa, Y., Hollnagel, E.: Enhancing operator control by adaptive alarm presentation. International Journal of Cognitive Ergonomics (Lawrence Erlbaum Associates) 5(3), 367–384 (2001)
5. Mulder, J.M.F.: Supporting the internal battle. In: Thirteenth International Ship Control Systems Symposium (SCSS) (2003)
6. Kruse, A.A., Schmorrow, D.D.: Session overview: Foundations of augmented cognition. In: Schmorrow, D.D. (ed.) Foundations of Augmented Cognition, pp. 441–445. Lawrence Erlbaum Associates, Mawah (2005)
7. Dickson, B.T.: Closed Loop Systems - Stability and Predictability. In: Schmorrow, D.D. (ed.) Foundations of Augmented Cognition, pp. 617–620. Lawrence Erlbaum Associates, Mawah (2005)
8. Dorneich, M.C., Whitlow, S.D., Mathan, S., Carciofini, J., Ververs, P.M.: The communications Scheduler: A task scheduling mitigation for a Closed Loop Adaptive System. In: Schmorrow, D.D. (ed.) Foundations of Augmented Cognition, pp. 132–141. Lawrence Erlbaum Associates, Mawah (2005)
9. Diethe, T.: The Future of Augmentation Managers. In: Schmorrow, D.D. (ed.) Foundations of Augmented Cognition, pp. 631–640. Lawrence Erlbaum Associates, Mawah (2005)

10. Fuchs, S., Berka, C., Juhnke, J., Hale, K.S., Levendowski, D.: Physiological Sensors Cannot Effectively Drive System Mitigation Alone. In: Foundations of Augmented Cognition, 2nd edn. pp. 193–200 (2006)
11. Schnell, T., Macuda, T., Poolman, P.: Toward the Cognitive Cockpit: Flight Test Platforms and Methods for Monitoring Pilot Mental State. In: Foundations of Augmented Cognition, 2nd edn. pp. 268–278 (2006)
12. Boer, L.C.: Workload-watch as an element of human engineering testing and evaluation. In: Eleventh Ship Control Systems Symposium, 2nd edn., Computational Mechanics Publications, Southampton, Boston (1997)
13. TMS International. Mobi 8. 200. TMS International, Oldenzaal, the Netherlands
14. Tobii Technology AB. Tobii (2006)
15. Noldus. Observer XT. [6.0] (2006)
16. Boersma, P.: Praat, a system for doing phonetics by computer. Glot. International 5(9/10), 341–345 (2001)
17. Uyl, M.J.d., Kuilenburg, H.v.: FaceReader: an online facial expression recognition system. In: Proceedings of the 5th international conference on methods and techniques in behavorial reseearch, pp. 589–590 (2005)
18. Mathworks. Matlab 7.1. 200
19. Scherer, K.R., Grandjean, D., Johnstone, T., Klasmeyer, G., Bänziger, T.: Acoustic correlates of task load and stress. In: Proceedings of ICSLP2002 (2002)
20. Rothkrantz, L.J.M., Wiggers, P., Wees, J.v., Vark, R.J.v.: Voice stress analysis. In: International conference on text, speech and dialogue, vol. 3206, pp. 449–456 (2004)
21. Ekman, P., Friesen, W.V.: Facial action coding system: A technique for the measurement of facial movement, Consulting Psychologists Press (1978)
22. Truong, K.P., van Leeuwen, D.A., Neerincx, M.A.: Unobtrusive Multimodal Emotion Detection in Adaptive Interfaces: Speech and Facial Expressions. In: Schmorrow, D.D., Reeves, L.M. (eds.) FAC 2007, vol. 4565, (This Volume) Springer, Heidelberg (2007)
23. Grootjen, M., Neerincx, M.A., Veltman, J.A.: Cognitive Task Load in a Naval Ship Control Centre: from identification to prediction. Ergonomics 49(12-13), 1238–1264 (2006)
24. Grootjen, M., Bierman, E.P.B., Neerincx, M.A.: Optimizing cognitive task load in naval ship control centres: Design of an adaptive interface, IEA 16th World Congress on Ergonomics (2006)
25. Grootjen, M., Neerincx, M.A., Passenier, P.O.: Cognitive task load and support on a ship's bridge: Design and evaluation of a prototype user interface. In: INEC, Conference Proceedings, 2002, pp. 198–207 (2002)
26. Wilson, G.F., Russel, C.A.: Psychophysiologically Versus Task Determined Adaptive Aiding Accomplishment, Foundations of Augmented Cognition, 2nd edn., pp. 201–207 (2006)
27. Harkness-Regli, S., Tremoulet, P.D., Hastie, H., Stibler, K.: Mitigation Strategy Design for Optimal Augmented Cognition Systems. Foundations of Augmented Cognition, 2nd edn., pp. 208–214 (2006)
28. Nicholson, D., Stanney, K., Fiore, S., Davis, L., Fidopiastis, C., Finkelstein, N., Arnold, R.: An Adaptive System for Improving and Augmenting Human Performance. Foundations of Augmented Cognition, 2nd edn., pp. 215–222 (2006)
29. Greef, T.E.d., Dongen, C.J.G.v., Grootjen, M., Lindenberg, J.: Augmenting Cognition: Reviewing the Symbiotic Relation Between Man and Machine. In: Schmorrow, D.D., Reeves, L.M. (eds.) FAC 2007, vol. 4565, (This Volume) Springer, Heidelberg (2007)

Measuring Spatial Factors in Comparative Judgments About Large Numerosities

Catherine Sophian

Department of Psychology, University of Hawaii, Honolulu, HI 96822 USA
csophian@hawaii.edu

Abstract. Numerical information is crucial to successful performance on many tasks. Accordingly, as a basis for developing augmented cognition applications, it is important to understand how people apprehend numerical information and whether there are systematic limitations on their ability to do so accurately. This paper reports research on the role of non-numerical spatial information and of numerical representations in adults' judgments about large-numerosity spatial arrays. Arrays that contained more open space tended to be perceived as less numerous than ones with less open space. Further, the accuracy with which viewers estimated the arrays' numerosities bore little relation to their success in identifying the more numerous array in each pair. Numerical judgments thus are heavily influenced by spatial information that is not necessarily a reliable cue to numerosity. While some information about absolute numerosity is extracted in making numerical comparisons, it appears to be very imprecise.

1 Introduction

The ability to discriminate large numerosities, like discriminations between continuous quantities such as area and duration, is a function of the ratio between the quantities. Even infants successfully discriminate between 8 and 16 items, but they fail when the contrast is 8 versus 10 [1]. Research with adults has led to estimates that the degree of contrast at which they are able to attain a 75% success rate on a two-choice discrimination task is one in which the ratio of the smaller to the larger numerosity is about .86, corresponding to the discrimination of 25 from 29.

Understanding the cognitive processes underlying numerical judgments is important to the development of augmented cognition systems for any application in which the evaluation of numerical quantities is vital to sound decision-making. A particularly important issue to consider is whether the ways in which people normally process numerical information may introduce systematic biases that could be compensated for via an augmented cognition system.

One reason to suspect that such biases are likely to exist is that numerical contrasts often are associated with in continuous properties of stimuli, such as their aggregate surface areas or contour lengths. Moreover, the same ratio properties that control numerical discriminations also control discrimination on non-numerical dimensions such as area and duration (cf., [2]). The covariation that is often present between

D.D. Schmorrow, L.M. Reeves (Eds.): Augmented Cognition, HCII 2007, LNAI 4565, pp. 157–165, 2007.
© Springer-Verlag Berlin Heidelberg 2007

number and other quantitative dimensions raises the possibility that in making numerical discriminations people may utilize non-numerical information such as aggregate stimulus area, and that possibility is consistent with the observation that numerical discriminations vary with stimulus parameters in precisely the same way that non-numerical discriminations do. The trouble is, that if stimuli that need to be compared numerically differ on other dimensions that enter into discriminative processing—for instance, if one array is composed of larger items than the other—those differences can introduce biases into the numerical judgments that are generated.

Studies with infants have obtained strong evidence that what appear to be numerical discriminations are in fact based on non-numerical properties, at least under some circumstances. These studies rely on the phenomenon of habituation—a decrease in responding over repeated presentations of the same or similar stimuli, followed by renewed responding when the stimuli are changed in ways that the infant notices. Clearfield and Mix habituated infants to arrays that were identical in both numerosity and either contour length [3] or aggregate area [4], after which they showed the infants two kinds of test arrays: (a) arrays that matched the previous stimuli in number but differed in either contour length or area, and (b) arrays that matched the previous stimuli in contour length or area but differed in number. The important finding was that the infants looked more at the arrays that differed from the habituation arrays in contour length or area than at those that differed in numerosity.

The classic adult research on numerosity discrimination (e.g., [5], [6]) used arrays of dots without attempting to control item size, so that numerical discriminations might well have been a function of with differences between the stimuli in continuous extent (e.g., total stimulus area or contour length). More recently, Whalen, Gallistel, and Gelman [7], and Shuman and Kanwisher [8], using sequences of dot as stimuli, controlled for total sequence duration but not for the cumulative duration of dot exposure.

Results obtained by Barth, Kanwisher, and Spelke [9] raise the possibility that dependence on non-numerical information in making numerical judgments may be a function of the fineness of the discrimination that is required. Barth et al. controlled for non-numerical forms of quantity comparison by using a cross-format (spatial vs. temporal) task, reasoning that since spatial and temporal quantities do not share non-numerical dimensions such as area or duration, successful cross-format discrimination could only be based on numerosity. They found that performance was as good on these problems as on corresponding single-format problems, suggesting that even in the single-format condition adults did not rely on non-numerical forms of quantity information. However, their task differed from other studies of numerical discrimination in that participants had to discriminate same-numerosity pairs (e.g., a 20-tome sequence and an array of 20 dots) from different-numerosity pairs, and within the different-numerosity problems the ratio of the smaller to the greater numerosity one was .67 or smaller, corresponding to comparisons such as 20 vs. 30. As this is a substantially more marked contrast than that at which previous research has obtained evidence of successful numerical discrimination, Barth et al.'s results are entirely consistent with the possibility that finer numerical discriminations involve substantial use of non-numerical cues.

2 Experiment 1

In my research, I have been examining the role of non-numerical information in relative magnitude judgments for pairs of numerosities in which the numerical contrast is quite small. An initial experiment, conducted with 14 undergraduate students, varied the sizes of the items comprising the arrays to be compared in such a way that the more numerous array was equally often composed of smaller items and of larger items than the less numerous one. Examples of the problems are shown in Figure 1. The problems varied in a variety of ways other than the relation between item size and relative numerosity, but most of them did not have a significant impact on performance, so I won't explain them in detail. One variable that did matter was the numerical contrast in a problem: performance was poorer, at 68% correct, on the contrast 21 versus 24 than on contrasts of either 18 versus 21 (81% correct) or 24 versus 28 (78% correct), corresponding to the fact that the ratio of smaller to larger numerosity is a bit closer to 1 for the 21 versus 24 contrast (a ratio of .875) than for the others (each of which correspond to a ratio of .857). The relation between item size and numerosity had an even more marked effect on performance, and it was in the opposite direction to what might be expected if judgments were based on contour length or aggregate stimulus area: Participants correctly identify the more numerous array when that array was composed of smaller items than its counterpart (so that the correct array was smaller than its counterpart in contour length and stimulus area) than when it was composed of larger items (and thus was greater than its counterpart in contour length and stimulus area). Overall, 85% of the problems on which the more numerous array was composed of smaller items were answered correctly, as compared to just 67% of those on which the more numerous array was composed of larger items than the other array. An analysis of variance confirmed that this effect was statistically reliable, $F(1,13) = 7.13$, $MSe = .096$, $p < .05$, as was the effect of numerical contrast, $F(2,26) = 10.07$, $MSe = .012$, $p < .001$.

Although not consistent with the idea that adults compare continuous quantity properties of arrays such as contour length or stimulus area as a basis for making relative numerosity judgments, the effects of item size in this study do support the more general notion that people can and do use a variety of non-numerical information in making judgments of relative numerosity. One possible explanation for the inverse effect of item size observed in Experiment 1 is that participants' experiences with everyday objects, which very often vary in size inversely with number, biased them toward choosing arrays composed of smaller items as the more numerous. Smaller items are very often packaged in large numerosities than larger ones, so that, for instance, a single-serving package of candies contains more pieces when the individual candies are small than when they are larger. Experience with this inverse relation may have led to the impression that, of two arrays that differed only slightly in numerosity, the one comprised of smaller items was the more numerous.

Notwithstanding the bias toward choosing the alternative composed of smaller items, the participants in Experiment 1 were able to identify the correct array more often than not even when it in fact consisted of larger items than its counterpart. The question remains, therefore, how these numerical discriminations were made. Inspection of Figure 1 suggests another non-numerical cue that might have contributed to correct performance. It is the presence of unfilled space, either within

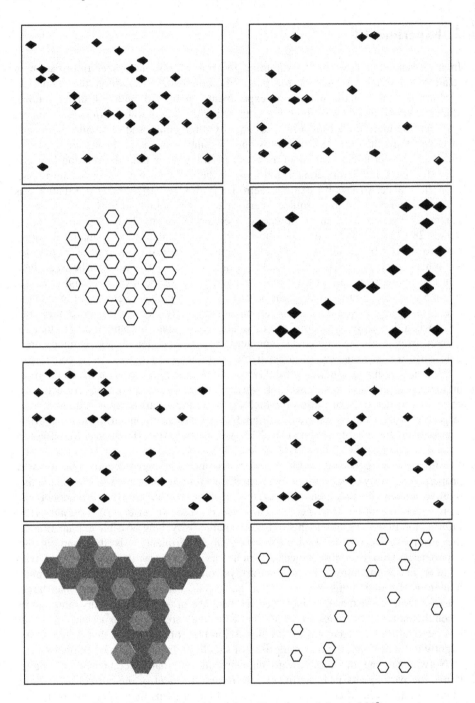

Fig. 1. Examples of problems from Experiment 1 (rotated 90°)

an array or at its edges. A second experiment examined the impact of this kind of information on judgments of relative numerosity.

3 Experiment 2

Specifically, Experiment 2 varied two spatial properties of arrays: (a) the degree to which the array as a whole filled the page, and (b) the amount of empty space between items within an array, by varying whether the items were evenly spaced or arranged in clusters, creating larger gaps between the clusters. In addition to investigating the effects of these variables on discrimination performance, the experiment also assessed the accuracy with which participants had encoded numerical information about the arrays they compared and how that related to their discrimination performance. Upon completion of the discrimination task, participants were asked to estimate the numerosities of the arrays they had just seen. Insofar as adults make relative numerosity judgments by forming representations of the numerosities of each array and comparing those (rather than by comparing non-numerical properties of the arrays), variation in the accuracy of viewers' estimates would be expected to correlate fairly well with their success in identifying the more numerous arrays.

20 undergraduate students (6 men and 14 women) participated in this experiment. Examples of the problems presented to them are shown in Figure 2. Half of the problems involved arrays containing small outline drawings of triangles or crescent shapes, which were evenly spaced and arranged in either an oval configuration that left the corners of the page empty or a rectangular configuration that filled the page more completely. The remaining problems involved arrays containing larger outline drawings of the same shapes, which were either evenly spaced or arranged in pairs or clusters of four, creating larger spaces between clusters. Each problem pitted an array of triangles against an array of crescent shapes; and the two arrays differed both in numerosity and, orthogonally, in layout. Thus, the more numerous array was equally often the one with more open space and the one with less. Two numerical contrasts were used: 40 versus 45 and 42 versus 48.

Consider first how performance was affected by variations in how the small-item arrays filled the page. The data from these problems are summarized in the upper portion of Table 1. Participants' judgments were significantly more accurate when the more numerous array was the one that filled the page more completely ($M = .86$) rather than the one that left empty space at the corners ($M = .59$). An analysis of variance (ANOVA) on the data confirmed that this effect was statistically reliable, $F(1,19) = 11.27, MSe = .131, p < .01$.

Variations in the spacing of items within arrays also affected performance. The data from the large-item arrays in which item spacing was varied are summarized in the lower portion of Table 1. Participants' judgments were significantly more accurate when the more numerous array was the one in which items were evenly spaced ($M = .83$) than when its items were clustered, leaving extra empty space between the clusters ($M = .70$). This effect, too, was statistically reliable, $F(1,19) = 7.90, MSe = .044, p = .01$.

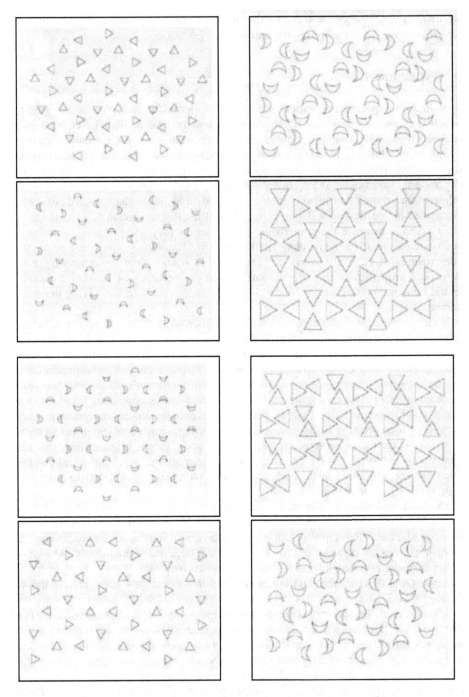

Fig. 2. Examples of problems from Experiment 2 (rotated 90°)

Table 1. Mean Proportions of Correct Responses as a Function of Spatial Layout

	Numerical Ratio	
Spatial Variable	40 v 45	42 v 48
I. Array Configuration		
More numerous array fills page more completely than less numerous array	.856	.863
Less numerous array fills page more completely than more numerous array	.557	.619
II. Spacing of items		
Items in more numerous array are evenly spaced while those in less numerous array are clustered	.819	.850
Items in more numerous array are clustered while those in less numerous array are evenly spaced	.672	.731

The estimates participants gave for the largest number of items in the arrays they had seen ranged from 20 to 110, with a median of 50. The estimates for the smallest number of items in the arrays they had seen ranged from 10 to 65, with a median of 27.5. Estimation accuracy, measured by the average deviation of viewers' estimates of the smallest and largest numerosities from the correct values, correlated only a non-significant .147 with performance across all of the discrimination problems combined. In contrast, the correlation between discrimination scores for the two major subsets of problems in the experiment—those involving small items arranged to more or less completely fill the page, and those involving larger items arranged either in clusters or evenly—was a statistically significant .541; and the correlation between scores on subsets of problems that were essentially replications of one another was .944.

In short, the results of Experiment 2 again support the idea that numerical discriminations are often based on non-numerical properties of the stimuli to be compared. Consistent with the expectation that viewers would interpret open space as an indication of relatively low numerosity, performance was more accurate when the array with more open space was the less numerous one than when it was the more numerous one.

An even more compelling finding from Experiment 2 was inaccuracy of viewers' verbal estimates of the numerosities of the arrays they had seen and its lack of relation to their accuracy in making relative numerosity judgments. If viewers had been generating numerical estimates as they viewed the arrays it seems unlikely that immediately upon completion of a task in which they formed approximate numerical representation of 128 arrays (two on each of 64 trials), every one of which contained between 40 and 48 items, their memory of those approximate numerical representations would be so poor as to result in estimates that differed so greatly from the actual numerosities. Additionally, the lack of significant correlation between the accuracy of viewers' verbal estimates and their discrimation performance strongly suggests that numerical representations of the sort needed to make the verbal estimates were not the basis for the relative numerosity judgments. Instead, it seems likely that viewers judged relative numerosity on the basis of cues that did not require determining, even approximately, how many items were in either of the arrays they were comparing. Indeed, many participants expressed surprise and a sense of unpreparedness when asked for their verbal estimates, as if they would have processed the arrays quite differently had they known they would be asked about the absolute numerosities of the arrays.

4   Conclusions

There are many ways of arriving at a judgment as to which of two arrays is more numerous, some specifically numerical (such as counting) and others not, such as comparing the sizes of items or the amount of empty space in the arrays. While the present results show that numerical discriminations are strongly influenced by spatial factors, they certainly do not rule out the use of specifically numerical comparison strategies as well, under appropriate circumstances. A more reasonable conclusion is that adults draw upon a variety of different processes in making judgments about numerosity. While this idea may seem unparsimonious, in fact it is only an instantiation of the well-established idea that much of mathematical cognition, like other kinds of cognition, is strategically adapted to the particulars of the problems to be solved. Brazilian children selling produce in the marketplace use heuristic combinations of additions and subtractions to arrive at the total cost for a specified number of items [10]; and competent U.S. students use a variety of strategies to evaluate the equivalence or ordinal relations among pairs of rational numbers [11].

The resourcefulness adults exhibit in finding different ways of thinking about which array is the more numerous is likely what makes possible the impressive degree of success they attain in discriminating among very similar numerosities, even when there are too many items to count. At the same time, the use of non-numerical information introduces biases in numerical judgments—biases that are adaptive in that they reflect ways in which number often covaries with other information but that can also lead to error. Among the biases that should be taken into account in the development of augmented cognition systems are a bias toward judging small items as more numerous than a comparable number of larger ones and a bias toward judging arrays in which there is salient empty space as less numerous than ones which appear more full.

References

1. Lipton, J.S., Spelke, E.S.: Origins of number sense: Large-number discrimination in human infants. Psych. Sci. 14, 396–401 (2003)
2. Walsh, V.: A theory of magnitude: common cortical metrics of time, space and quantity. Trends Cognit. Sci. 7, 483–488 (2003)

3. Clearfield, M.W., Mix, K.S.: Number versus contour length in infants' discrimination of small visual sets. Psych. Sci. 10, 408–411 (1999)
4. Clearfield, M.W., Mix, K.S.: Amount versus number: Infants' use of area and contour length to discriminate small sets. J. Cognit. and Devel. 2, 243–260 (2001)
5. Buckley, P.B., Gillman, C.B.: Comparisons of digits and dot patterns. J. Exper. Psych. 1103, 1131–1136 (1974)
6. van Oeffelen, M.P., Vos, P.G.: A probabilistic model for the discrimination of visual number. Percep. and Psychophys. 32, 163–170 (1982)
7. Whalen, J., Gallistel, C.R., Gelman, R.: Nonverbal counting in humans: The psychophysics of number representation. Psych. Sci. 10, 130–137 (1995)
8. Shuman, M., Kanwisher, N.: Numerical magnitude in the human parietal lobe: Tests of representational generality and domain specificity. Neuron 44, 557–569 (2004)
9. Barth, H., Kanwisher, N., Spelke, E.: The construction of large number representations in adults. Cognit. 86, 201–221 (2003)
10. Carraher, T.N., Carraher, D.W., Schliemann, A.D.: Mathematics in the streets and in schools. Brit. J. Devel. Psych. 3, 21–29 (1985)
11. Smith III, J.P.: Competent reasoning with rational numbers. Cognit. and Instruc. 13, 3–50 (1995)

Augmented Metacognition Addressing Dynamic Allocation of Tasks Requiring Visual Attention

Tibor Bosse[1], Willem van Doesburg[2], Peter-Paul van Maanen[1,2], and Jan Treur[1]

[1] Department of Artificial Intelligence, Vrije Universiteit Amsterdam
De Boelelaan 1081a, 1081HV Amsterdam, the Netherlands
{tbosse, treur}@cs.vu.nl
[2] TNO Human Factors, P.O.Box 23, 3769ZG Soesterberg, the Netherlands
{willem.vandoesburg,peter-paul.vanmaanen}@tno.nl

Abstract. This paper discusses the use of cognitive models as augmented metacognition on task allocation for tasks requiring visual attention. In the domain of naval warfare, the complex and dynamic nature of the environment makes that one has to deal with a large number of tasks in parallel. Therefore, humans are often supported by software agents that take over part of these tasks. However, a problem is how to determine an appropriate allocation of tasks. Due to the rapidly changing environment, such a work division cannot be fixed beforehand: dynamic task allocation at runtime is needed. Unfortunately, in alarming situations the human does not have the time for this coordination. Therefore system-triggered dynamic task allocation is desirable. The paper discusses the possibilities of such a system for tasks requiring visual attention.

Keywords: Visual attention, cognitive modeling, augmented metacognition.

1 Introduction

The term *augmented cognition* [6, 10] was used by Eric Horvitz at the ISAT Woods Hole meeting in the summer of 2000 to define a potentially fruitful endeavor of research that would explore opportunities for developing principles and computational systems that support and extend human cognition by taking into explicit consideration well-characterized limitations in human cognition, spanning attention, memory, problem solving, and decision making. This paper focuses on extending human cognition by the development of principles and computational systems addressing task allocation of tasks requiring visual attention. In previous work [2], cognitive models of visual attention were part of the design of a software agent that supports a naval warfare officer in its task to compile a tactical picture of the situation in the field. In the domain of naval warfare, the complex and dynamic nature of the environment makes that the warfare officer has to deal with a large number of tasks in parallel. Therefore, in practice, (s)he is often supported by software agents that take over part of these tasks. However, a problem is how to determine an appropriate allocation of tasks: due to the rapidly changing environment, such a work division cannot be fixed beforehand [1]. Task allocation has to take place at runtime,

D.D. Schmorrow, L.M. Reeves (Eds.): Augmented Cognition, HCII 2007, LNAI 4565, pp. 166–175, 2007.

dynamically. For this purpose, two approaches exist, i.e. *human-triggered* and *system-triggered* dynamic task allocation [3]. In the former case, the user can decide up to what level the software agent should assist her. But especially in alarming situations the user does not have the time to think about such task allocation [7]. In these situations it would be better if a software agent augments the user's metacognitive capabilities by means of system-triggered dynamic task allocation. This paper discusses the usage of cognitive models of visual attention that can be incorporated within assisting software agents offering augmented metacognition in order to obtain such a system-triggered dynamic task allocation,

In Section 2 a further elaboration on the motivational background for augmented metacogntion is given. Section 3 a generic design of augmented metacogntion based on cognitive models of visual attention is described. In Section 4 some applications of the framework are introduced and discussed. The paper is concluded with a general discussion and some future research.

2 Augmented Metacognition: Motivational Background

Support of humans in critical tasks may involve a number of aspects. First, a software agent can have knowledge about the task or some of its subtasks and, based on this knowledge, contribute to task execution. Usually, performing this will also require that the software agent has knowledge about the environment. This situation can be interpreted as a specific form of augmented cognition: *task-content-focused augmented cognition*. This means that the cognitive capabilities to do the task partly reside within the software agent, external to the human, and may extend the human's cognitive capabilities and limitations. For example, if incoming signals require a very fast but relatively simple response, in speed beyond the cognitive capabilities of a human, a software agent can contribute to this task, thus augmenting the human's limited reaction capabilities. Another example is handling many incoming stimuli at the same time, which also may easily be beyond human capabilities, whereas a software agent can take care of it.

If the software agent provides task-content-focused augmented cognition, like in the above two examples, it may not have any knowledge about the coordination of the subtasks and the process of cooperation with the human. For example, task allocation may completely reside at the human's side. However, as discussed in the introduction, when the human is occupied with a highly demanding task, the aspect of coordination may easily slip away. For example, while working under time pressure, humans tend to spend less attention to reflection on their functioning. If the software agent detects and adapts to those situations it will have a beneficial effect; e.g., [8]. This type of reflection is a form of metacognition: cognitive processes addressing other cognitive processes. A specific type of support of a human from an augmented cognition perspective can also address such reflective aspects: *augmented metacognition*. This is the form of augmented cognition that, in contrast to task-content-focused augmented cognition, addresses the support or augmentation of a human's limitations in metacognitive capabilities. The type of augmented metacognition discussed in this paper focuses on dynamic task allocation.

Augmented metacognition can be provided by the same software agent that provides task-content-focused augmented cognition, or by a second software agent that specialises on metacognition, for example the task allocation task. The former case results in a reflective software agent that has two levels of internal processing: it can reason both about the task content (object-level process) and about the task coordination (meta-level process); e.g., [9]. The latter case amounts to a specific case of a reflective multi-agent system: a multi-agent system in which some of the agents process at the object level and others at the meta-level.

The distinction made between task-content-focused augmented cognition and augmented metacognition provides a designer with indications for structuring a design in a transparent manner, either by the multi-agent system design, or by the design of a reflective software agent's internal structure. This paper focuses on the latter, the design of the reflective internal structure of the software agent. An implementation of such an agent has been evaluated for two case studies.

3 Augmented Metacognition Design

In this section, first the generic design of the proposed augmented metacognition is presented in Section 3.1. After that, Section 3.2 describes how principles of Signal Detection Theory (SDT) can be applied within this design.

3.1 Prescriptive and Descriptive Models

The present design is based on the idea that the software agent's internal structure augments the user's metacognitive capabilities. This structure is composed of two maintained models of the user's attention. The first is called a *descriptive model*, which os a model that estimates the user's actual attentional dynamics. The second is called a *prescriptive model*, which prescribes the way these dynamics should be. In Figure 1 a conceptual design of such a software agent is shown. Depending on the user's and the agent's own attentional levels, the agent decides whether the user (or the agent itself) is paying enough attention to the right tasks at the right time. This is determined by checking whether the difference between described attention and prescribed attention is below a certain threshold. In Figure 1 this comparison is depicted in the middle as the *compare* process. Based on this, the agent either adapts its support or it does not, i.e. the *adapt* process in Figure 1.

From the perspective of the agent, the runtime decision whether to allocate a task to itself or to the user comes down to the decision whether to support this task or not. The question remains what the agent could use as a basis for deciding to take over responsibility of a task, i.e. by exceedance of a certain threshold, using both descriptive and prescriptive models of user attention. An answer to this is that the agent's decision to support can be based on several performance indications: (PI1) a performance indication of the user concerning her ability to appropriately allocate attention (to the right tasks at the right time), (PI2) a performance indication of the agent concerning its ability to soundly prescribe the allocation of attention to tasks, (PI3) a performance indication of the system concerning its ability to soundly describe the user dynamics of the allocation of attention to tasks, and (PI4) a performance indication of the agent concerning its ability to soundly decide to support the user in her task to allocate attention to tasks.

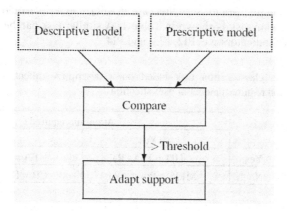

Fig. 1. Conceptual model of the attention allocation system

3.2   Some Principles of SDT

On of the ways to let the agent estimate the performances of the user and the agent itself from the previous paragraph is by using the principles of *Signal Detection Theory*, or simply SDT [5]. In this subsection a theoretical framework based on SDT is defined, including a method that constitutes a means for identifying when to trigger attention allocation support.

To let a software agent reason about the performance of the user concerning her ability to appropriately allocate attention (PI1), a formal framework in SDT terms is needed in which it can describe it. These terms are mainly based on a mathematical description of the following situations:

1) The descriptive model of user attention indicates that attention is paid (A) to the tasks that are required by the prescriptive model (R). This situation is also called a *hit* (HIT).
2) The descriptive model of user attention indicates that attention is not paid (not A) to the tasks that are not required by the prescriptive model (not R). This situation is also called a *correct rejection* (CR).
3) The descriptive model of user attention indicates that attention is paid (A) to the tasks that are not required by the prescriptive model (not R). This situation is also called a *false alarm* (FA).
4) The descriptive model of user attention indicates that attention is not paid (not A) to the tasks that are required by the prescriptive model (R). This situation is also called a *miss* (MISS).

The task to discriminate the above situations can be set out in a table as a 2-class classification task. The specific rates of HITs, FAs, MISSs, and CRs, are calculated by means of probabilities of the form P(X|Y), where X is the estimate of certain behaviour and Y is the estimate of the type of situation at hand. The descriptive and prescriptive models mentioned earlier can be seen as the user's attentional behaviour (A or not A) in a specific situation that either requires attention (R) or does not (not R). A HIT, for example, would be in this case P(A|R), and a FA would be P(A|not R), etc. This classification task is shown in Table 1. A similar task can be defined for the other performance indicators, i.e. PI2, PI3, and PI4.

Table 1. A 2-class classification task based on a descriptive (attention allocated) and prescriptive (attention required) model of user attention

		Attention required?	
		Yes	No
Attention	Yes	HIT = P(A | R)	FA = P(A | not R)
allocated?	No	MISS = P(not A | R)	CR = P(not A | not R)

In SDT, the measure of sensitivity (d') is commonly used as an indicator for various kinds of performances. The measure is a means to compare two models, in this case descriptive and prescriptive models. Hence the calculation of such sensitivities can be used by the agent to determine whether to support the user or not. For instance. low sensitivities (< threshold) may result in the decision to adapt support. The calculation of sensitivity in terms of the above mentioned HIT, FA, MISS, and CR, can be done by using the following formula:

$$d' = HIT - FA = CR - MISS$$

As can be seen in the formula, to calculate sensitivity, the measurement of HIT and FA are sufficient. No estimates of CR or MISS are needed, since HIT – FA is equal to CR – MISS.[1] Furthermore, sensitivity is dependent on both HIT and FA, rather than on HIT or FA alone. A user that has a high sensitivity as a result of attending to all tasks all the time (high HIT rate), is not only impossible due to the maximum capacity of human attention, but also very inefficient. Think of the very limited attention each task probably will receive due to unneeded FAs. The other way around, a low FA rate as a result of attending to nothing, is obviously not desired as well.

4 Applications

This section discusses two applications of the presented framework for task allocation based on visual attention. In Section 4.1, a pilot study is described, of which the main aim was to establish a (descriptive) model of a person's visual attention in the execution of a simple task in the warfare domain. For this pilot study, a simplified version of an Air Traffic Control (ATC) task was used. Next, Section 4.2 addresses a more realistic case: the task of Tactical Picture Compilation (TPC) by a naval warfare

---

[1] This is due to the fact that HIT = 1 – MISS and therefore a high HIT results in a low MISS, and vice versa (the same holds for CR = 1 – FA).

officer. For both cases, it is explained how descriptive models of visual attention may be used for task allocation, using the design introduced in Section 3.

4.1 Multitask

In order to test the ideas presented in the previous sections, a pilot study has been performed. The setup of this pilot study consisted of a human participant executing a simple warfare officer-like task [2]. To create such a setup, the software Multitask [4] was used (and slightly altered in order to have it output the proper data). Multitask was originally meant to be a low fidelity ATC simulation. In this study, it is considered to be an abstraction of the cognitive tasks concerning the compilation of the tactical picture, i.e. a warfare officer-like task. A screenshot of the task is shown in Figure 2.

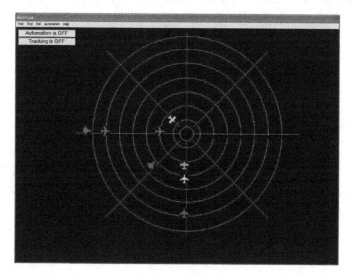

Fig. 2. The interface of the used environment based on MultiTask [4]

In the pilot case study, the participant (controller) had to manage an airspace by identifying aircrafts that all are approaching the centre of a radarscope. The centre contained a high value unit (HVU) that had to be protected. In order to do this, airplanes needed to be cleared and identified to be either hostile or friendly to the HVU. The participant had to click on the aircraft according to a particular procedure depending on the status of the aircraft. Within the conducted pilot study, three different aircraft types were used, which resulted in different intervals of speed of the aircrafts. The above dynamic properties of the environment were stimuli that resulted in constant change of the participant's attention. The data that were collected consist of all locations, distances from the centre, speeds, types, and states (i.e., colours). Additionally, data from a Tobii x50 eye-tracker[2] were extracted while the participant was executing the task. All data were retrieved several times per second (10-50 Hz).

---

[2] http://www.tobii.se.

Based on such data, a cognitive model has been implemented that estimates the distribution of the user's attention over the locations of the screen at any moment during the experiment [2]. This model uses two types of input, i.e., *user-input* and *context-input*. The user-input is provided by the eye-tracker, and consists of the (x, y)-coordinates of the gaze of the user over time. The context-input is provided by the Multitask environment, and consists of the variables speed, distance to the centre, type of aircraft, and aircraft status. The output of the model is represented in the form of an dynamically changing 3D image. An example screenshot of this is shown in Figure 3 at an arbitrary time point.[3] The x- and y-axis denote the x- and y-coordinates of the grid, and the z-axis denotes the level of attention. In addition, the locations of all tracks, the status of the tracks, the location of the gaze, and the mouse clicks are indicated in the figure by small dots, colour, a star, and a big dot, respectively. Figure 3 clearly shows that at this time point there are two peaks of attention (locations (12,10) and (16,9)). Moreover, a mouse click is performed at location (16,9), and the gaze of the subject is also directed towards that location.

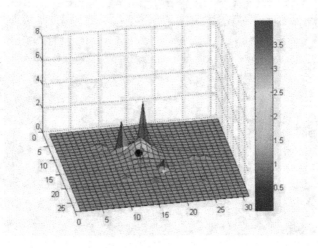

Fig. 3. Example Output of the Cognitive Model of Visual Attention [2]

In terms of Section 3, the presented model is a descriptive model of the task. If, in addition to this a prescriptive model is created, both models can be used for dynamic task allocation, using the principles of Signal Detection Theory. Hence the presented model of visual attention can be used for augmented metacognition purposes: the system maintains a cognitive model of the attentional dynamics of an user, and accordingly, extends the user's metacognitive capabilites. By introducing a threshold, a binary decision mechanism can be established, which decides for each location whether it receives (enough) attention or not ("A" or "not A" in Table 1). The idea is to use such a mechanism for dynamic task allocation for the type of tasks in the naval domain as considered in this paper. For example, in case an user is already allocated to some task, it may be better to leave that task for him or her, and allocate tasks to the system for which there is less or no commitment from the user (yet).

---

[3] See http://www.few.vu.nl/~pp/attention for a complete animation.

4.2 Tactical Picture Compilation Simulator

The characterizations of different attentional states in relation with adaptive task allocation was investigated in another case study, namely one in the naval surface warfare domain. In Figure 4 a snapshot of the interface of the Tactical Picture Compilation (TPC) Simulator, used in this study, is shown. Similar to the case study in the previous section, this study was also conducted in an effort to augment the metacognitive capabilities of the user in naval operations in naval operations and to leverage cognitive models of attention. However, the present study focused on a more realistic domain: its goal was to establish an implicit work division between a naval officer and a supportive agent based on a cognitive model of the TPC task. TPC is a critical task in naval surface warfare. It is continuously performed by naval warfare officers during operations at sea. The main goal is to create an accurate tactical picture of the immediate surroundings of the ship using the ship's sensors. Changes in the tactical picture can occur either extremely slow or very rapidly depending on the traffic density at sea.

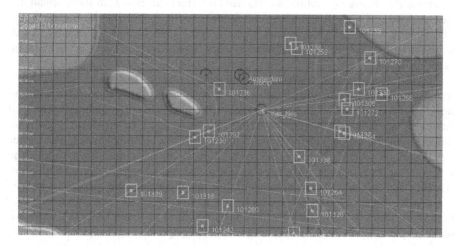

Fig. 4. Tactical picture compilation simulation that was used to implement a dynamic task allocator based on a cognitive model of attention

The application contained a TPC agent that supported the officer's interpretation of the behaviour of ships in the area. The officer observes the behaviour of the ships in the area over time in order to deduce if they have hostile intent or not. The attentional capacity of the officer may come under stress during transitional periods from low traffic densities to high traffic densities or during intense tactical action. During these periods of high cognitive workload, the officer is supported by the TPC agent. The question is how to determine the optimal division of workload without adding to the workload of the officer by letting him or her decide what the division should be. Instead, the main region of interest on the radar screen is determined by using a cognitive model of attention. The model is similar to the one used for the study mentioned in Section 4.1. It deduces the region of interest based on an interpretation of eye gaze behaviour of the officer as well as information about the properties of the objects and spaces visible on the radar screen. The various symbols and lines are not equally visually salient and the model must correct for this. The regions that are not covered by the modeled attention of the officer are then assigned to the TPC agent for processing. The officer therefore *implicitly* communicates the metacognitive decision which radar tracks are desired to be handled by the TPC agent.

This implicit communication is based on the assumption that the user's cognitive performance in determining threat is better than that of the TPC agent. This means that no prescriptive variant of the TPC model was used to determine the work division between the TPC agent and the officer. A prescriptive model of the TPC task, as described in Section 3, may be used to inform the work division decision, by checking if the officer pays attention to the radar tracks that represent the greatest threat. If not, then the optimal work division may need to be re-assessed. The TPC agent will automatically be assigned those tracks that fall outside the scope of attention of the officer. In future versions of this application, a prescriptive model can be implemented to enhance performance in situations where threat is ambiguous or situations that contains multiple threats from different directions. In those situations, the most optimal work division may consist of the officer covering one threat and the TPC agent covering another, instead of just keeping track of nominal radar tracks. A prescriptive TPC model is then required to detect threats outside the scope of attention of the officer.

This form of decision support is implicit in the sense that there is no explicit communication between officer and agent about the decisions supported. Both the work division decision and task related decisions happen automatically. An interesting question is to determine whether the acceptance of this form of decision support by naval officers can be enhanced if the system communicates to the officer the reasons on which it bases its decisions. This might cause the officer to trust the system more, because the reasons on which decisions are made inspire confidence. On the other hand, situations might develop in which the officer generates expectations about the decisions made by the supporting agent. This might lead to a form of paranoia in which the officer is distracted from the main task (TPC) because of the desire to check the decisions of the supporting agent.

5 Discussion

The Augmented Cognition International Society defines augmented cognition as 'an emerging field of science that seeks to extend a user's abilities via computational technologies, which are explicitly designed to address bottlenecks, limitations, and biases in cognition and to improve decision making capabilities.' The Society also formulated a goal: '.. to develop computational methods and neurotech tools that can account for and accommodate information processing bottlenecks inherent in human-system interaction (e.g., limitations in attention, memory, learning, comprehension, visualization abilities, and decision making).' Augmented cognition is a wide area, that is applicable to various types of cognitive processes. As the area develops further, it may be useful to differentiate the field a bit more, for example, by distinguishing more specific classes of application.

In this paper, such a distinction is put forward: augmented cognition focusing on task content versus augmented cognition focusing on task coordination. As the latter is considered a form of metacognition, this suggests augmented metacognition as an interesting subarea of augmented cognition. The paper discussed applications to the metacognition used for dynamic task allocation within this area. It has been pointed out how functioning of human-computer systems can be improved by incorporating augmented metacognition in them. Especially in tasks involving multiple stimuli that require fast responses, this concept is expected to provide a substantial gain in effectiveness of the combined system.

Acknowledgments. This research was partly funded by the Royal Netherlands Navy under program number V524.

References

1. Bainbridge, L.: Ironies of automation. Automatica 19, 775–779 (1983)
2. Bosse, T., van Maanen, P.-P., Treur, J.: A Cognitive Model for Visual Attention and its Application. In: Proceedings of the 2006 IEEE/WIC/ACM Int. Conf. on Intelligent Agent Technology (IAT-06), IEEE Computer Society Press, Hong Kong (2006)
3. Campbell, G., Cannon-Bowers, J., Glenn, F., Zachary, W., Laughery, R., Klein, G.: Dynamic function allocation in the SC-21 Manning Initiative Program, Naval Air Warfare Center Training Systems Division, Orlando, SC-21/ONRS&T Manning Affordability Initiative (1997)
4. Clamann, M.P., Wright, M.C., Kaber, D.B.: Comparison of performance effects of adaptive automation applied to various stages of human-machine system information processing. In: Proceedings of the 46th Ann. Meeting of the Human Factors and Ergonomics Soc. pp. 342–346 (2002)
5. Green, D., Swets, J.: Signal detection: theory and psychophysics. Wiley, New York (1966)
6. Horvitz, E., Pavel, M., Schmorrow, D.D.: Foundations of Augmented Cognition. Washington, DC, National Academy of Sciences (2001)
7. Inagaki, T.: Adaptive automation: Sharing and trading of control. Handbook of Cognitive Task Design, 147–169 (2003)
8. Kaber, D.B., Endsley, M.R.: The effects of level of automation and adaptive automation on human performance, situation awareness and workload in a dynamic control task. Theoretical Issues in Ergonomics Science 5(2), 113–153 (2004)
9. Maes, P., Nardi, D.: Meta-level Architectures and Reflection, North-Holland, Amsterdam (1988)
10. Schmorrow, D.D., Kruse, A.A.: Augmented Cognition. In: Bainbridge, W.S. (ed.) Berkshire Encyclopedia of Human-Computer Interaction. Great Barrington, MA: Berkshire Publishing Group, pp. 54–99 (2004)

Highly Configurable Software Architecture Framework for Acquisition and Visualization of Biometric Data

Jan Stelovsky

University of Hawaii, Department of Information and Computer Sciences
1680 East-West Road, Honolulu, Hawaii 96816, USA

Abstract. The research in augmented cognition and its practical applications rely heavily on the acquisition and evaluation of biometrics data. We propose software architecture that offers unified approach to the integration of emerging hardware and evaluation technologies. In this paper we focus on the software layers that combine the data events and offer visual representations of the results. In particular, we show that the common evaluation of the collected data as well as the commonly used graphical depictions of the results can be achieved using a fully modular and extendible software architecture.

Keywords: software architecture, visualization, biometrics, eye-tracking.

1 Introduction

Acquisition of biometrics data, its evaluation and visualization of the results are key components of the research on human cognition. One of the main reasons that after years of basic and applied research the current technology is still far from being integrated into practical applications is that experiments are very time-consuming to design, administer and evaluate. While new biometric sensors are being developed and new visualization techniques are proposed, the software environment needed to analyze the data is typically highly sensor-dependent and hard-coded. Moreover, the visualizations tend to be complex in order to depict the experimental data in various perspectives and thus less suitable in practical applications where simpler user interfaces are customary, e.g. a set of gauges that aggregate several data dimensions.

To simplify the task of integrating all aspects of data collection, processing, and visualization for experimental purposes, we have been developing EventStream software framework that satisfies the following objectives:

- Incorporates various sensors, e.g., equipment measuring temperature, heart rate and skin resistance, pressure on the mouse case and buttons, eye-tracker, oximeter, interactive events (keyboard events, mouse movement and clicks).
- Supports various data sources and sinks, such as file, LAN and Internet (TCP/IP) streams, serial ports, interactive and software-generated events.
- Incorporates common data evaluation and display methodologies.
- Is based on unified software architecture that offers higher level abstractions, atomic building blocks as well as commonly used composite functionality.
- Is highly extendible with Java modules that can be combined and reconfigured.

D.D. Schmorrow, L.M. Reeves (Eds.): Augmented Cognition, HCII 2007, LNAI 4565, pp. 176–185, 2007.
© Springer-Verlag Berlin Heidelberg 2007

The software architecture that defined the input and output functionality, i.e. the support for the existing and emerging sensors and data sinks was described in detail in [1] and [2]. One of the challenges was to unify the real-time visualization of incoming data from interactive events with the replay of the experimental session that used data read from a data stream. Instead of converting this particular type of data into events or developing two display modules, we developed a generic solution – a set of conversion modules that can convert arbitrary events into data that can be deposited onto a stream or send data retrieved from a stream to listeners in the form of events. The time intervals in between two consecutive events were proportional to the time span originally recorded and the scaling factor could be freely chosen. The design and implementation of this facility was described in [3]. The data processing code and the implementation of various graphical representations of the results remained, however, hardwired and tailored specifically to each case.

In this article we shall first analyze the common visualization techniques and then propose a software architecture that extends the unification and extensibility effort to the data processing and visualization modules and describe a prototype implementation of the architecture's core elements.

2 Common Graphical Visualizations of Experimental Data

The evaluation and visualization of eye tracking data is one of the more complex endeavors in biometric experiments because of the magnitude of the data obtained as well as its referential complexity. Let us therefore look at some implemented and proposed graphical representations as they were collected and presented in [4].

A common presentation of event-based data is a 2-dimensional graph where one of the axes represents the elapsed time. While measurement data forms a discrete function, a polyline connecting the samples is an adequate visualization. For example, the 2-dimensional graph in Fig. 1 shows the pupil size during an eye-tracking session.

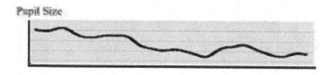

Fig. 1. A 2-dimensional graph depicting the *pupil size* with respect to *time axis*

The raw eye tracking data has to be analyzed in terms of fixations – numerous eye gaze points falling into the same area – and saccades – the rapid eye movements. Even though there is general agreement that visual information is processed only during the fixations, graphs that combine saccades and fixations are common in literature as they convey the impression of a continuous gaze path. Such combined Fixation Path graph is depicted in Fig. 2. The dynamic version of Fixation Path graph where the sequence of fixations is shown as a (possibly slowed down) movie is also very useful as it indicates where and for how long the subject looked.

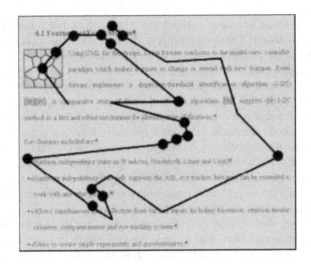

Fig. 2. A Fixation Path graph with *fixations* (*black circles*) and *saccades* (*lines*) on a *background image* that shows the text presented to the subject

The Transition Matrix graph in Fig. 3 identifies areas of interest, determines the probabilities of a transition between consecutive fixations in different areas. These probabilities are then depicted as oriented arrows between the areas of interest labeled with the percentage numeric values corresponding to the probabilities.

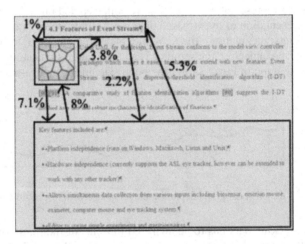

Fig. 3. A Transition Matrix graph with *areas of interest (rectangles)* and *transition probabilities (arrows with percentages)* superimposed on a *background image*

Another often used visualization is the Heatmap graph shown in Fig. 4. It depicts the overall hotspots of fixations as ovals whose color and size indicate the frequency of fixations within the underlying area.

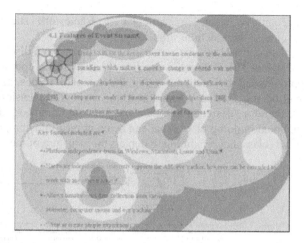

Fig. 4. A Heatmap graph with *fixations hotspots (colored ovals)* on a *background image*

Other graphical representations of biometric data are commonly used, among them those that use surfaces in 3-dimensional space, which are just extensions of curves within a 2-dimensional graph into 3-dimensional space in our context.

The above discussed visualizations were not selected according to their usefulness for the analysis of eye movement data. Instead, we tried to choose a wide spectrum of visually different representations.

3 Function Framework

Before the biometric data can be visualized, it needs to preprocessed. For instance, raw eye gaze data must be condensed into fixations. For the purposes of augmented cognition experiments, several dimensions of the data are typically combined to obtain indication of the subject's mental state and cognitive capabilities. For instance, higher heart rate and increased pressure on the mouse case may indicate stress levels that impede cognitive abilities. The schema in Fig. 5 shows how a function $F(x_1,...,x_n)$ can aggregate the data vector into one value which is then shown on a gauge.

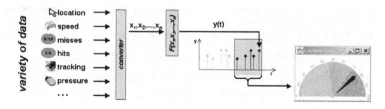

Fig. 5. Schematic data flow coalescing in a *cognitive gauge*

A more general schema may aggregate data over a recent time span in individual dimensions before combining them or employ several gauges to show different aspects of the cognitive state. In particular, a framework should allow the experimenter can choose the functions arbitrarily.

The biometric data consists of time-stamped events that form a discrete function in multidimensional space. This function is a series of samples of a continuous function that can be approximated by interconnecting the sampled values. In general, the preprocessing can be regarded as a function from one multidimensional space into another. We have therefore designed an extensible function framework that allows for definition of functional building blocks that can be combined into complex composite functions. The UML class diagram in Fig. 6 depicts the structure of the framework.

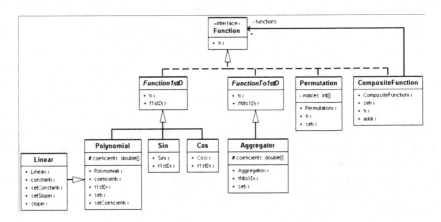

Fig. 6. UML class diagram of the function framework

At the heart of the framework is an interface contract that prescribes that a function must return a multidimensional point f(x) given a multidimensional point x. (The spaces may have different dimensions.)

```
public interface Function {
   public Point f (Point x);
}
```

We define a special case for one-dimensional functions. To be able to treat them the same way as the generic multidimensional functions we postulate that they change only the first coordinate of the given point and leave the other dimensions untouched.

```
public abstract class Function1stD implements Function {

   public abstract double f1stD (double x);

   public Point f (Point x) {
     x.vector [0] = f1stD (x.vector [0]);
     return x;
   }
}
```

To give an example, let us demonstrate the implementation of a particularly common one-dimensional function – the polynomial function.

```java
public class Polynomial extends Function1stD {

  protected double coeficients [];

  public double f1stD (double x) {
    double value = 0;
    for (int i = coeficients.length - 1; i >= 0; i--) {
      value = value * x + coeficients [i];
    }
    return value;
  }

}
```

The implementation of a `Linear` function is trivial as a subclass of `Polynomial` with a constructor that has the two parameters `slope` and `constant`.

Finally, let us demonstrate the implementation of function composition. (We present a simplified version without the accessor methods for the properties.)

```java
public class CompositeFunction implements Function {

  private ArrayList<Function> functions;

  public CompositeFunction (Function... functions) {
    for (Function function : functions) {
      this.functions.add (function);
    }
  }

  public Point f (Point x) {
    for (Function g : functions) {x = g.f (x);}
    return x;
  }

}
```

We support other useful functions as well. For instance, we define the basis for aggregate functions that can combine the values in several dimensions. Functions that filter the data or reduce the number of dimensions are trivial extensions of this framework. (The class `Point` itself provides for the composition of two points, one N-dimensional and the other M-dimensional, into a point in N+M-dimensional space.)

The architecture presented above provides for an extremely simple, yet powerful framework. Together with the standard mathematical functions, this framework can accommodate a large variety of data-processing functions. As we will see later, graphical visualization methods can, for instance, use a composition of `Linear` functions with a function that permutates the coordinates of a point to scale the data to fit the drawing specifications and screen constraints. Obviously, the applications of the functional framework extend beyond the evaluation and visual representation of data as the framework provides a basis amenable to further mathematical treatment.

4   Visualization Framework

Closer analysis of the graphs in Fig. 1 through Fig. 4 reveals that these visualizations have a common basis – there is some "background graphics" such as graph axes, an image, or potentially continuous media such as sound or video. Superimposed on this media is some representation of points: as a sequence of line segments (Fig. 1 and Fig. 2), circles (Fig. 2), rectangles (Fig. 3), ovals (Fig. 4), arrows (Fig. 3), or textual labels (numbers in Fig. 3). Every Java programmer will associate these geometrical shapes immediately with the methods for drawing primitive shapes in her preferred graphical support package. Furthermore, we observe that the shapes tend to have more parameters than the x and y coordinates, e.g., the size and color of the ovals in the heatmap in Fig. 4 or the numeric values in Fig. 3. Also, each of the lines or arrows needs an additional point, i.e. another pair of x and y coordinates. Moreover, some graphs combine several representations, such as lines and circles in Fig. 2. Despite these complexities the implementation of the graphs is fairly straightforward.

Can the implementation of such visualizations be facilitated even more by a common underlying framework? Probably every programmer will write common software modules for drawing the axes and scaling the x and y coordinates. But further commonalities emerge if we treat a visualization as the representation of a sequence of points in a multidimensional space. (It is of course no coincidence that the function framework discussed in the previous section provides us exactly with such points.) The responsibility of a graph is therefore to provide such a sequence of points. Then each of the points can be drawn by a specific "painter". (Notice that the "background graphics" in the last paragraph can be also interpreted as one of the coordinates – then a frames number of a continuous media can be represented as a coordinate value and the painter will paint the corresponding frame.) The UML class diagram in Fig. 7 shows the basic structure of the proposed visualization framework.

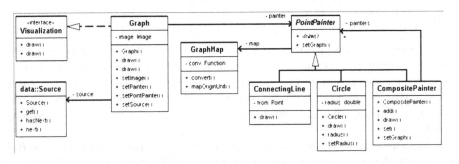

Fig. 7. UML class diagram representation of the graphical visualization framework

The core of the framework is the `Graph` class that supplies one `draw()` method that draws the entire sequence of points and another `draw()` method that the paints the "current" point. It requests the points from the `Source` of data and uses a `PointPainter` to draw each of them. Again, let us illustrate this with a simplified version of the code:

```java
public class Graph implements Visualization {

    private Source source;
    private PointPainter painter;

    public Graph (Source source) {this.source = source;}

    public void setPointPainter (PointPainter painter) {
        this.painter = painter;
        painter.setMap (new GraphMap (new Point(0,100)
            , new Point(10,0)));
    }

    public void draw (Graphics graphics) {
        while (source.hasNext ()) {
            painter.draw (graphics, source.next ().get ());
        }
    }

    public void draw (Graphics graphics, Point point) {
        painter.draw (graphics, point);
    }
}
```

Notice that the while the `source` is responsible for preparing the `Point` data, the `painter` can convert it to the actual screen coordinates using the class `GraphMap`:

```java
public class GraphMap {

    private Function conversion;

    public void mapOriginUnit (Point o, Point u) {
        Linear lx = new Linear (o.x(), u.x() - o.x());
        Linear ly = new Linear (o.y(), u.y() - o.y());
        Permutation pm = new Permutation (0, 1);
        conversion = new CompositeFunction (lx, pm, ly, pm);
    }

    public Point convert (Point point) {
        return conversion.f (new Point (point));
    }
}
```

The convenience method `mapOriginUnit()` illustrates how this framework can be used to quickly prototype the scaling and transition needed to map a data point to the actual position on a screen pane – otherwise a quite error-prone operation due to the fact that the y axis on the screen runs in the opposite direction than we are used to see in a book. Suppose that the origin and unit points contain the screen coordinates of the (0,0) and (1,1) points in the data space. Then the conversion to the screen point is given by two linear functions as defined in the above code. We can use a composition of these functions if we interchange the coordinates before we apply the second linear function and interchange them again at the end. The application of this composite function within the `convert()` method then becomes trivial.

Needless to say, this code is not a masterpiece of efficiency as four functions will be applied every time a point is drawn. On the other hand, the overhead will be typically negligible compared to the effort needed to draw the pixels of a line or an oval, and the clarity of the code (once the coordinate interchanges become second nature) is a clear advantage. Moreover, the above code can be easily modified into a more efficient version.

Finally, as an example of a `PointPainter`, let us present a simplified version of a class that draws a circle:

```
public class Circle extends PointPainter {

    private int radius = 10;
    private GraphMap map;

    public Circle (int radius) {this.radius = radius;}

    public void setMap (GraphMap map) {this.map = map;}

    public void draw (Graphics graphics, Point point) {
      Point p = map.convert (data);
      graphics.gc ().fillOval (Graph.round(p.x()-radius),
          Graph.round(p.y()-radius), 2*radius, 2*radius);
    }
}
```

Note that instead of letting the painter convert the data into screen coordinates, our function framework would allow us to incorporate the conversion functions into the data-processing by appending them to the end of the function composition. While we opted to leave them as a responsibility of the graph's functionality, we could also let the graph pass them to the source for integration.

A careful reader may ask: What if our circles needed to vary their radius and color to reflect additional dimensions of the source data? Then the source will have to add other two dimensions to our points and the painter will need to convert these coordinates into the appropriate values of the corresponding data types. This is simple with numeric data such as the circle radius and can be incorporated into the conversion within the `GraphMap` class. Similarly, a grayscale value can be accommodated within the point's conversion. One could also imagine converting data into the RGB value for color definition or even introducing three separate dimensions for either the proportion of primary colors or – probably more suitably for visualization purposes – the hue, saturation and brightness components of a color. The more general solution, however, is to supply separate conversion functions that map the data points into the appropriate data type.

The visualization framework also incorporates a composite pattern to accommodate representations where one point is visualized in multiple fashions. The implementation of the pattern in `CompositePainter` is almost identical to that of `CompositeFunction`. To give an example, the saccades and fixations in the Fixation Path graph shown in Fig. 2 can be drawn using the composition of a `ConnectingLine` and `Circle` painters.

4 Conclusion

The functional and visualization frameworks present a simple solution that unifies a wide variety of commonly used data processing functions and visualizations. Both frameworks are very extendible. New data processing functions can be constructed either as a composition of existing ones or, if this is not possible, by writing a Function subclass in Java. Similarly, complex visualizations can be composed from basic shapes and new painters can be implemented as Java subclasses. Moreover, specifications of function parameters and function compositions can be provided separately from Java code – e.g. in the form of XML configuration files – and the corresponding classes can be dynamically loaded. Parameterization and composition can be even made part of the user interface thus allowing the experimenter to choose the best preprocessing and visual representation of the data.

There is an additional benefit of our approach: the visualization in real time and the replay of an experimental session is a natural extension that does not require any coding effort. Whether the data is generated as a sequence of events in real time or whether it is read from a stream, our EventStream software can provide it to the data processing layer in either fashion. And since the graph drawing layer does not depend on whether the points arrive with or without delay, a replay is generated simply by pausing by a given time span before prompting the graph to draw the next point. Even if the graph insist on getting the consecutive points "immediately" – i.e. within a while loop – the data source can block the drawing thread for the necessary span of time. Note however that this replay facility works only in the forward fashion and more elaborate state "undo/memento" facility would be needed to go backward in time without having to reconstruct the entire session.

A prototype of the proposed frameworks has been implemented in Java using Eclipse and its SWT toolkit. We plan to incorporate an enhanced version into the software visualization project that we are currently developing.

Acknowledgments. Fig. 1 through Fig. 4 courtesy of C. Aschwanden.

References

1. Stelovsky, J., Aschwanden, C.: Measuring Cognitive Load with EventStream Software Framework. In: Sprague, R. (ed.) Proceedings of the 36th Hawaii International Conference of System Sciences (CD-ROM), IEEE Computer Society, Washington (2003)
2. Stelovsky, J.: An Extendible Architecture for the Integration of Eye Tracking and User Interaction Events of Java Programs with Complex User Interfaces. In: Bullinger, H.-J., Ziegler, J. (eds.) Human-Computer Interaction: Ergonomics and User Interfaces, vol. 1, pp. 861–865. Lawrence Erlbaum Associates, Mahwah (1999)
3. Stelovsky, J., Aschwanden, C.: Software Architecture for Unified Management of Event Notification and Stream I/O and its Use for Recording and Analysis of User Events. In: Proceedings of Hawaii International Conference on System Sciences, p. 138 (2002)
4. Aschwanden, C.: EventStream Experimenter Workbench: From Data Collection to Integrated Visualization Techniques to Facilitate Eye Movement Research. Ph.D. Dissertation, University of Hawaii at Manoa (2005)

Simulation Fidelity Design Informed by Physiologically-Based Measurement Tools

Jack M. Vice[1], Corinna Lathan[1], Anna D. Lockerd[1], and James M. Hitt, II[2]

[1] AnthroTronix, Inc., 8737 Colesville Rd, L203
Silver Spring, MD 20910, USA
{jvice,clathan,alockerd}@atinc.com
[2] Independent Consultant, 110 Cherrywood Drive
Gaithersburg, MD 20878, USA
jameshitt@verizon.net

Abstract. Virtual environments (VE's) and simulations are being employed for training applications in a wide variety of disciplines, both military and civilian. The common assumption is that the more realistic the VE, the better the transfer of training to real world tasks. However, some aspects of task content and fidelity may result in stronger transfer of training than even the most high fidelity simulations. A physiologically-based system capable of dynamically detecting changes in operator behavior and physiology throughout a VE experience and comparing those changes to operator behavior and physiology in real-world tasks, could potentially determine which aspects of VE fidelity will have the highest impact on transfer of training. Thus, development of training assessment and guidance tools that utilize operator behavior and physiology to determine VE effectiveness and transfer of training are needed.

Keywords: virtual reality, simulation, transfer of training, physiology, behavior, training effectiveness.

1 Introduction

Virtual environments (VE's) and simulations are being employed for training applications in a wide variety of disciplines, both military and civilian. Technological advances are enhancing the ability of developers to create VE's with visual, auditory, haptic, and even olfactory realism. Such VE's allow the military to train skills that are too costly, too dangerous, or are otherwise impossible to practice. The common assumption is that the more realistic the VE, the better the transfer of training to real world tasks. However, some aspects of task content and fidelity may result in stronger transfer of training than even the most high fidelity simulations. This has traditionally been determined by performance measurements compared before and after design iterations. Each time design modifications are made, end users are tested on the VE and their performance is compared to performance on the prior VE design. In such study, improved performance is assumed to be related to improved design. However, the specific aspects of design improvement that directly relate to transfer of

D.D. Schmorrow, L.M. Reeves (Eds.): Augmented Cognition, HCII 2007, LNAI 4565, pp. 186–194, 2007.
© Springer-Verlag Berlin Heidelberg 2007

training improvements have yet to be identified. Furthermore, this method of design focuses on trial and error, and is therefore, time consuming, undirected, and may result in false associations between performance and VE parameters. For example, unless each aspect of the new simulator design is introduced separately, it will not be known which design improvements bear the strongest significance to performance improvements. Thus, a more comprehensive assessment of the quality of interaction with a simulation based on changes in recordable brain and peripheral bioelectrical signals is needed to effectively identify the specific aspects of simulation that bare relevance to real world tasks.

2 Simulation Fidelity

One of the major questions simulation designers must address is the notion of "how much fidelity is enough?" Advances in sensor technology, automated data collection techniques, and the increased number of research and training questions requiring answers have helped drive the simulation industry to increased simulation fidelity. In theory, the notion is that the higher the simulation fidelity the more likely an operator is to behave in a similar fashion within the simulation as they would in the real world. Researchers using simulation techniques are *limited in practice to the potential benefits of increased simulation fidelity due to:*

- Cost and practical restrictions
- Simulation development resources (e.g. hardware, software, space requirements, etc)
- No guarantee that a particular level of simulation fidelity is sufficient enough to accurately depict the operating environment
- A limited understanding of the trade-offs between increases in simulation fidelity and operator behavior

2.1 Cost and Practical Restrictions

Simulation costs vary widely depending on the simulation requirements. Simulation costs can include those related to development; recruitment and compensation of operators; test plan development, management; simulation training; data collection, refinement, and analysis; and simulation validation and testing. Almost all of these factors increase overall project costs in conjunction with simulation fidelity increases. Very often higher fidelity simulations allow researchers to collect large amounts of data (e.g. terabytes in the case of physiological data). The complexity of these high fidelity simulations increases the requirements on data collection, refinement, and analyses of such projects.

2.2 Simulation Development Resources

Another factor potentially affecting the use of simulation design is the required developmental resources. Independent of the type of simulation (e.g. virtual environment (VE), human-in-the-loop (HITL) simulation, or fast-time simulation), it is most likely that the higher levels of simulation fidelity will require increases in development resources to run the simulation. These resources might include simulation hardware, software, training materials, confederates, simulation management, and/or simulation planning activities.

2.3 Simulation Fidelity Metrics

Historically, simulation fidelity has been described in subjective terms such as high, medium, or low which may or may not be related to the effectiveness of the simulation. For example, you can have low fidelity simulations which are highly effective for training and you can have high fidelity simulations which are ineffective for training purposes. Inherent within the use of simulations is the fact that simulations are just that – simulations, and therefore one can never simulate all aspects of the operating environment.

2.4 Limited Understanding of Simulation Trade-Offs and Operator Behavior

Today's simulations can include a very high level of realism based on technological advances in the areas of visual, auditory, haptic (e.g. motion), and olfactory systems. The research community is just beginning to understand the relationships between these simulation factors and the effects on operator behavior. In many cases, changes in simulated environments occur via trial and error and include multiple changes across any number of these perceptual and sensory systems. While this haphazard method might be justified within any single simulation, experimental confounds are created which limit the ability of researchers to determine the individual effects of any one simulation system change. For example, if a simulator's visual and haptic systems are "upgraded" to increase simulation realism, it is impossible to determine if operator performance changes (e.g. behavior, transfer of training, etc.) can be accounted for by the changes in the visual system, the haptic system, or both. The only valid conclusion that can be drawn from this example is that the operator performance changes occurred when both systems were altered. There is also evidence to support the notion that a sensitive change in a simulation system is required to elicit changes in operator behavior. For example, Burki-Cohen et al. (2003) reported that while an initial study of the potential benefits of adding motion to flight simulators had no effect with respect to pilot training and evaluation, a subsequent study reported that if the motion was of a particular type (enhanced hexapod motion), benefits of motion were observed.

3 Physiological Measures

The use of physiological measures in understanding human behavior has made significant progressions over the last few decades. The ability to collect multiple sources of physiological data, the advances in computing power, the decrease in physical size of apparatuses, and the ability to tie the scientific knowledge represented in the areas of human physiology with behavior and cognitive functioning have all contributed to these advances. Physiological measures can be categorized with respect to the particular human nervous system with which they are associated. Table 1 provides a breakdown of some of the more common physiological measures and their associated nervous system (Andreassi, 1995).

Table 1. Common Physiological Measures

Central Nervous System	Somatic Nervous System	Autonomic Nervous System
EEG (electroencephalogram)	EMG (electromyogram)	Heart Rate
ERP (event-related potential)	EOG (electroculography)	Blood Pressure
		Electrodermal Activity
		Pupil Response
		Blood Volume

To overcome some of the simulation fidelity issues discussed in Section 2, we propose the use of physiological measures to support the determination of simulation fidelity requirements. Many of the approaches used to date have focused on attempting to maximize the transfer of training during simulations based on the ability to elicit desired behaviors from operators during simulations with the notion that these behaviors would transfer to the real world applications. Our approach hypothesizes that transfer of training will be maximized and simulation fidelity requirements best determined by trying to match operator's physiological responses in the simulated environment with those collected in the real environment.

3.1   Characteristics of Physiological Measures

There are several important characteristics of physiological measures which can affect their use in both real-world and simulated environments. These include:

- Invasiveness – to what degree can the physiological measure be collected in a noninvasive manner?
- Cost – what is the cost of data collection? Required equipment? Data reduction and analysis?
- Sensitivity – how sensitive is the measure to changes in the environment? Operator behavior? Artifacts?
- Validity – does the physiological measure have validity (face, construct, etc.)?
- Practicality – can the physiological measure be accurately measured in both the real-world and simulated environments?
- Reliability – does the physiological measure provide repeatable results?

Each of these characteristics must be considered when collecting data using physiological measures. Any measure which is significantly lacking a desired level of even one of these factors should be used with caution during research.

3.2   Use of Physiological Measures in Simulated and Real-World Environments

Scientists and researchers have been collecting physiological measures in a variety of simulated environments at an increasing rate. These studies speak not only to the ability to reliably collect such data but also the feasibility within simulated environments.

A recent effort (Meehan et al., 2002) was conducted to determine which physiological measures could induce presence within a virtual environment. Participants were placed into a virtual environment which induced a particular level of stress associated with the fear of falling through a hole in the floor. The authors hypothesized that this stressful environment should evoke significant changes in the three physiological measures monitored during their experience in the virtual environment (heart rate, skin conductance, and skin temperature) compared to the training room (baseline condition). In this study, heart rate was the most effective objective physiological measure for detecting changes in presence. Another study, by Baumgartner et al (2006), recorded the EEGs of adolescents and adults searching for changes in brain activity associated with being placed in a virtual environment. Differences in brain activity and reported spatial presence levels were higher for the children than for the adults based on differences in brain development between the two groups.

NASA has been conducting research using physiological measures for the application of adaptive automation for pilots. The notion is that measurement of EEG can be correlated with attention levels. This research also has been extended to include the measurement of ERPs (Prinzel et al, 2001). Backs (1999) has conducted work examining heart period changes between low- and high-workload flight tasks to determine which physiological measures of cardiovascular activity are most related to changes in pilot performance. Ahlstrom and Friedman-Berg (2006) recorded eye movement activity for air traffic controllers during simulation to predict cognitive workload levels. Specifically, this effort examined two different weather-display designs and measured blink rate and pupil diameter to determine which display design was causing increases in cognitive workload.

Based on the difficulty of collecting physiological measures outside of the lab, there has not been as much reported data for real-world physiological studies as there has been for simulation studies. One exception is the work conducted by Healey and Picard (2004) in which drivers' stress levels were recorded using electrocardiogram (EKG), electromyogram (EMG), skin conductance and respiration measures as drivers followed a set route. The results found that skin conductivity and heart rate correlated best with stress levels. Results from real-world studies such as this can help simulation designers determine which physiological measures are best correlated between simulated and real-world environments to maximize the likelihood of transfer of training and to aid in determining simulation acquisition decisions.

One of the large programs related to this area of work is called Augmented Cognition or AugCog. The AugCog program, initially funded by DARPA in 2001, focuses on determining an operator's cognitive state in real-time through continuous physiological measures. The development of systems to detect an operator's cognitive state through physiological measures can provide researchers with an understanding of when operator's are stressed, overloaded, or receiving information in a medium (visual, auditory, tactile, etc) which is not optimal for task completion. The notion is the computer can adapt based on the operator's physiological state and adjust its operations to best support the operator. This might be in the form of automating a task, allocating a task to another operator, or altering the information flow or medium in which the data is conveyed to the operator. One contractor is working with the US Army and has begun to test the augmented cognition concept in the field. One field study monitored 8 soldiers as they performed three tasks. These tasks, identifying targets, monitoring mission tasks, and maintaining radio counts of mission participants, were completed under three conditions (low workload, high workload with no aiding, and high workload with the communications scheduler). The communications scheduler was a decision aid designed to present pre-programmed messages to the soldiers based on their cognitive state measured by physiological indices. Early findings illustrated that use of the communications scheduler was responsible for a 94% increase in monitoring mission tasks and a 36% increase in recalling radio counts of mission participants (Lawlor, 2006). Readers who are interested more in the AugCog program and its related concepts are directed to see Schmorrow (2005).

4 SISO Simulation Framework

SISO (Simulation Interoperability Standards Organization) met in 1999 to discuss how to address issues associated with simulation fidelity and its historically subjective nature. The group aimed at developing more objective measures by which simulation fidelity could be defined, measured, and discussed. One of the outputs from the SISO Fidelity Experimentation Implementation Study Group (Roza, Gross, and Harmon, 2000) was a conceptual framework for understanding and applying fidelity. This original framework is presented in Figure 1.

Roza et al. point out some interesting facts regarding this framework which are worth mentioning.

- The framework is centered on the notion that a physical reality is the basis from which all of the known reality can be obtained.
- The known reality is the source from which simulation requirements are known and is the source from which the simulation's fidelity is known.

These two facts highlight the fact that the current framework is based on concepts that are primarily related to the physical features of the simulation and the ability of the simulation designers to understand both the physical reality and known reality to best determine the appropriate level of simulation fidelity required. It also highlights the separation of the simulation requirements and the simulation capabilities. As will be explained in the next section, our approach marries these two together to maximize the likelihood that the simulation requirements and simulation capabilities are equivalent – thus reducing the risk that the simulation designers spent resources on simulation capabilities that are not required.

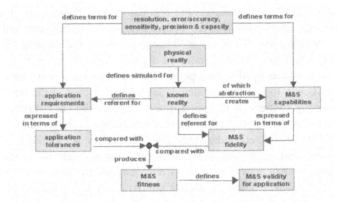

Framework for Understanding & Applying Fidelity

Fig. 1. Simulation Fidelity (from Roza et al., 2000)

4.1 Current Simulation Design Approach Versus Physiological-Based Simulation Design Approach

Table 2 provides both a linear breakdown of the general steps involved in current simulation design and requirements definition and our proposed approach based on physiological measurement. There are some very major differences between these two approaches beyond the obvious stated difference between simulation design based on physical characteristics only and simulation design based on operator physiology. These inherent pros and cons are provided in Table 3 for the two approaches.

Table 2. Comparison on Current Simulation Design Approach and Proposed Physiological-Based Simulation Design Approach

Current Simulation Design Approach	Physiological-Based Simulation Design Approach
• Observe real-world environment	• Measure physiology in real world environment under varying conditions
• Design simulated environment as close to real-world as possible	• Design simulated environment as close to real-world environment as feasible focusing on both physical and physiological aspects
• Validate simulated environment through testing (primarily face validity)	• Validate simulated environment through operator testing
• Conduct simulations	• Determine which simulation characteristics are correlated with physiological measures
• Measure operator performance differences in simulation	• Redesign simulation as needed
• Measure transfer of training to real world	• Conduct simulations
• Redesign simulation as needed	• Measure transfer of training to real world

Table 3. Pros and Cons of Two (2) Simulation Design Approaches

	Pros	Cons
Current Simulation Design Approach	• Design based on observable physical characteristics • High face validity	• Simulator redesign is costly • Based on trial-and-error approach • Relationship of simulation design to transfer-of-training is unknown • Easy to alter behavior
Physiological-Based Simulation Design Approach	• Design based on observable physical characteristics and physiological measurements • High face and construct validity • Outcome of simulation redesigns is known • Relationship of simulation design to transfer-of-training is known • Allows for better allocation of simulation resources • Difficult to alter physiological responses results in more accurate data	• More difficult to measure physiology in the real world • Data collection complexity is increased

5   Summary

This paper outlines a new approach to determining fidelity simulation design using physiological-based measures. A physiologically-based system capable of dynamically detecting changes in operator behavior and physiology throughout a VE experience and comparing those changes to operator behavior and physiology in real-world tasks, could potentially determine which aspects of VE fidelity will have the highest impact on transfer of training. We have outlined many of the pros and cons to using the current simulation design approach compared to a physiological-based approach. We understand that a comparative analysis between the two simulation design approaches is required to measure the actual differences in performance outcomes. Such performance outcomes could include: 1) cost, 2) transfer of training, 3) return on investment (ROI), 4) program risk, and 5) reliability and validity measures.

The development of training assessment and guidance tools that utilize operator behavior and physiology to determine VE effectiveness and transfer of training are needed. Successful development of the proposed training assessment technologies have application within commercial and industrial training facilities where a decreased time to transition untrained employee to trained employee has significant cost savings, as well as training positions in which performance errors could result in injury to a human, such as the medical field (i.e. surgical simulation training) and jobs involving operation of dangerous or expensive equipment. Similarly, provided the developed system is affordable and easy to use, students at all levels would benefit from an accelerated learning system.

References

1. Ahlstrom, U., Friedman-Berg, F.: Controller scan-path behavior during severe weather avoidance (DOT/FAA/TC-06/07). Atlantic City International Airport, NJ: Federal Aviation Administration William J. Hughes Technical Center (2006)
2. Andreassi, J.L.: Psychophysiology: Human Behavior & Physiological Response, 3rd edn. Lawrence Erlbaum Associates, Hillsdale (1995)
3. Backs, R.W., Lenneman, J.K., Sicard, J.L.: The Use of Autonomic Components to Improve Cardiovascular Assessment of Mental Workload in Flight. International Journal of Aviation Psychology 9(1), 33–47 (1999)
4. Baumgartner, T., Valko, L., Esslen, M., Jancke, L.: Neural Correlate of Spatial Presence in an Arousing and Noninteractive Virtual Reality: An EEG and Psychophysiology Study. Cyberpsychology and Behavior 9(1), 30–45 (2006)
5. Bürki-Cohen, J., Go, T.H., Chung, W.W., Schroeder, J., Jacobs, S., Longridge, T.: Simulator Fidelity Requirements For Airline Pilot Training And Evaluation Continued: An Update On Motion Requirements Research. In: Proceedings of the 12th International Symposium on Aviation Psychology (April 2003)
6. Healy, J.A., Picard, R.W.: Detecting Stress During Real-World Driving Tasks Using Physiological Sensors. Cambridge Research Laboratory, HP Laboratories Cambridge, MA. HPL-2004-229 (2004)
7. Lawlor, M.: Human-computer interface gets personal (2006). Signal, July 2006 issue. Accessed on Feb 15th, 2007 at http://www.afcea.org/signal/articles/templates/SIGNAL_Article_Template.asp?articleid=1159& zoneid=188
8. Meehan, M., Insko, B., Whitton, M., Brooks, F.P.: Physiological measures of presence in stressful virtual environments. In: Proceedings of the 29th Annual Conference on Computer Graphics and Interactive Techniques, San Antonio, TX (2002)
9. Prinzel, L.J., Pope, A.T., Freeman, F.G., Scerbo, M.W., Mikulka, P.J.: Empirical Analysis of EEG and ERPs for Psychophysical Adaptive Task Allocation. NASA-Langley Technical Report No. TM-2001-211016 (2001)
10. Schmorrow, D.D. (ed.): Foundations of Augmented Cognition. Lawrence Erlbaum Associates, Hillsdale (2005)
11. Roza, Z.C., Gross, D.C., Harmon, S.Y.: Report Out of the Fidelity Experimentation Implementation Study Group, 00S-SIW-151. In: 2000 Spring Simulation Interoperability Workshop (SIW), Simulation Interoperability Standards Organization (SISO), Orlando, FL (2000)

Reverse Engineering the Visual System Via Genetic Programs

Diglio A. Simoni

Bioinformatics Program, Research Computing Division
RTI International, Research Triangle Park, NC 27709 USA
dsimoni@rti.org

Abstract. We propose a datamining based method for automated reverse engineering of search strategies during active visual search tasks. The method uses a genetic program (GP) that evolves populations of fuzzy decision trees and selects an optimal one. Previous psychophysical observations of subjects engaged in a simple search task result in a database of stimulus conditions and concomitant measures of eye gaze information and associated psychophysical metrics that globally describe the subjects search strategies. Fuzzy rules about the likely design properties of the components of the visual system involved in selecting fixation location during search are defined based on these metrics. A fitness function that incorporates both the fuzzy rules and the information in the database is used to conduct GP based datamining. The information extracted through the GP process is the internal design specification of the visual system vis-à-vis active visual search.

Keywords: active visual search, eye tracking, psychophysics, fuzzy logic, datamining, knowledge discovery, genetic programming, reverse engineering.

1 Introduction

A fuzzy logic control process is proposed that automatically selects the next fixation location during the target discovery periods of active visual search. This paper describes an automated procedure for extracting from a database the rules that drive this control process in the form of an optimal fuzzy decision tree.

Section 2 provides the motivation of the work within the context of active visual search. Section 3 briefly introduces a *perception-based* model that incorporates the decision tree structure. Section 4 briefly discussed the ideas of fuzzy logic and the decision tree approach. Section 5 describes how genetic programs can be used to obtain an optimal decision tree for active visual search. Finally Section 6 provides a summary.

2 Active Visual Search

Visual search is accomplished through a cycle of fixations and visual scene analysis interrupted by saccades. A saccade produces a rapid shift of gaze, redirecting the

D.D. Schmorrow, L.M. Reeves (Eds.): Augmented Cognition, HCII 2007, LNAI 4565, pp. 195–200, 2007.

fovea onto a new point in the visual scene. As the visual system reacquires the image data, the visual scene is remapped onto primary visual cortex governed by the physical limits imposed by the retinal photoreceptor layout and the cortical magnification factor. These limits constrain the representational power of cortex and, therefore, also constrain the computational capabilities of the visual system. Given that the results of these visual computations lead to the behaviors that we observe, it is important to understand how these and other physical constraints affect performance. Previous search studies have generated many insights into this question using various visual search tasks [1][2][3][4][5][6][7][8][9]. Although some of these studies permitted eye movements, the focus of the studies has been to characterize processes that occur during a fixation. More recent studies have specifically addressed what processes characterize visual search when the eye is allowed to move freely about the image [10][11][12][13][14][15][16][17][18][19].

With each new fixation, the amount of cortical machinery associated with the various stimuli, as well as the linear distances between their cortical representations, varies as the image information is mapped in a nonlinear fashion onto primary visual cortex to reflect the new foveal direction in the visual scene. Previous studies of active visual search in the monkey have shown that target detection probability is invariant with respect to set size after applying a proper scaling for stimulus density. This has been shown by appropriately normalizing the probability functions for different set sizes using a metric constructed from an average measure of local stimulus density obtained from each set size [16]. This observation, together with those obtained from lateral masking or crowding studies that describe the severe degradation in identification performance that results from the introduction of flanking distractors around a given target [20][21][22], suggests the importance of local stimulus density upon target detection. In addition, evidence exists from monkey studies that active, feature-selective, attentive mechanisms can adjust the effective stimulus density. Under conditions where the display can be segmented by color differences, the nearest neighbor distances and/or cortical separations that account for performance are determined by stimuli containing the target color—essentially discounting the remaining stimuli from consideration [16][23].

3   *Perception-Based* Model of Active Visual Search

A characterization of these types of constraints has been used to derive an extensible *perception-based* model of visual search that incorporates a novel selection mechanism for new fixation location based on hybrid neural network and fuzzy logic representations. The system's design principles are derived from psychophysical observations of human search performance during active visual search tasks via the use of real-time infrared eye trackers [24]. Psychophysical experiments [25] were used to obtain probabilistic measures of both stimulus and neuroanatomical features that constrain the human visual system's real-time selection of image regions during the target discovery periods of active visual search. Mathematical precisiation tools were used to recast the psychophysical metrics as fuzzy predicates in order to develop a rule set which drives a robust model of human search performance that takes into account the intrinsic uncertainty of sensory processing. The final result is a search mechanism composed of a bottom-up neural network-based sensory processing model (which computes a saliency across the image) coupled to a top-down fuzzy expert system (FES) model of search decision processes which can help both test as well as predict human search performance given precisely controlled sets of visual stimuli [26].

A question that remains is whether the search model optimally describes the eye movement strategies that the human foveated visual system uses when faced with the problem of finding a target in a visual scene. One method for assessing performance is to compare the computational model against an ideal Bayesian observer model [27][28][29][30] for search tasks. An ideal observer model uses precise knowledge about the statistics of the visual stimuli that contain the same spectral characteristics as natural scenes, and about its own sensory constraints, to make eye movements that gain the most information about target location. It has been found that humans achieve nearly optimal search performance when compared with a Bayesian ideal observer [17]. Ideally, a computational model of visual search should approach the same level of performance. In this paper we describe a genetic programming approach to evolve populations of fuzzy decision trees and select an optimal model that reverse engineers the search strategies employed by humans engaged in visual search tasks.

4 Datamining a Fuzzy Decision Tree

The particular approach to fuzzy logic used by the *perception-based* model is the fuzzy decision tree [31]. Fuzzy decision trees are extension of the classical AI concept of decision trees. The leaf nodes (those with degree one) are labeled with co-called root concepts. Nodes of degree greater than one are labeled with composite concepts, which are constructed from the root concepts using logical operations like "AND", "OR" and "NOT". Each root concept has a fuzzy membership function associated with it. These membership functions are derived from examination of the psychophysical metrics obtained during visual search task experiments. The membership functions for composite concepts are constructed from those assigned to the root concepts using fuzzy logic connectives and modifiers. The structure of the decision tree determines its function. This structure is equivalent to determining the rules that characterize the control process that drives the selection of fixation location during active visual search. Discovering this structure can be recast as a datamining problem because it is equivalent to efficiently extracting valuable non-obvious information embedded in a large quantity of data [32]. Data mining consists of three steps: a) the construction of a database that represents truth which in this case consists of the list of stimuli presented to subjects during active visual search tasks and their behaviors, including eye gaze information and associated psychophysical measures; b) the use of a data mining function to extract the valuable information which in this paper is a genetic program; and c) the determination of the value of the information obtained in the second step, which in our case is the comparison of the resulting model against both the ideal observer model and human performance measures.

5   Discovering the Fuzzy Decision Tree's Structure Using a Genetic Program

A genetic program is a problem independent method for automatically creating graphs that represent computer programs, mathematical expressions, digital circuits, and the like. The procedure evolves a solution using Darwin's principle of survival of the fittest. The method is based on an optimization procedure that manipulates a string of numbers in a manner loosely similar to how chromosomes are modified in biological evolution [33]. An initial population made up of strings of numbers is selected arbitrarily, perhaps at random. A string of numbers is a "chromosome" and each number in the string is a "gene." A set of chromosomes forms a population. Each chromosome represents parameters that optimize a "fitness function". In our case the chromosomes are the fuzzy predicates of a decision tree that describes search strategies during active visual search. The fitness function is a performance index that is to be maximized. In our case the fitness function is a comparison of the performance of the decision tree, given a particular stimulus display and a current fixation location in that display, with the behavioral data recorded during experiments using the same experimental conditions.

The operation of the genetic algorithm proceeds in steps. Beginning with the initial population, "selection" is used to choose which chromosomes should survive to form a "mating pool." Chromosomes are chosen based on how fit they are relative to the other members of the population. More fit individuals end up with more copies of themselves in the mating pool so that they will more significantly effect the formation of the next generation. Next, two operations are taken on the mating pool. First, "crossover" (which represents mating, the exchange of genetic material) occurs between parents. In crossover, a random spot is picked in the chromosome, and the genes after this spot are switched with the corresponding genes of the other parent. In our case, this is equivalent to sub-tree exchange between two decision trees. Following this, "mutation" occurs. Mutation is a change of the value of a randomly selected gene. After the crossover and mutation operations occur, the resulting strings form the next generation and the process is repeated. Another process known as "elitism" is also employed. Elitism consists of copying a certain number of fittest individuals into the next generation to make sure they are not lost from the population. Finally, a termination criterion is used to specify when the algorithm should stop, e.g., when a preset maximum number of generations has been reached or the fitness has not changed significantly in a certain number of generations.

6   Summary

A fuzzy logic based algorithm for optimal construction of decision trees that describe search strategies during active visual search is under is under development. A method for automatically determining fuzzy decision tree structure, and hence the related fuzzy if-then rules from a large behavioral database is discussed. This method uses a genetic program, an algorithm that automatically evolves other computer programs or mathematical expressions.

References

1. Cameron, E.L., Tai, J.C., Eckstein, M.P., Carrasco, M.: Signal detection theory applied to three visual search tasks—Identification, yes/no detection and localization. Spatial Vision 17, 295–325 (2004)
2. Duncan, J., Humphreys, G.W.: Visual search and stimulus similarity. Psychological Review 93, 433–458 (1989)
3. Eckstein, M.P., Thomas, J.P., Palmer, J., Shimozaki, S.S.: A signal detection model predicts the effects of set size on visual search accuracy for feature, conjunction, triple conjunction, and disjunction displays. Perception & Psychophysics 62, 425–451 (2000)
4. Palmer, J., Verghese, P., Pavel, M.: The psychophysics of visual search. Vision Research 40, 1227–1268 (2000)
5. Strasburger, H., Harvey, L.O., Harvey Jr., L.O., Rentschler, I.: Contrast thresholds for identification of numeric characters in direct and eccentric view. Perception & Psychophysics 49, 495–508 (1991)
6. Treisman, A.: Features and objects: The fourteenth Bartlett memorial lecture. Quarterly Journal of Experimental Psychology: A Human Experimental Psychology 40, 201–237 (1988)
7. Treisman, A.M., Gelade, G.: A feature-integration theory of attention. Cognitive Psychology 12, 97–136 (1980)
8. Wolfe, J.M., Cave, K.R., Franzel, S.L.: Guided search: An alternative to the feature integration model for visual search. Journal of Experimental Psychology: Human Perception and Performance 15, 419–433 (1989)
9. Wolfe, J.M., O'Neill, P., Bennet, S.C.: Why are there eccentricity effects in visual search? Visual and attentional hypotheses. Perception & Psychophysics 60, 140–156 (1998)
10. Findlay, J.M., Brown, V., Gilchrist, I.D.: Saccade target selection in visual search: The effect of information from the previous fixation. Vision Research 41, 87–95 (2001)
11. Findlay, J.M., Gilchrist, I.D.: Eye guidance and visual search. In: Underwood, G. (ed.) Eye guidance in reading, driving and scene perception, pp. 295–312. Elsevier, Oxford (1998)
12. Geisler, W.S., Chou, K.L.: Separation of low-level and high-level factors in complex tasks: Visual search. Psychological Review 102, 356–378 (1995)
13. Hooge, I.T., Erkelens, C.J.: Adjustment of fixation duration in visual search. Vision Research 38, 1295–1302 (1998)
14. Maioli, C., Benaglio, I., Siri, S., Sosta, K., Cappa, S.: The integration of parallel and serial processing mechanisms in visual search: Evidence from eye movement recording. European Journal of Neuroscience 13, 364–372 (2001)
15. Motter, B.C., Belky, E.J.: The guidance of eye movements during active visual search. Vision Research 38, 1805–1815 (1998)
16. Motter, B.C., Belky, E.J.: The zone of focal attention during active visual search. Vision Research 38, 1007–1022 (1998)
17. Najemnik, J., Geisler, W.S.: Optimal eye movement strategies in visual search. Nature 434, 387–391 (2005)
18. Shen, J., Reingold, E.M., Pomplun, M., Williams, D.E.: Saccadic selectivity during visual search: The influence of central processing difficulty. In: Hyönä, J., Radach, R., Deubel, H. (eds.) The mind's eyes: Cognitive and applied aspects of eye movement research, pp. 65–88. Elsevier, Amsterdam (2003)
19. Zelinsky, G.J., Rao, R.P.N., Hayhoe, M.M., Ballard, D.H.: Eye movements reveal the spatiotemporal dynamics of visual search. Psychological Science 8, 448–453 (1997)

20. Bouma, H.: Interaction effects in parafoveal letter recognition. Nature 226, 177–178 (1970)
21. Pelli, D.G., Palomares, M., Majaj, N.J.: Crowding is unlike ordinary masking: Distinguishing feature integration from detection. Journal of Vision, 4 12(12), 1136–1169 (2004)
22. Toet, A., Levi, A.: The two-dimensional shape of spatial interaction zones in the parafovea. Vision Research 32, 1349–1357 (1992)
23. Motter, B.C., Holsapple, J.W.: Cortical image density determines the probability of target discovery during active search. Vision Research 40, 1311–1322 (2000)
24. Simoni, D.A., Motter, B.C.: Human search performance is a threshold function of cortical image separation. Journal of Vision 3(9), 228 (2003)
25. Motter, B.C., Simoni, D.A.: The roles of cortical image separation and size in active visual search performance. Journal of Vision, 7 2(6), 1–15 (2007)
26. Simoni, D.A.: Augmented Search for Clinical and Research Images. In: Dylan, D., Morrow, K., Stanney, M., Reeves, L. (eds.) Foundations of Augmented Cognition, 2nd edn., pp. 329–332. Strategic Analysis, Inc. (2006)
27. Green, D.M., Swets, J.A.: Signal Detection Theory and Psychophysics. Wiley, New York (1966)
28. Burgess, A.E., Ghandeharian, H.: Visual signal detection. II. Effect of signal-location identification. Journal of the Optical Society of America A 1, 906–910 (1984)
29. Geisler, W.S., Diehl, R.L.A: A Bayesian approach to the evolution of perceptual and cognitive systems. Cognitive Science 27, 379–402 (2003)
30. Kersten, D., Mamassian, P., Yuille, A.L.: Object perception as Bayesian inference. Annual Review of Psychology 55, 271–304 (2004)
31. Tsoukalas, L.H., Uhrig, R.E.: Fuzzy and Neural Approaches in Engineering (Chapter 5). John Wiley and Sons, New York (1997)
32. Bigus, J.P.: Data Mining with Neural Nets (Chapter 1). McGraw-Hill, New York (1996)
33. Goldberg, D.E.: Genetic Algorithms. In: Search, Optimization and Machine Learning, Addison-Wesley, London (1989)

EEG-Based Estimation of Mental Fatigue:
Convergent Evidence for a Three-State Model

Leonard J. Trejo[1], Kevin Knuth[2], Raquel Prado[3], Roman Rosipal[4], Karla Kubitz[5],
Rebekah Kochavi[6], Bryan Matthews[7], and Yuzheng Zhang[3]

[1] Quantum Applied Science and Research, 999 Commercial Street, Suite 205, Palo Alto,
CA 94303, USA
ltrejo@quasarusa.com
[2] Department of Physics, University at Albany, Albany, NY, 12222 USA
kknuth@albany.edu
[3] Department of Applied Mathematics and Statistics, University of California, 1156
High Street, Santa Cruz, CA 95064, USA
raquel@ams.ucsc.edu
[4] Austrian Research Institute for Artificial Intelligence, Freyung 6/6, A-1010 Vienna, Austria
roman.rosipal@ofai.at
[5] Dept. of Kinesiology, Towson University, Towson, MD, 21252 USA
kkubitz@towson.edu
[6] QSS Group, Inc., MS269-3, Moffett Field, CA 94035-1000 USA
rkochav@mail.arc.nasa.gov
[7] Mission Critical Technologies, Inc., MS269-3, Moffett Field, Ca 94035-1001 USA
bmatthews@mail.arc.nasa.gov

Abstract. Two new computational models show that the EEG distinguishes
three distinct mental states ranging from alert to fatigue. *State 1* indicates
heightened alertness and is frequently present during the first few minutes of
time on task. *State 2* indicates normal alertness, often following and lasting
longer than State 1. *State 3* indicates fatigue, usually following State 2, but
sometimes alternating with State 1 and State 2. Thirty-channel EEGs were recorded from 16 subjects who performed up to 180 min of nonstop computer-
based mental arithmetic. Alert or fatigued states were independently confirmed
with measures of subjects' performance and pre- or post-task mood. We found
convergent evidence for a three-state model of fatigue using Bayesian analysis
of two different types of EEG features, both computed for single 13-s EEG epochs: 1) kernel partial least squares scores representing composite multichannel
power spectra; 2) amplitude and frequency parameters of multiple single-
channel autoregressive models.

Keywords: EEG, mental fatigue, alertness, computational models, situation
awareness, performance monitoring, augmented cognition.

1 Introduction

There are countless high-risk occupations today, such as in aviation, transportation,
aerospace, military, medicine, and industrial settings, in which fatigued individuals

D.D. Schmorrow, L.M. Reeves (Eds.): Augmented Cognition, HCII 2007, LNAI 4565, pp. 201–211, 2007.
© Springer-Verlag Berlin Heidelberg 2007

routinely operate complex, automated systems. This undesirable state of affairs has contributed to more than a few well publicized—and many not so well publicized—disasters [1]. Recent analyses of crash data confirm that fatigue and inattention pose the greatest known risks to automobile driver and passenger safety, surpassing all other known risks including alcohol and secondary tasks such as cell-phone usage [2]. Accordingly, there continues to be much scientific interest in assessing, monitoring, and predicting fatigue [3],[4],[5],[6].

The risk of errors or accidents in such jobs could be reduced with the aid of automated systems that detect, diagnose and mitigate occupational fatigue. Designs for such automated fatigue-monitoring systems, or AFMS, have been proposed, and their accuracy in research settings has increased dramatically in the last few years. It is highly probable that AFMS will soon be reliable enough for general deployment. Future AFMS may even predict the likelihood of fatigue seconds to minutes before its onset. Most AFMS designs combine physiological or behavioral measures, such as brain activity (EEG), cardiac measures, eye-tracking, pupil size, lid closure, head tilt, or muscle activity (EMG), with intelligent computational systems to estimate present levels of fatigue. Of all these measures, the EEG may be the most informative measure of fatigue, because it is directly related to neuronal activity in the cerebral cortex and is also the key clinical method used for automated classification of sleep stages, which are related to some aspects of fatigue.

Researchers interested in using EEG features to classify mental activity have typically administered a stimulus, recorded EEG, and then applied statistical or machine-learning algorithms to classify EEG features into one or more 'states' (e.g., fatigued/ not fatigued/ high mental workload/ low mental workload). Gevins et al. [7] were among the first to attempt to develop an online, EEG-based drowsiness detector. Based on automated sleep scoring research, they developed a computer program which did a spectral analysis on the EEG data and calculated the ratios of delta to alpha, and theta to alpha activity. Calculated ratios were compared to 'drowsiness threshold' ratios previously calculated and these comparisons were used to estimate operator state. Gevins et al. tested their computerized drowsiness detector on EEG recordings from 31 individuals and found that 84% of testing, epochs were identified as drowsy both by expert scorers and by the drowsiness detector.

We consider the success of drowsiness detection to be akin to sleep staging, which has also been successfully performed by automated systems [8]. However, we are primarily concerned here with *mental fatigue in awake subjects*, which we define as the unwillingness of alert, motivated subjects to continue performing mental work [9]. In this way, mental fatigue differs from the other factors that also impair operator functioning, including sleepiness, lack of motivation, monotony, lack of training, and physical fatigue. The most consistent finding in prior EEG studies is that mental fatigue-related manipulations are associated with increased theta band power at the midline frontal location (i.e., Fz) and decreased alpha band power at one or more parietal locations (e.g., P7 and P8) [10],[11],[12],[13],[14].

As in other studies, we measured continuous EEG during a task, segmented the EEG, and analyzed the power spectral density of the segments to produce features that could be used to assess the effects of mental fatigue on ongoing brain activity. For overall tests of fatigue effects, we focused our measurements on the frontal midline theta band (4-8 Hz) activity and parietal alpha band (8-13 Hz) because these bands respond systematically to changes in operator state [15]. However, we used the power spectral density estimates at all EEG frequencies and electrodes to create algorithms which accurately classify mental fatigue using single EEG epochs in individual subjects. More specifically, we developed and cross-validated algorithms for classifying 13-s long segments of EEG activity according to fatigue. Indeed, such classifiers were highly successful, usually between 90% and 100% accurate in classifying EEG epochs [16],[17].

Our initial hypothesis was that a classifier could be trained to recognize features of EEG recordings made during periods known to be alert or fatigued by using independent measures of fatigue. These measures included mood estimates, performance and time on task. We examined the hypothesis that the application of such a classifier to EEG epochs from states in which the fatigue level was not known would produce an orderly output, with values of EEG features lying in the range between those of the known fatigued and alert EEG epochs used to train the classifier. Indeed the output of such classifiers indicated an orderly progression of classification scores from alert to fatigued states over time on a task known to induce fatigue [17].

In this paper, we consider the hypothesis that transitions from alert to fatigued states may not be entirely smooth or continuous, much like the quasi-categorical stages of sleep. To do this we examine two different feature extraction methods and statistical models to describe EEG features over a wide range of time, spanning from initial alert conditions to final fatigued conditions. In particular we consider whether the distributions of classification features are more consistent with two-state or three-state models of fatigue and alertness. We find that in a majority of subjects, the data appear to be more consistent with a three-state model than a two-state model.

2 Methods

2.1 Summary of Methods from the Prior Study

A detailed description of experimental and analytical methods for the prior study, from which the current study data were obtained, has been submitted for publication and is available on line [18]. Briefly, data were collected from 16 participants recruited from the San Francisco Bay Area community. The participants included 12 males and 4 females with a mean age of 26.9 y (SD = 7.4 y). Subjective moods were indexed by the Activation Deactivation Adjective Checklist (AD-ACL [19]) and the Visual Analogue Mood Scales (VAMS [20]). Observed behavior included ratings of activity and alertness from videotaped recordings of each participant's performance. The performance measures were response time (RT) and response accuracy. The physiological measures were derived from spontaneous EEGs and EOGs.

Participants sat in front of a computer with the right hand resting on a 4-button keypad and performed arithmetic summation problems, consisting of four randomly generated single digits, three operators, and a target sum (e.g., 4+7–5+2=8), which were displayed on a computer monitor continuously until the subject responded. The participants: a) solved the problems, b) decided whether their 'calculated sums' were less than, equal to, or greater than the target sums provided, c) indicated their decisions by pressing the appropriate key on the keypad. The keypad buttons were labeled "<," "=," and ">," respectively. Subjects were told to answer as quickly as possible without sacrificing accuracy. After a response, there was a 1 s inter-trial interval, during which the monitor was blank. Participants performed the task until either they quit from exhaustion or 3 h had elapsed. All participants performed the task for at least 90 min and eleven participants completed the maximum 3-h period.

During the task, the EEG was recorded continuously using 32 Ag/AgCl electrodes embedded in a Quik-Cap™ (Compumedics USA, El Paso, TX). The reference electrodes were averaged mastoids and the ground electrode was located at AFz. Vertical and horizontal electrooculograms (VEOG and HEOG) were recorded using bipolar pairs of 10 mm Ag/AgCl electrodes (i.e., one pair above and below the left eye; another pair to the right and to the left of the orbital fossi). Impedances were maintained at less than 5 kΩ for EEG electrodes and less than 10 kΩ for EOG electrodes. The EEG was amplified and digitized with a calibrated 64-channel Synamps™ system (Compumedics USA, El Paso, TX), with a gain of 1,000, sampling rate of 500 s^{-1} and a pass band of 0.1 to 100 Hz, then digitized and stored on magnetic and optical media.

Participants: a) were given an orientation to the study, b) read and signed an informed consent document, c) completed a brief demographic questionnaire (age, handedness, hours of sleep, etc.), d) practiced the arithmetic task for 10 minutes, and e) were prepared for EEG and EOG data collection. They then completed the pretest self-report measures (i.e., the AD-ACL and VAMS) and performed the mental arithmetic task until either three hours had elapsed or they were unwilling to continue. After the task, they completed post-test self-report measures and were debriefed.

The EEGs were: a) submitted to an algorithm for the detection and elimination of eye-movement artifact, b) visually examined and blocks of data containing artifact were manually rejected, c) epoched around the stimulus (i.e., from −5 s pre-stimulus to +8 s post -stimulus), d) low pass filtered (50 Hz; zero phase shift; 12 dB/octave roll off), and e) submitted to an automated artifact rejection procedure (i.e., absolute voltages > 100 μV). The overall single-epoch rejection rate was 47%. The 'cleaned and filtered' epochs were decimated to a sampling rate of 128 Hz. EEG power spectra were estimated with Welch's periodogram method at 833 frequencies from 0-64 Hz.

2.2 Prior Classification Procedures

We classified single EEG epochs using kernel partial least squares decomposition of multichannel EEG spectra coupled with a discrete-output linear regression classifier (KPLS-DLR [21]). Through extensive side-by-side testing of EEG data, Rosipal et al. found that KPLS-DLR was just as accurate as KPLS-SVC, which uses a support vector classifier for the classification step. KPLS selects the reduced set of orthogonal basis vectors or "components" in the space of the input variables (EEG spectra) that maximizes covariance with the experimental conditions. DLR finds the linear hyperplane in the space of KPLS components that separates the classes. In a pilot study, and in our present data, we found that the first 15 minutes on task did not produce mental fatigue, whereas mental fatigue was substantial in the final 15 minutes. So we randomly split EEG epochs from the first and last 15-min periods into equal-sized training and testing partitions for classifier estimation. Only the training partition was used to build the final models. The number of KPLS components in the final models was set by five-fold cross-validation. The criterion for KPLS-DLR model selection was the minimum classification error rate summed over all cross-validation subsets.

2.3 Statistical Modeling Procedures

The first model we tested was an extension of our earlier work with the KPLS-DLR classifiers trained using multichannel EEG spectra to distinguish alert and fatigue states [16],[17]. The features of this classifier are components that linearly combine the set of multi-channel EEG power spectral densities and represent each EEG epoch with a single score, much like the components of factor analysis or principal components analysis. The KPLS component scores of consecutive 13-s EEG epochs recorded during the mental arithmetic task were analyzed using Bayesian optimal data-based binning methods [22]. To make the problem computationally stable with the limited data available, we used only the scores of the first KPLS component (the component of greatest covariance with the fatigue states identified in the training set of EEG epochs).[1]

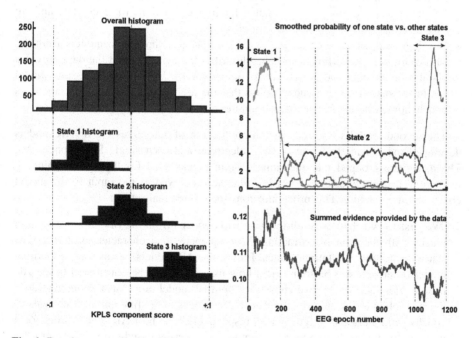

Fig. 1. Development of optimal binning classifier for 3-state model in Subject 13. From upper left to lower left: Overall histogram of KPLS scores across all 15-min blocks. Histogram and evidence (bar graph under histogram) for each of three states. Upper right to lower right: Smoothed quality of evidence for each state vs. the other two states for single EEG epochs spanning the entire session (time also increases from left to right). Summed evidence provided by the data as a function of EEG epochs.

---

[1] In prior tests, we had already found that most of the discriminatory power for mental fatigue lies in the first KPLS component and that often, only a single component is necessary.

The specific procedure involved four main steps (also illustrated in Fig. 1):

1. First, the optimal histogram of the entire task session was computed, and this served to delineate the number of histogram bins, and their positions for further analysis.
2. The data were then broken into blocks of 15-min duration, and optimal bins were computed for each block. For two-state models, a characteristic set of blocks was chosen as exemplars for each state: State 1 (alert) and State 3 (fatigued). For three-state models an additional characteristic set of blocks was chosen as exemplars for State 2 (normal). The set for State 2 was chosen by eye, and the first and last blocks were always included in the sets of blocks for States 1 and 3 respectively. There are ways we could automate the choice of blocks for each state in the future.
3. Then for each set of exemplar data, another histogram-style density model was generated to be used as a model of the likelihood function. Note that this is not exactly a histogram, since empty bins are given some probability mass, i.e., no bin may have a probability of zero. We used the optimal bins derived from the KPLS scores and some heuristics to generate likelihood functions for either two or three fatigue states. We now have estimated likelihood functions for each state and we assume equal a priori probabilities for all states.
4. We then computed the evidence for the two-state or three-state models from the sum of the likelihood functions. This describes the evidence that the data provides about a given state and allows for a comparison of the two- or three-state model fits to the data. Low evidence implies that the algorithm cannot be sure about its conclusions, whereas high evidence implies confidence.

The second model we tested was an application of autoregressive or AR models developed independently for each EEG electrode and each single EEG epoch [23]. The data were grouped into the same 15-min blocks used for the optimal binning method. The 13-s epochs of the EEG time series served as the input to the model construction procedure. This procedure consists of three main steps:

1. We first fit AR models to all the 13-s EEG epochs from the first and last 15-min blocks with the goal of extracting the frequencies that characterize alert/fatigue states or alert/normal/fatigue states. Fitting the AR models means that an optimal model order needs to be found (i.e., how many lags will be considered in the AR model). For each subject we chose the "optimal model order" as the one that does the best job in terms of correctly classifying epochs in the first and last intervals as epochs from alert and fatigue states, respectively. The best AR model order for a given individual is chosen using an optimality criterion based on which order does the best in terms of discriminating fatigue and alert states, i.e., discriminating between epochs from the first and final blocks in the EEG frequency range averaging over all the EEG channels recorded.
2. We then proceeded to select which channels do best in terms of correctly classifying alert and fatigue epochs in the first and last blocks. This was done by applying the k-means clustering method with two (or three) classes to all the frequencies and

moduli[2] of the AR models fit to the EEG epochs from the 15-min blocks. Specifically, we used data from the first and last 15-min blocks and grouped them into 3 clusters using k-means. We labeled the alert cluster as the one that had the best performance in terms of classifying epochs from the first 15-min and the "fatigue cluster" as that that had the best performance (measured as classification accuracy). The remaining cluster was labeled as the normal cluster. We hypothesize that some epochs recorded after the first 15-min and prior to the last 15-min would belong to this new cluster. Then, the accuracy of this classification method is computed for each channel. Finally we retained only the channels that had a minimally acceptable accuracy of $X\%$, where X varied with the subject. Different values of X were considered; based on our analyses across subjects, $X \in (60; 85)$ was suggested.

3. Once the channels were selected, we ran the classifier for the remaining epochs and for each epoch computed the probability of fatigue and alert (or fatigue, alert, and normal) states using the combined information provided for the channels chosen in Step 2. This was done by giving the same weight to all the channels.

3 Results

3.1 Relevant Results in the Prior Study

Detailed results and statistics in the prior study appear in a preceding report [18]; only summaries of the most relevant results will appear here. The AD-ACL data indicated that time on task led to decreased general activation (i.e., self-reported energy) and preparatory arousal (i.e., self-reported calmness) and increased general deactivation (i.e., self-reported tiredness). The VAMS subscale scores (i.e., afraid, confused, sad, angry, energetic, tired, happy, and tense) did not significantly change with time on task (i.e., pretest vs. posttest), suggesting that time on task, despite its effects on activation and arousal, did not influence moods. Significant effects of time on task for behavioral observations indicated that there was a linear decrease in alertness and a linear increase in activity. Within-subjects contrasts also showed a significant linear increase in RT with time on task. There were no significant effects of time on task for response accuracy. Our prior analysis showed that time on task was linked with progressive increases in frontal midline theta and parietal midline alpha power.

3.2 KPLS Classification Results from the Prior Study

We applied the KPLS-DLR classification procedure to EEG recordings from 14 of the 16 subjects (two subjects had too few EEG epochs for model estimation). The EEG epochs were synchronized with the onset of each math problem, extending from –5 s to +8 s relative to each stimulus onset. We also reduced the likelihood of electromyogram artifacts by low-pass filtering the EEG with either an 11-Hz or 18-Hz cutoff. For each subject we constructed a KPLS-DLR model using either linear or nonlinear kernel functions and selected the best model as described above. Classification accu-

---

[2] The characteristic roots of the AR model are described in terms of their frequencies and moduli. The amplitude of each frequency in the power spectrum is a function of the moduli. We fitted an AR model to each epoch and computed the roots of the characteristic AR polynomial at the posterior mean of the AR coefficients.

racies across both classes for 18-Hz filtered EEG ranged from 91.12 to 100% (mean = 98.30%). The corresponding range for 11-Hz filtered EEG was 89.53 to 98.89% (mean = 98.30%). The number of KPLS components ranged from 1 to 4 (mean 2.77) for 18-Hz EEG and from 1 to 5 (mean 3.76) for 11-Hz EEG.

3.3 Optimal Binning Classification Results

We applied the optimal binning procedure to the KPLS scores for each subject and compared the histograms and quality of evidence for 2-state and 3-state models (Fig. 1). In every case (n=14) the evidence for the three-state model was greater than the evidence for the two state model (Fig. 2).

3.4 AR Model Classification Results

We applied the AR classifier construction method to the EEG epochs across all 15-min blocks for each subject, comparing the model fits and classification accuracy for 2-state and 3-state models. Subjects 2 and 14 were not included due to insufficient EEG epochs for the analyses. In 9 of the 12 remaining cases, a 3-state model was superior to a 2-state model (Fig. 3).

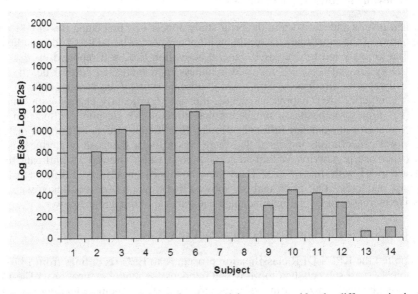

Fig. 2. The quality of 3-state models vs. 2-state models was gauged by the difference in the log of the evidence for the models. In all subjects tested, this difference was large, ranging from 60.8 log units for Subject 13 to 1795.3 log units for Subject 5. Subjects are ordered 1 to 14 by the log evidence for their 2-state model. Subjects 7-14 had relatively high baseline evidence for a 2-state model. For these subjects, the range for improvement that could be obtained with a 3-state model was more limited than for the Subjects 1-6, who had relatively less 2-state model evidence.

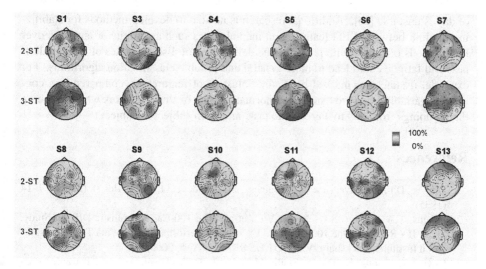

Fig. 3. Accuracies of 2-state and 3-state AR-model based classifiers for 12 subjects (S2 and S14 were omitted). Each topographical plot depicts the accuracy of classification as a function of electrodes. The overall accuracy may be controlled by exclusion of channels that do not meet minimal accuracy criteria. In 9 of the 12 subjects, the accuracy of the 3-state model exceeded that of the 2-state model.

4 Discussion

We considered the main hypothesis that EEG features drawn from a long and tiring mental arithmetic task are better explained by three-state models of mental fatigue than by two-state models. Previously, we had found that the accuracy of a two-state KPLS-DLR classification of single-trial EEG epochs ranged from 90% to 100% with a mean of 97% to 98% [18]. While the performance of these classifiers was highly accurate for single EEG epochs and may serve as the basis for monitoring mental fatigue in operational settings, they do not fully illuminate the underlying structure of fatigue states over time. In this study we found that both optimal binning methods and AR-model based classifiers of EEG features distinguish three distinct states: State 1 appears to be one of brief, but heightened alertness, being present when subjects were fresh, but giving way to State 2 after 15 to 45 minutes on task. State 2 typically lasted longer than State 1, and corresponded to the main body of time on the task. We provisionally consider State 2 to be a state of "normal" alertness, which is distinct from heightened alertness. State 2 is also distinct from State 3, which appeared later in the task, and overlapped with the end-state of fatigue.

Some important implications for future studies are underscored by our results. First, as others have found [24],[25], EEG classification algorithms benefit greatly by being both individualized and multivariate. The development of more general models, which apply to a broad set of subjects or tasks, will require considerable additional research. For example, a well-known problem in the applied EEG community is that the performance of classification algorithms from day to day, or at different times of day is unstable [26]. Additional research is needed to develop methods for stabilizing the link between EEG features and mental states such as fatigue or alertness over long periods of time. Quite possibly, the delineation of discrete states of mental alertness and fatigue could lead to more general and reliable classification algorithms. For example, if states are marked by distinct clusters of features, as compared to a continuous variable, then we can devise normalizations of those features which preserve the groupings from day to day, task to task, and even subject to subject.

References

1. Dinges, D.F.: An overview of sleepiness and accidents. J. Sleep Res. 4 (Suppl), 4–14 (1995)
2. Dingus, T.A., Klauer, S.G., Neale, V.L., et al.: The 100-Car Naturalistic Driving Study, Phase II - Results of the 100-Car Field Experiment Performed by Virginia Tech Transportation Institute, Blacksburg, VA, DOT HS 810 593 (April 2006)
3. Gevins, A., Leong, H., Du, R., Smith, M.E., Le, J., DuRousseau, D., et al.: Towards measurement of brain function in operational environments. Biol. Psychol. 40, 169–186 (1995)
4. Kennedy, J.L.: Some practical problems of the alertness indicator. In: Floyd, W.F., Welford, A.T. (eds.) Symposium on Fatigue. Oxford, England: H. K. Lewis & Co (1953)
5. Wilson, G.F., Fisher, F.: The use of cardiac and eye blink measures to determine flight segment in F4 crews. Aviation, Space and Environmental Medicine 62, 959–962 (1991)
6. Russo, M.B., Stetz, M.C., Thomas, M.L.: Monitoring and predicting cognitive state and performance via physiological correlates of neuronal signals. Aviation, Space, and Environmental Medicine 76, C59–C63 (2005)
7. Gevins, A.S., Zeitlin, G.M., Ancoli, S., Yeager, C.L.: Computer rejection of EEG artifact. II. Contamination by drowsiness. Electroencephalography and Clinical Neurophysiology 42, 31–42 (1977)
8. Agarwal, R., Gottman, J.: Computer-assisted sleep staging. IEEE Trans. Biomed. Eng. 48, 1412–1423 (2001)
9. Montgomery, L.D., Montgomery, R.W., Guisado, R.: Rheoencephalographic and electroencephalographic measures of cognitive workload: analytical procedures. Biological Psychology 40, 143–159 (1995)
10. Fairclough, S.H., Venables, L., Tattersall, A.: The influence of task demand and learning on the psychophysiological response. Intl. J. of Psychophysiology 56, 171–184 (2004)
11. Gevins, A., Smith, M.E.: Detecting transient cognitive impairment with EEG pattern recognition methods. Aviation, Space and Environmental Medicine 70, 1018–1024 (1999)
12. Gevins, A., Smith, M.E., McEvoy, L., Yu, D.: High-resolution EEG mapping of cortical activation related to working memory: Effects of task difficulty, type of processing, and practice. Cerebral Cortex 7, 374–385 (1997)
13. Hankins, T.C., Wilson, G.F.: A comparison of heart rate, eye activity, EEG and subjective measures of pilot mental workload during flight. Aviation, Space, and Environmental Medicine 69, 360–367 (1998)
14. Smith, M.E., McEvoy, L.K., Gevins, A.: The impact of moderate sleep loss on neurophysiologic signals during working-memory task performance. Sleep 25, 784–794 (2002)
15. Gevins, A., Smith, M.E., Leong, H., McEvoy, L., Whitfield, S., Du, R., et al.: Monitoring working memory load during computer-based tasks with EEG pattern recognition methods. Human Factors 40, 79–91 (1998)

16. Trejo, L.J., Kochavi, R., Kubitz, K., Montgomery, L.D., Rosipal, R., Matthews, B.: Measures and models for estimating and predicting cognitive fatigue. In: Forty-fourth Annual Meeting of the Society for Psychophysiological Research, Santa Fe, New Mexico, USA (October 20-24, 2004)

17. Trejo, L.J., Kochavi, R., Kubitz, K., Montgomery, L.D., Rosipal, R., Matthews, B.: Measures and models for predicting cognitive fatigue. In: Caldwell, J.A., Wesensten, N.J. (eds.) Biomonitoring for Physiological and Cognitive Performance During Military Operations. In: Proceedings of Symposium OR05 Defense and Security, 28 March-1 April 2005, Kissimmee, FL, Proceedings of SPIE, 5797, pp. 105–115 (2005)

18. Trejo, L.J., Kochavi, R., Kubitz, K., Montgomery, L.D., Rosipal, R., Matthews, B.: EEG-based estimation of mental fatigue (2006). Available on-line at: http://publications.neurodia.com/Trejo-et-al-EEG-Fatigue-2006-Manuscript.pdf

19. Thayer, R.E.: Activation-Deactivation Adjective Check List: Current overview and structural analysis. Psychological Reports 58, 607–614 (1986)

20. Stern, R.A.: Visual Analogue Mood Scales. Odessa, FL: P.A.R. Inc. (1997)

21. Rosipal, R., Trejo, L.J., Matthews, B.: Kernel PLS-SVC for Linear and Nonlinear Classification. In: Proceedings of ICML-2003, Washington, DC, pp. 640–647 (2003)

22. Knuth, K.H.: Optimal data-based binning for histograms. Manuscript submitted (2006)

23. Prado, R., Zhang, Y.: AR-based probabilistic EEG classifier. Technical report prepared for the ERTAS Project. NASA Ames Research Center, Moffett Field, CA (2005). Available online at http://www.ams.ucsc.edu/ raquel/cognitive

24. Galbraith, G.C., Wong, E.H.: Moment analysis of EEG amplitude histograms and spectral analysis: Relative classification of several behavioral tasks. Perceptual and Motor Skills 76, 859–866 (1993)

25. Smith, M.E., Gevins, A., Brown, H., Karnik, A., Du, R.: Monitoring task loading with multivariate EEG measures during complex forms of human-computer interaction. Human Factors 43, 366–380 (2001)

26. Wilson, G.F., Russell, C.A.: Operator functional state classification using multiple psychophysiological features in an air traffic control task. Human Factors 45(3), 381–389 (2003)

Augmenting Task-Centered Design with Operator State Assessment Technologies

Karl F. Van Orden[1], Erik Viirre[1], and David A. Kobus[2]

[1] Naval Health Research Center
[2] Pacific Science and Engineering

Abstract. Task-Centered Design (TCD) of human-system interfaces focuses on supporting the user throughout all phases of tasks, from initiation to completion. TCD typically requires software that monitors aspects of system information to trigger tasks, develop user-friendly information sets, propose task solutions and actions, and confirm actions as directed and approved by the operator. The operator monitors tasks awaiting completion on a Task Manager display. We demonstrate that moment-to-moment operator workload monitoring is greatly facilitated by TCD. Workload estimates were obtained every 2-min over the course of a 35-min test session during an air defense command and control scenario. Workload was readily modeled by the task loading, and the density of track icons on the display. A second study related the unitary workload estimates to NASA TLX workload subscales. Unpublished data from our laboratory indicated that eye activity measures (e.g., blink frequency and duration, pupil diameter, fixation frequency and dwell time) did not improve the estimation of workload. These findings indicate that at least for well-executed TCD systems, eye tracking technologies may be best employed to monitor for fatigue and incongruities between the focus of attention and task requirements. Recent findings using EEG hold promise for the identification of specific brain signatures of confusion, orientation, and loss of situational awareness. Thus the critical element of human directed systems is good initial design. Understanding of the task will lead to system automation that can balance the workload of the operator, who is functioning in a normal state. However, physiological monitoring will be most useful if operators veer beyond their normal conditions and are confused, overloaded, disoriented or have other impairments to their abilities. By detecting the operator's loss of function early, inappropriate operator inputs can potentially be avoided.

1 Introduction

The purpose of this paper is twofold. The first is to describe how using appropriate design strategies can improve user performance and significantly mitigate task overload conditions. The second purpose is to describe how psychophysiological and augmented cognition methods can best be employed when "task management" design principles are used. There has been a plethora of studies examining how psychophysiological variables (e.g., electro-encephalogram, eye activity, heart rate and variability) change as a function of task workload (see Craven et al., 2006;

D.D. Schmorrow, L.M. Reeves (Eds.): Augmented Cognition, HCII 2007, LNAI 4565, pp. 212–219, 2007.
© Springer-Verlag Berlin Heidelberg 2007

Poythress et al., 2006; Wilson & Russell, 2003), and how these measures might be used to monitor human operators for task overload and/or used to trigger automated processes. Using a Task-Centered Design approach, where an operator's job is broken down into tasks, and subsequently decomposed into sub-tasks, provides an opportunity to accurately measure moment-to-moment workload fluctuations (see Campbell et al., 2003; Osga & Van Orden, 2000). Without the requirement to monitor for workload, the application of operator state monitoring technologies can focus on issues such as confusion, stress, drowsiness, and forms of loss of spatial and situational awareness. Some recent findings are discussed which suggest that neural markers for some of the aforementioned cognitive states may be detected when they are not consciously perceived.

The main tenet of Task Centered Design (TCD) is supporting the user through all task phases. This involves not only presenting the typical "alert" to the user, but building information sets specific to the task, recommending a course of action, and confirming that the task was completed upon approval of the actions by the system. For example, within the air traffic control domain, specific tasks might be triggered when automation detects aircraft within distances appropriate to begin descent for landing, when aircraft are on courses that will result in violated spatial separation, or when spacing for approach controllers could be improved. In such instances, a task icon could appear on a task manager display, which when selected, would open a task information set window. The information set pertinent for the task would contain background information and, more importantly, a recommended course of action for approval. For a spacing task, the recommended course of action might be to reduce the speed of a particular aircraft. Upon operator approval of the course of action, the system would generate an electronic voice command to the aircraft (or alternative data link) with new air speed guidance.

Several benefits of task managed design include an active (vice passive) control of the processes by the user, support through most or all phases of the task, and the potential ability of automation to forecast critical events and time tasks so that they occur sooner than would otherwise. In other words, tasks could be forecasted by the system and presented to the user prior to their typical trigger points as potential backlogs are detected. This form of task management is important, as it is well know that operators have a poor sense of time management under high workload conditions.

2 Task Centered Design and Workload Assessment

Van Orden (2001) examined how workload correlated with task loading and other variables in a 40-minute simulated air defense task hosted upon a TCD work station. Tasks included reporting new air contacts, reporting identification changes to air contacts, and sending messages to aircraft entering restricted areas. The participants provided subjective workload estimates every two minutes, and these were matched with the number of tasks appearing on a task manager display, and the number of air contacts present on the display. Results indicated that the number of air contacts present on the display combined with the number of tasks present correlated significantly with the subjective workload measure. For several participants, psychomotor activity (mouse clicks to reveal information about specific air contacts) was also included, in order to capture work associated with gaining awareness of the air contacts on the display. Data for one such participant is included in Figure 1. (Not shown are number of air contacts on the display, which varied between 15 and 30, and increased steadily over the duration of each experimental session.). Combined measures of contact density, number of tasks to be performed, and psychomotor activity accounted for 70 percent of the variance in subjective workload estimates for this participant. Interpolating subjective workload from the aforementioned variables produced a moment-to-moment workload series, shown in Figure 2.

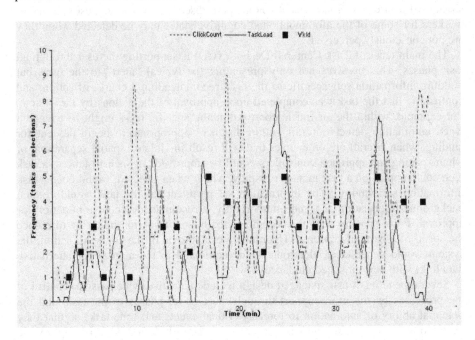

Fig. 1. Plot of frequency of mouse click activity (dashed line), task load (solid line) and subjective workload estimates (filled squares) over time in minutes for the test session

The preceding description on deriving a moment-to-moment workload time series from data easily obtained from system and user activity measures underscores two points: First, that task data from a TCD implementation is an important factor in the determination of workload. The second point is *that psychophysiological data would add little to improving the workload estimates*. However, data on the operator state could be very beneficial if applied for other purposes. It has been previously demonstrated that psychophysiological data would be useful for the determination of drowsiness (Van Orden, K.F., Jung, T-P., & Makeig, 2000;; Makeig & Jung, 1996) and loss of attentional focus (Makeig, Jung & Sejnowski, (2000). Recent findings suggest that brain activity and electroencephalographic (EEG) measures might provide information on cognitive states such as false memories (Garoff-Eaton, Slotnick, & Schacter, 2006; Schacter, Reiman, Curran et al., 1996) or spatial disorientation (Viirre et al., 2006). These findings indicate that similar measures

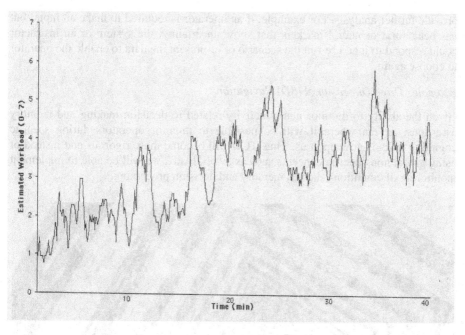

Fig. 2. Subjective workload for one participant based upon a regression model using psychomotor activity, task loading, and the number of aircraft on the display as input

might be capable of identifying such operator states as self-deception or loss of situation awareness; conditions beyond the normal scope of performance of trained operators. This type of monitoring could serve as a safe-guard, or used as a training tool, especially under grueling or stressful operating conditions, or in advanced training scenarios.

3 Uncertainty, Disorientation, and Self Deception

Schacter, Reiman, Curran et al., (1996) demonstrated that positron emission tomography (PET) recordings differed as a function of whether participants had accurately or falsely remembered words from a previously studied list. The PET activation differences between these conditions were greatest in the pre-frontal cortical regions of the brain. There were clear differences between correct assertions and incorrect ones. A rudimentary interpretation of this result was that in the incorrect assertion state, there was detectable neural activity reflecting uncertainty in the decision. Thus, as the subject was forced to make an assertion, there were clear differences between assertions that were made that were accurate and those that were wrong. The disconcordance of brain activation from conscious actions and underlying unconscious decision making has far reaching ramifications. An important practical application is that operator confusion or uncertainty can likely be detected. Thus, situations where an operator implements an input, but is uncertain about it, the operator, and their human or automated supervisors can be alerted to that state and provide further analysis. For example, if an operator is required to make an input, but has behavioral or neural markers that show uncertainty, the system or an instructor could respond to it and re-run the scenario or re-present the data to enable the operator to choose again.

Example: Three Dimensional (3D) Navigation

Given the ability to monitor neural activity related to decision making and memory assertions, an era where it will be possible to monitor operators during specific cognitive tasks is now upon us. Thus TCD will become more rigorous and instead of using global non-specific concepts such as "work load", we will be able to implement monitoring of conditions such as memory and decision processing.

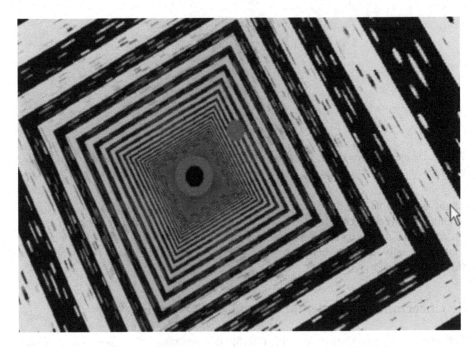

Fig. 3. Three Dimensional scene used during visual tracking task

Data from neural monitoring during a navigation task suggests an example. In Strychacz et. Al (2005), we had subjects carry out a tracking task while virtually traveling through a three-dimensional scene (See figure below). We then had subjects view another 3 dimensional scene that resulted in the onset of motion sickness. Monitoring neural patterns using high density EEG demonstrated a strong signature of Alpha wave and alpha harmonic peaks in the posterior mid-parietal region (See figure X below). These peaks were eliminated when the motion sickness appeared.

Further, we found similar neural activity changes in the same region during a navigation task where we implemented Schacter's paradigm (Viirre, et. al. 2006). Participants were asked to observe a rectilinear virtual environment on a computer screen (See Figure 3). The point of view of observer was randomly shifted and rotated

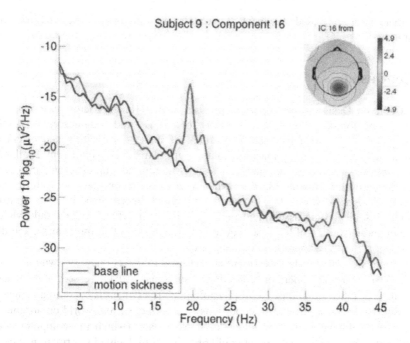

Fig. 4. Prominent power peaks at 20 and 40 Hz in ventral midline sources during the tracking (light colored line) that are suppressed during motion sickness (darker line)

and the subject was asked to keep track of their apparent compass heading. Randomly, the scene movement would stop and the subject was presented with a compass rose and a "lost button". They indicated which heading they believed they were facing or, if they were not confident of the heading, they pushed the "lost" button. Continuous EEG and eye movement data were recorded during the trials on 128 scalp and 2 eye channels. EEG activities were labeled "correct" (heading fashion to the data presented above in Figure 4. Similar to word recall tasks, frontal midline sources were found to show significant differences between correct and incorrect in the interval 500 ms after the button press, indicated within +/- 45 degrees), "incorrect" or "lost". Subjects were found to make incorrect heading assertions approximately 20-30% of the time, even though they were given the option to indicate they were lost. Significant differences between "correct" and "incorrect" responses were apparent in neural activity in ventral posterior midline sources in all subjects in the time interval 500 ms prior to the button response. These differences occurred in the alpha EEG frequency range in similar.

These results suggest that it may be possible to detect in near real-time neural activity markers of operator task attention to a three dimensional task and to the loss of that attention. Thus when training pilots to perform instrument maneuvers or when training radiologists to interpret moving three-dimensional images such as ultra sound, an automated augmented cognition system or an instructor would be able to detect when the operator was not on task. This information could be used to enhance task performance by notifying the trainee pilots to re-orient using navigation instruments; or provided feedback to trainee radiologists to re-establish their orientation.

4 Conclusion

Task Centered Design is an important process in the Human Factors component of systems development. The combination of TCD and augmented cognition technologies – used to detect neurophysiological state -- is exciting and offers the potential to improve human-machine interactions. However, significant challenges remain with regard to how an operator's state is monitored, and different approaches should be carefully examined in the earliest phases of system design. Careful task-centered design review of a system will yield more benefit than grafting neurophysiological state assessment onto an existing interface. TCD should yield a thorough understanding of the vast majority of system states that might arise, and then reveal opportunities to appropriately manage them.

Neurophysiological state assessment is best used to detect operators who are "out-of-range" for normal operator conditions: such as - overstressed, over-loaded, disoriented or other situations. Neurophysiological assessment is becoming refined in the ability to detect specific state conditions in a variety of real-world environments. Instead of a pilot being in a state of "high workload" (which the computer could already determine), state assessment could provide more detailed information such as; they are not correctly monitoring their three dimensional orientation. Such state assessments would provide greater opportunity for detecting and mitigating human-system failures.

As the technological advances occur, the difficulty in using these technologies will become designing paradigms for identifying the appropriate neural signals. For example, the operational aviation environment is vastly different from a laboratory setting. Two technologies that may offer some promise for real-time detection during operations on moving platforms: advanced electro-encephalography (EEG) and functional near infrared (fNIR) recording. EEG systems now incorporate miniature amplifiers at the electrode that greatly enhance signal to noise and reject local interference sources. Portable wireless EEG sets now exist. FNIR is a newer technology that can measure regional blood oxygenation changes in the outer layers of the cerebral cortex using infrared light. EEG and fNIR have been used to look for signatures related to GLOC and related phenomena. It provides reliably repeatable measures that are empirically useable if not perfectly correlated to known physiologic changes. Further, limited studies relevant to target detection and loss of SA can be carried out in functional magnetic resonance imaging (fMRI) systems. FMRI can be used with some simulations of disorienting conditions, but can not be applied to operational conditions. Fortunately, with its fine spatial resolution, it can greatly assist in identification of specific brain areas involved in motion processing and thus be used to compare data across subjects and further refine operational tools and measures.

References

1. Campbell, N., Osga, G., Kellmayer, D., Lulue, D., Williams, E.: A Human-Computer Interface Vision for Naval Transformation, SSC San Diego Technical Document 3183, (June 2003)
2. Craven, P.L., Belov, N., Tremoulet, P., Thomas, M., Berka, C., Levendowski, D., Davis, G.: Cognitive workload gauge development: comparison of real-time classification methods. In: Schmorrow, D.D., Stanney, K.M., Reeves, L.M. (eds.) Foundations of Augmented Cognition, pp. 75–84. Arlington, Virginia: Strategic Analysis (2006)
3. Garoff-Eaton, R.J., Slotnick, S.D., Schacter, D.L.: Not all false memories are created equal: The neural basis of false recognition. Cerebral Cortex 16, 1645–1652 (2006)
4. Makeig, S., Jung, T._P.: Tonic, phasic, and transient EEG correlates of auditory awareness during drowsiness. Cognitive Brain Research 4, 15–25 (1996)
5. Makeig, S., Jung, T.-P., Sejnowski, T.J.: Awareness during drowsiness: Dynamics and electrophysiological correlates. Can J Exp Psychol. 54(4), 266–273 (2000)
6. Osga, G.A, Van Orden, K.F.: Key User Support Technologies to Optimize Future Command Crew Efficiency, Naval Command, Control and Ocean Surveillance Center, RDT&E Division, August, San Diego, CA (2000)
7. Poythress, M., Berka, C., Levendowski, D.J., Chang, D., Baskin, A., Champney, R., Hale, K., Milham, L., Russell, C., Seigel, S., Tremoulet, P.D., Craven, P.: Correlation between expected workload and EEG indices of cognitive workload and task engagement. In: Schmorrow, D.D., Stanney, K.M., Reeves, L.M (eds.) Foundations of Augmented Cognition, pp. 75–84. Arlington, Virginia: Strategic Analysis (2006)
8. Schacter, D.L., Reiman, E., Curran, T., Sheng Yun, L., Bandy, D., McDermott, K.B., Roediger, H.L.: Neuroanatomical correlates of veridical and illusory recognition memory: Evidence from positron emission tomography. Neuron 17, 1–20 (1996)
9. Strychacz, C., Viirre, E., Wing, S.: The use of EEG to measure cerebral changes during computer-based motion sickness-inducing tasks. In: Proceedings of the SPIE vol. 5797, pp. 139–147 (2005)
10. Van Orden, K.F.: Monitoring Moment-to-Moment Operator Workload Unising Task Load and System-State Information. SSC Technical Report No. 1864. Space and Naval Warfare Systems Center, June, San Diego, CA (2001)
11. Van Orden, K.F., Jung, T-P., Makeig, S.: Combined eye activity measures accurately estimate changes in sustained visual task performance. Biological Psychology 52, 221–240 (2000)
12. Viirre, E., Wing, S., Huang, R-S., Strychacz, C., Koo, C., Stripling, R., Cohn, J., Chase, B., Jung, T-P.: EEG markers of spatial disorientation. In: Schmorrow, D.D., Stanney, K.M., Reeves, L.M (eds.) Foundations of Augmented Cognition, pp. 75–84, Arlington, Virginia: Strategic Analysis (2006)
13. Wilson, G.F., Russell, C.A.: Real-time assessment of mental workload using psychophysiological measures and artificial neural networks. Human Factors 45, 635–643 (2003)

Augmented Cognition and Cognitive State Assessment Technology – Near-Term, Mid-Term, and Long-Term Research Objectives

Leah M. Reeves[1], Dylan D. Schmorrow[2], and Kay M. Stanney[3]

[1] Potomac Institute for Policy Studies, 901 North Stuart Street, Suite 200, Arlington, VA 22203
[2] Office of Naval Research, 875 North Randolph Street, Suite 1425, Arlington, VA 22203-1995
[3] Universtiy of Central Florida, 4000 Central FL Blvd, Orlando, FL 32816-2993
lreeves@potomacinstitute.org, schmord@onr.navy.mil, kstanney@cfl.rr.com

Abstract. The 1st Augmented Cognition International (ACI) conference was held in July 2005 in conjunction with the HCI International conference in Las Vegas, Nevada. A full day working group session was held during this inaugural ACI conference to facilitate the development of an Augmented Cognition R&D agenda for the near- (1-2 years), medium- (within 5 years) and long-term (> 5 years). Working group attendees included scientists, developers, and practitioners from government, academia, and industry who were invited to participate based on their numerous years of experience and expertise in the Augmented Cognition and related fields. This article highlights key results of the workshop discussions that were focused on Cognitive State Assessment (CSA) R&D objectives, particularly with regard to the design and implementation of CSA tools and techniques.

Keywords: Augmented Cognition, human factors, cognitive state assessment, sensors, design, neuroergonomics, neurotechnologies, neurophysiological.

1 Introduction

In conjunction with the HCI International conference in Las Vegas, Nevada, the Augmented Cognition International (ACI) Society [1] held its first ACI Conference. During this inaugural ACI conference [3], a full day working group session was held to facilitate the development of an Augmented Cognition R&D agenda for the near- (1-2 years), medium- (within 5 years) and long-term (> 5 years). Working group attendees included scientists, developers, and practitioners from government, academia, and industry. Participants were invited based on their numerous years of experience and expertise in the Augmented Cognition and

D.D. Schmorrow, L.M. Reeves (Eds.): Augmented Cognition, HCII 2007, LNAI 4565, pp. 220–228, 2007.

related fields. The workshop was focused on three key Augmented Cognition science and technology (S&T) areas: Cognitive State Assessment (CSA), Mitigation Strategies (MS), and Robust Controllers (RC). This article highlights key results that emanated from the portion of the workshop discussions that were focused on CSA S&T research objectives, particularly with regard to the design and implementation of CSA tools and techniques. Future articles will highlight the overall results of the workshop with respect to all three Augmented Cognition S&T areas-- CSA, MS, and RC [8].

During the CSA portion of the workshop, attendees discussed, debated, and agreed upon a final definition of what constitutes a cognitive state sensor—*A cognitive state sensor (or suite of sensors) acquires physiological and behavioral parameter(s) that can be reliably associated with specific cognitive states, which can be measured in* <u>*real-time*</u> *while an individual or team of individuals is engaged with a system, where:*

- cognitive state is anything needing to be measured to base design decisions on it;
- cognitive or "functional" state is the moment-to-moment dynamic and functional capabilities (e.g., capacity, bottlenecks) of the human brain, and;
- cognitive or "functional" state has a causative / moderating / predictive relationship to a performance variable.

The following sections highlight the workshop's findings with regards to the identification of:

- the most important impediments government, academic, and industry scientists and practitioners must overcome in Augmented Cognition CSA research and development;
- the most important challenges to the effective design, use, and adoption of CSA tools and techniques;
- CSA design, development, and implementation successes that have been accomplished to date, and;
- future directions in the design and use of CSA tools and techniques.

2 Key CSA-Focused Results That Emanated from the Workshop

At the heart of Augmented Cognition applications is the ability to capture 'cognitive state' or 'operator functional state' as a source for driving system adaptation in real time and thus 'closing the loop' around the human [1], [2], [3], [4], [5], [6], [9]. Table 1 summarizes CSA technologies that have thus far been explored and successfully implemented by Augmented Cognition researchers and developers via proof-of-concept (e.g., small n, restricted tasks) prototypes of operational applications (e.g., unmanned aerial vehicle control station, smart vehicle system, fast mover jet simulation, and dismounted-mobile soldier operations) [2], [3], [5], [7].

Table 1. Summary of Maturing Augmented Cognition Technologies and Proven Implementations to Date (reprinted and adapted with permission [5])*

Sensors/Gauges (developed by who)	Use (Measures What / Implemented How)	Appropriateness for Mobile Applications
EDA (Electrodermal Activity)/GSR (galvanic skin response)-based Arousal & Cognitive Workload Gauge (Anthrotronix, Inc.)	*Provides estimates of arousal & general cognitive workload* • Implemented by Lockheed Martin Advanced Technology Laboratories (LMATL) in a command & control closed-loop application domain	Most appropriate for stationary users; not yet tested in mobile application domains or with mobile users
Electrocardiography (EKG, ECG)-based Arousal & Cognitive Workload Gauge (Anthrotronix, Inc.)	*Uses heart rate variability (HRV) measures to provide estimates of arousal & general cognitive workload* • Implemented by LMATL in a command & control closed-loop application domain	Most appropriate for stationary users; not yet tested in mobile application domains or with mobile users
Body Position/Posture Tracking (University of Pittsburgh)	*Posture shift data, head position, & head velocity are used to gauge levels of attention (i.e., engagement)* • Implemented by LMATL & Boeing in 2 different command & control closed-loop application domains • Implemented by DaimlerChrysler in a vehicular closed-loop application domain	Appropriate for stationary users in stationary or mobile application domains; not yet tested with mobile users & most likely would not be appropriate for such
Stress Gauge (Institute for Human and Machine Cognition [IHMC])	*Uses Video Pupillometry (VOG), High Frequency Electrocardiogram (HFQR ECGS), & Electrodermal Response (EDR) to track autonomic response to time-pressured, high workload tasks & to detect moment-to-moment cognitive stress related to managing multiple competing tasks & is thus good for measuring attention HIP bottleneck effects* • Implemented by Honeywell in closed-loop dismounted soldier application domains	May be appropriate for mobile users & stationary or mobile application domains

Table 1. (*continued*)

Arousal Meter Gauge (Clemson University)	*Uses interbeat interval (IBI) derived from ECG to track decrements in performance due to low arousal states in divided attention & vigilance tasks & is thus a good measure of attention human information processing (HIP) bottleneck effects* • Implemented by Honeywell in closed-loop dismounted soldier application domains • Implemented by Boeing in a command & control closed-loop application domain	May be appropriate for mobile users & stationary or mobile application domains
eXecutive Load Index (XLI Gauge) (Human Bionics, Inc.)	*Uses electroencephalography(EEG) measures to assess ability to allocate attentional resources during high workload, competing tasks & is thus a good measure of attention HIP bottleneck effects & general cognitive workload* • Implemented by Honeywell in closed-loop dismounted soldier application domains	May be appropriate for mobile users & stationary or mobile application domains
P300 Novelty Detector Gauge (City College New York [CCNY] / Columbia University)	*Uses EEG auditory P300 signals from frontal & parietal electrodes to track attentional resources used to attend to novel stimuli & is thus a good measure of attention HIP bottleneck effects* • Implemented by Honeywell in closed-loop dismounted soldier application domains	May be appropriate for mobile users & stationary or mobile application domains
Engagement Index Gauge (NASA/CCNY/ Honeywell)	*Uses EEG-based measures to track how cognitively engaged a person is in a task (level of alertness) & is effective at assessing attention HIP bottleneck effects associated with both sustained & divided attention tasks, particularly during low workload conditions* • Implemented by Honeywell in closed-loop dismounted soldier application domains	May be appropriate for mobile users & stationary or mobile application domains
New Workload Assessment Monitor	*Uses combined sensors to gauge general workload levels & estimate*	Most appropriate for stationary users; not

Table 1. (*continued*)

(NuWAM) combined EEG, ECG, EOG sensors (Air Force Research Laboratory [AFRL])	*executive function & attention HIP bottleneck effects* • Implemented by Boeing in a command & control closed-loop application domain	yet tested in mobile application domains or with mobile users
Fast functional near infrared (fNIR) device (Drexel University)	*Measures brain blood oxygenation & volume changes & is an effective tool for assessing spatial & verbal working memory HIP bottleneck effects* • Implemented by LMATL in a command & control closed-loop application domain	Most appropriate for stationary users but shows promise for mobile users & mobile application domains
Whole Head fNIR (Archinoetics)	*Measures brain blood oxygenation & volume changes & is an effective tool for assessing spatial & verbal working memory HIP bottleneck effects* • Implemented by Boeing in a command & control closed-loop application domain	Most appropriate for stationary users; not yet tested in mobile application domains or with mobile users
Pupillometry (EyeTracking, Inc.'s [ETI] Index of Cognitive Activity [ICA] system)	*Uses proprietary & patented techniques for estimating cognitive activity based on changes in pupil dilation & gaze & is a good measure of general cognitive workload & sensory input, attention & executive function HIP bottleneck effects* • Implemented by LMATL & Boeing in 2 different command & control closed-loop application domains	Most appropriate for stationary users; not yet tested in mobile application domains or with mobile users
Low Density EEG (Advanced Brain Monitoring, Inc.'s [ABM] 3, 6, or 9 channel cap)	*Uses a portable EEG cap, wireless transmitter, & B-Alert software to effectively estimate various types of cognitive states, namely: vigilance/arousal, workload, engagement, distraction/drowsiness, & working memory levels* • Implemented by LMATL in a command & control closed-loop application domain	May be appropriate for mobile users & stationary or mobile application domains
High density EEG	*Uses an event-related potential*	Appropriate for

Table 1. (*continued*)

(ElectroGeodesics, Inc.'s [EGI] 128 or 256 electrode net)	*(ERP) EEG-based system to estimate which & to what degree particular brain regions are invoked during task performance; may be an effective tool for assessing both verbal & spatial working memory & general cognitive workload* • Evaluated but not implemented by LMATL in their command & control closed-loop application	stationary users; not yet tested in mobile application domains or with mobile users & may be too cumbersome for such applications
DaimlerChrysler's EEG system (FIRST of Berlin, Germany)	*Uses EEG combined with EOG & electromyography (EMG) to assess low versus high workload levels & is effective at assessing sensory memory bottleneck effects* • Implemented by DaimlerChrysler in a vehicular closed-loop application domain	Appropriate for stationary users in stationary or mobile application domains; not yet tested on mobile users
Event Related Optical System [EROS] (University of Illinois)	*Uses fast optical imaging techniques to identify brain region signatures resulting from cued & non-cued attentional shifts during task performance & thus may be a good estimate of sensory, attention, & executive function HIP bottleneck effects* • Evaluated for potential implemented in Boeing's command & control closed-loop application domain	Appropriate for stationary users in stationary or mobile application domains; not yet tested with mobile users
Cognitive Monitor [CogMon] (QinetiQ)	*Uses behavioral measures from interactions with cockpit controls, EEG-based physiological measures, subjective measures, & contextual information to assess stress, alertness, & various workload levels & is effective at assessing all 4 HIP bottleneck effects* • Implemented in both a military fast-jet simulation & a command & control application environment • Planned for implementation efforts in support of Boeing's AugCog program in their command & control closed-loop application domain	Appropriate for stationary users in stationary or mobile application domains; not yet tested with mobile users

*Note: The above CSA technology list is by no means all-inclusive. For a thorough review of available sensors, see NATO report on Operator Functional State Assessment [10]. Further, many of these tools may be used individually or combined in various ways to assess multiple HIP bottlenecks, as well as other HCI task factors (e.g., context, environmental stress effects, etc.).

All of the workshop participants were in some way involved with one or more of the R&D efforts to develop and test the operational prototypes. Based on their experiences and lessons learned, the participants reported many varied issues regarding important challenges to the effective *design* of CSA tools and techniques, with a consensus being that basic sensor technology—a critical component of Augmented Cognition applications--will continue to require basic and applied research in many areas, including [5]:

- design of the sensors for ease of use, calibration, appropriate resolution/sensitivity, noise cancellation, and less invasiveness;
- better understanding of neurophysiological, psychological, and cognitive theories that should be driving sensor placement, data analysis, and subsequent 'cognitive load' and/or 'cognitive state' gauge derivation, and;
- determining appropriate experimental techniques in applied task settings to assess effectiveness of sensors to accommodate both general use settings and individual differences across task domains.

When discussing important challenges to the effective *use* of CSA technology, many of the above issues were reiterated, with additional points of concern being: wearability, ability to account and accommodate for day-to-day and individual user variability, and the development of appropriate signal processing algorithms and their interpretations [5]. Many of these same issues were again noted when discussing important challenges to the effective *adoption* of CSA technology, with additional points of concern including: user acceptance (e.g., ease of use, comfort, safety, trust, control) and fieldability, with value-added performance benefits and objectively measurable return on investments.

2.1 Short-, Medium-, and Long-Term CSA R&D Objectives

The workshop attendees identified the following short-term objectives as future directions to pursue in CSA technology R&D:

- Facilitate collaboration across agencies, institutions, and companies to identify challenges that have been overcome and the variety of approaches that have proven successful / unsuccessful – identify best practices.
- Address calibration issues–can use pure task classification be used or is complex task classification needed?
- How much tolerance to failure there be (e.g., high risk, high pay-off)?
- Need to develop step-wise approaches to the fidelity of CSA validation environments:
  - Identify what is the right/minimal amount of data needed to obtain reliable measures of cognitive state;

- Consider both central and peripheral physiological measures;
- Identify which sensors are appropriate for which tasks/ environments (i.e., scalable sensor suites);
- Consider next generation sensors;
- Identify potential sensor fusion issues (i.e., conflicting information from sensors) ;
- Need larger n and more experimentation to enhance reliability, validity, etc.

- How can such technology be implemented with teams of users (e.g., start developing proof-of-concept prototypes)?

The workshop attendees identified the following medium-term objectives as future directions to pursue in CSA technology R&D:

- Identify constraints on sensor technology by exploring the range of operational environments in which it can be feasibly and effectively implemented.
- Explore other domains such as usability testing, system design evaluation, learning/training, entertainment.
- Develop predictive models to complement real-time models; so Augmented Cognition systems can be proactive and not just reactive:

  - will require thorough understanding of task context and how to model too.

- Establish user models to understand issues of fatigue, individual differences and other human variables.
- Develop evaluation approaches that utilize months of data with the same users in efforts to improve classification and model building:

  - enough varied data will facilitate the building of more robust models for each individual;
  - models need to evolve over time (e.g., as person learns, fatigue, etc.)

- Develop tools and techniques that rely on less processing power and time for the analysis/classification of sensor data.
- How can we start validating CSA technology with teams of users?

Regarding long-term CSA R&D objectives, the main consensus was the need to truly operationalize CSA technologies and sensor technology in particular. The continued reduction in analysis/classification of sensor data (e.g., feature reduction) via validated tools and techniques will be needed to ensure CSA and supporting Augmented Cognition technologies are compact and light weight, minimally invasive, and easy to don/doff.

3 Conclusions

This article highlighted some key discoveries and challenges that may impact the future of CSA S&T. The results summarized here may be used as guidance for determining where present and future Augmented Cognition CSA R&D efforts should be focused to ensure the continued growth and maturity of the field and the robustness of its applications. These results may also be used as recommendations and suggested priorities for where national and supra-national institutions (e.g., DARPA, ONR, NIH, NSF) might focus additional funding resources to facilitate the development of new CSA research objectives. Such R&D will be necessary for operational Augmented Cognition S&T to realize its full potential in the near-, medium-, and long-terms.

References

1. Augmented Cognition International (ACI) Society: Official website, available at: http://www.augmentedcognition.org
2. Kobus, D.A., Brown, C.M., Morrison, J.G., Kollmorgen, G., Cornwall, R.: DARPA Improving Warfighter Information Intake under Stress–Augmented Cognition Phase II: The Concept Validation Experiment (CVE). DARPA/IPTO technical report submitted to CDR Dylan Schmorrow (October 31, 2005)
3. Schmorrow, D.D. (ed.): Foundations of Augmented Cognition, 1st edn. Lawrence Erlbaum Associates, Mahwah (2005)
4. Schmorrow, D.D., Kruse, A.A.: Augmented Cognition. In: Bainbridge, W.S. (ed.) Berkshire Encyclopedia of Human-Computer Interaction, pp. 54–59. Berkshire Publishing Group, Great Barrington (2004)
5. Schmorrow, D., Kruse, A., Reeves, L.M., Bolton, A.: Augmenting cognition in HCI: 21st century adaptive system science and technology. In: Jacko, J., Sears, A. (eds.) Handbook of human-computer interaction, 3rd edn. Lawrence Erlbaum Associates, New Jersey (in press) (2007)
6. Schmorrow, D., McBride, D. (eds.): Special Issue on Augmented Cognition. International Journal of Human-Computer Interaction, 17(2) (2004)
7. Schmorrow, D.D., Reeves, L.M.: 21st century human-system computing: augmented cognition for improved human performance. Aviat Space Environ Med (in press) (2007)
8. Schmorrow, D.D., Stanney, K.M., Reeves, L.M. (eds.): Foundations of Augmented Cognition, 4th edn. (in preparation)
9. Schmorrow, D., Stanney, K.M., Wilson, G., Young, P.: Augmented cognition in human-system interaction. In: Salvendy, G. (ed.) Handbook of human factors and ergonomics, 3rd edn. John Wiley, New York (in press) (2005)
10. Wilson, G.F., Schlegel, R.E. (eds.): Operator Functional State Assessment, NATO RTO Publication RTO-TR-HFM-104. Neuilly sur Seine, France: NATO Research and Technology Organization (2004)

Part II

Applications of Augmented Cognition

Augmented Cognition, Universal Access and Social Intelligence in the Information Society

Ray Adams and Satinder Gill

CIRCUA, Collaborative International Research Centre for Universal Access, School of
Computing Science, Middlesex University, Ravensfield House, The Burroughs, Hendon,
London NW4 4BT, United Kingdom
r.g.adams@mdx.ac.uk, s.gill@mdx.ac.uk

Abstract. The two concepts of universal access and augmented cognition have
both contributed significantly to providing the intended users of modern
information and communication technology with the necessary resources to
achieve enhanced interaction and performance. The two concepts share a
number of important features including; the improvement of user performance,
the use of concepts from cognitive psychology, a consideration of user
modelling, a user sensitive approach, support for customisation, personalisation,
adaptation and adaptive systems. They differentially emphasise; short term and
long term demands, ambient intelligence, ubiquitous computing, people with
disabilities, the Information Society and social skills. Since the present research
programme (CIRCUA) is focussed upon the design and evaluation of
universally accessible systems within a vocational context, the concepts of
universal access and augmented are both very relevant, though both need to
draw more upon the concept of social intelligence if they to tackle key issues of
the Information Society.

1 Introduction

The concept of universal access is presented in the following words [18] "In order for
these new technologies to be truly effective, they must provide communication modes
and interaction modalities across different languages and cultures, and should
accommodate the diversity of requirements of the user population at large, including
disabled and elderly people, thus making the Information Society universally
accessible, to the benefit of mankind". The concept of augmented cognition is
summarised as follows. "Augmented Cognition seeks to extend a user's abilities via
computational technologies that are explicitly designed to address and accommodate
bottlenecks, limitations, and biased in cognition, such as limitations in attention,
memory, learning, comprehension, visualization abilities, and decision making." [19].
Both universal access and augmented cognition draw upon currently developing
theories of human cognition that underpin both generic and specific cognitive user
models. The notion of cognitive overload is relevant to both universal access and
augmented cognition, as shown below, by means of user modelling approaches.
Conversely, user modelling is potentially a significant contributor to a better

D.D. Schmorrow, L.M. Reeves (Eds.): Augmented Cognition, HCII 2007, LNAI 4565, pp. 231–240, 2007.

understanding of both universal access and cognitive overload and can benefit from an involvement in both. However, though universal access explicitly states the need for a thorough consideration of the social aspects of the Inclusive Information Society, augmented cognition tends to focus more on the individual at work, though possessing the potential that is now being applied to social factors that mitigate or exacerbate overload [20]. Cognitive overload offers many possible ways to resolve problems of the Information Society. If that is so, then socially relevant concepts might support the application of augmented cognition to the solution of social or vocational problems within the context of universal access.

The present two goals are:

(a) the creation of accessible systems that support vocational and social effectiveness for people with special requirements and

(b) to build the joint contribution of cognitive and social factors into UA design methodologies for socially relevant systems.

2   The Concept of Universal Access

How will the concept of universal access support the achievement of these two goals? To create accessible systems to support vocational and social effectiveness for people with special requirements requires a number of contributory factors. The Universal Access framework provides (i) the motivation to achieve inclusivity in society, (ii) methods to model the key parameters of intended users, technology platforms, contexts of use and social contexts, (iii) evaluation methods for accessible, interactive systems, (iv) methodologies to design and build such systems and (v) the potential to include cognitive and social factors into UA design methodologies for socially relevant systems [1] [2] [3].

3   The Concept of Augmented Cognition

How will the concept of augmented cognition support the achievement of these two goals? Augmented cognition took the traditional concept of cognitive overload and revitalised it with the newer notion of augmented cognition, using sensors and gauges to identify and measure the cognitive states of an individual so that any overloads could be mitigated by the provision of computational technologies. Clearly, this is highly analogous to the case where individuals face accessibility problems and limitations that can be overcome, by the provision of appropriately designed, adaptive technology. Augmented cognition provides (i) a rational basis for the identification of different types of cognitive overload, (ii) ways to measure cognitive overloads, (iii) methods to identify and provide suitable methods of augmentation (Adams, 2006) and emerging ways to consider team and social factors that interact with overload problems [20]. If so, then there are clear synergies between these two user-centred concepts i.e. augmented cognition and universal access.

4   The Concept of Social Intelligence

The third and essential concept to introduce here is social intelligence. How can social intelligence contribute to the above two goals? How can social intelligence help us to develop the concepts of universal access and augmented cognition? The essence of social intelligence can be seen as knowledge in co-action [13]. These researchers define social intelligence as "the ability of actors and agents to manage their relationships with each other." These relationships would engage us with the different agents (the people, tools, artefacts and technologies in the environment).

5   The Improvement of User Performance

If the above considerations are correct, then universal access, augmented cognition and social intelligence can all contribute substantially to the performance of interactive systems in synergistic but distinct ways. But how do they interact in this context? Universal Access aims to provide the intended users with systems that are accessible to them in terms of their abilities and disabilities, their tasks, their hardware and software and context of use. Such systems should contain the capability for customisation, personalisation, adaptability (i.e. change before use) and adaptivity (i.e. change during use). Augmented Cognition provides systems that can actively adapt (i.e. change during use) on the basis of the detection and measurement of different types of cognitive overload. To do so, such augmentation technologies must have the capabilities to be adaptive and to learn about the users and their requirements proactively, providing projective guidance and support [20]. Since, performance enhancements can be seen as drawing upon both accessibility and cognitive overload, it is worth asking about the relationship between them. One way is to expand the notion of accessibility, as considered next, to envelop cognitive overload and social intelligence.

6   Accessibility and Cognitive Overload

Accessibility problems can occur in different ways. Here are five complementary ways to conceive of accessibility, including cognitive accessibility that is very closely related to cognitive overload and thus to augmented cognition.

There is the first level of accessibility (physical access). Consider that individuals or groups who are denied access face substantial disadvantage and are effectively on the wrong side of a massive digital divide in our societies, separating the haves from the have-nots. Denial of access to information resources, whether deliberate or accidental, occurs at a cost and occurs for a variety of reasons due, in part, to the multiple levels of accessibility that are required to function properly.

The second type of accessibility problem involves lack of access from local systems to the necessary resources and communications (connectivity access). Digital poverty may be associated with a lack of resources. Geographical or organizational location may be related to lack of connectivity or excessively high costs.

The third type of accessibility problem involves the design of the interface, an aspect of design that has been given more prominence by universal access. For people with disabilities (long term or short term), older adults and those with atypical perceptual skills, the present rash of interactive interfaces and Graphical User Interfaces (GUIs) often presents insurmountable accessibility problems.

The fourth type of accessibility problem (cognitive access) involves cognitive processes like navigation and comprehension. It is the nearest version of accessibility to cognitive overload. People will inevitably vary in levels of education, culture, IST experience etc. Such variations may render the navigability of a system problematic or the contents of such a system inaccessible. In addition, problems occur with attention, memory, learning, visualization abilities, and decision making." [19] will impair cognitive accessibility through cognitive overload. Thus, it is suggested that cognitive accessibility and cognitive overload are closely related, if not synonymous, terms.

Fifth, and perhaps most importantly, we sometimes act as if IST were an end in itself. It is not. If an IST system does not allow individuals to access their goals, that system will be little used. It will have been a commercial or social failure. On a positive note, we live in an age of considerable pressures that may encourage inclusive design based, inter alia, on; (a) the political will to create an inclusive society, (b) the substantial skills-shortages faced by modern societies and (c) the need of IST vendors to achieve better market share in order to be successful. I will leave it to the reader to decide which are the most important of these factors and whether the three factors will always work together. However, as social creatures, access to objectives is best seen as a social activity, within the context of the inclusive information society. As the following table shows, accessibility types can also be related to the well developed internet layered model [16], which provides an important cross-validation of the above, new five-level approach to accessibility.

Table 1. Accessibility and the Internet layered model

Comparing:	Accessibility types	Internet layered model
1	Hardware access	Physical
2	connectivity access	data link
3	interface access	Network
4	cognitive access	Transport
7	goal / social access	Application

7   The Importance of the Social Context

When considering human performance, social context is very important for many reasons, particularly as it can be seen to influence user behaviour when using Information Society Technologies (IST). For example, it has been found that social context and emotional tone (task-oriented vs. socio-emotional) influenced the use of emoticons in short internet chats [9]. Social intelligence is a major consideration in our everyday lives, at work, education or leisure. It is often undervalued by researchers who look at cognitive aspects of users [3] [12]. Social intelligence is a central aspect of the folk psychology of today's citizens and cannot be ignored when working within the context of the Information Society ([14]

The concept of social intelligence has at least two components i.e. the person' skills to handle social settings and also their knowledge of the social world and it implications for them. It is clear that cognitive user models can incorporate them within their existing architectures. Simplex Two [1] [4] [5] [15] can incorporate "to understand and manage other people" as an attribute of the executive function. "To engage in adaptive social interactions" can be incorporated as a function of the complex output module. The long term memory and mental models modules can be used to cover "the individual's fund of knowledge about the social world". On this basis, there is no need to postulate a distinct social intelligence module at the moment, though social intelligence may reflect a distinct domain of knowledge and skills within currently postulated cognitive modules.

8 Social Context, Skills and Social Intelligence

Social intelligence is a major aspect of the triarchic theory of human intelligence [22]. On this view, intelligence comprises analytical, creative, and practical abilities [22] [23] [24]. There are also three performance components of social intelligence i.e. (i) problem solving in social settings, (ii) executive functions to make plans and execute them and (iii) the ability to learn to develop these component skills. All forms of intelligence are predicted to be sensitive to the context of measurement, so performance in a social task (like negotiation) would not correlate perfectly with performance on an intellectual task (like syllogistic reasoning), because of the differential influence of context. Social intelligence can also be subdivided into two types, knowing what to say (declarative knowledge) and knowing how to do actions (procedural knowledge) [14]. The concept of social intelligence is of the most relevance to inclusion and accessibility within the Information Society.

The status of social intelligence is not completely clear. If it were a completely distinct faculty of the human brain then, when confounding factors (like overall speed of response) are controlled, any correlation between social and other forms of intelligence should be vanishingly small. However, if social intelligence is seen as based on a subset of knowledge and skills within common systems and processes like long term memory, then correlations may be low but never zero.

It is clearly difficult to distinguish empirically between these two views of social intelligence, since that would require the detection of true zero correlations. However, there is no current evidence for the complete independence of social intelligence. A recent substantial review paper [14] applied the dichotomy between fluid and crystallized intelligence to social intelligence. Thus, crystallized intelligence covers a person's knowledge of their social context. Fluid intelligence is skill based, i.e. a person's capability for social problem solving. Exploratory factor analyses found that crystallized social intelligence fluid social intelligence but was well correlated with academic intelligence. However, none of the correlations were zero. Parsimony would suggest that there is basis to postulate a distinct social intelligence module at the moment, though social intelligence may be based on distinct knowledge and skills within a more generic cognitive architecture, as shown in figure one.

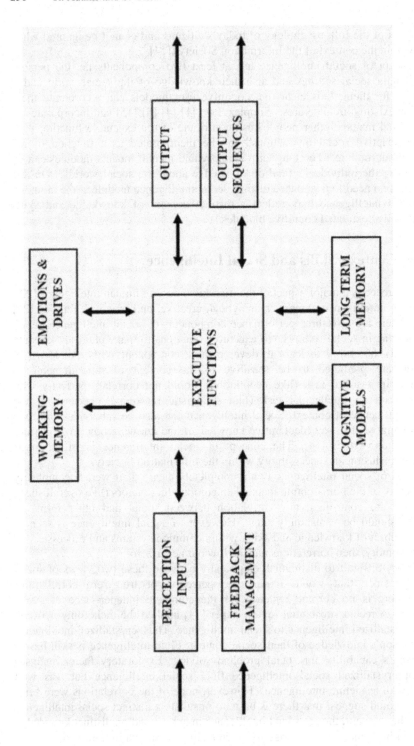

Fig. 1. Simplex two

9   Social Intelligence and Disability

If social intelligences cannot be dissociated completely from other forms of intelligence or cognition, on the basis between correlations between intelligence tests, then a consideration of cognitive disabilities, itself very relevant to universal access, could provide additional evidence. If social intelligence depends selectively on different regions of the brain, then certain brain injuries will be associated with the impairment of aspects of social intelligence but not other cognitive facilities. Some researchers [10] [11] have proposed that there are at least seven different types of intelligence, each with its own brain system. If so, then there could be evidence that specific brain injuries are associated with different intelligences. If social intelligence can be dissociated from other cognitive facilities, then some people with specific head injuries would retain their social intelligence but present with deficits in other functions and conversely, those with different head injuries could display the reverse pattern of impaired social intelligence with other cognitive functions intact. In psychoneurological case studies, injuries to the prefrontal lobes of the cerebral cortex can selectively impair personal and social intelligence, leaving other abilities intact [1] [4]. In contrast, injuries to the occipital and parietal lobes can be associated with the impairment of cognitive functions whilst social abilities remain unscathed. Similar evidence can be found when considering clinical conditions like Down syndrome and Alzheimer's disease. They are often associated with damaged cognitive sequelae but little or no impairment of social intelligence. By contrast, Pick's disease can spare some cognitive abilities while severely hitting a person's social skills. Autism spectrum disorder (ASD) and Asperger's syndrome are classically associated with a deficit in social intelligence and lack of empathy but not necessarily with learning difficulties, the so-called "theory of mind" explanation [17] [7] [8]. There is some suggestion that they do not find traditional ways to learn social skills to be conducive and so acquire them badly [8]. Infantile autisms, like Kanner's syndrome and Williams' syndrome, are associated with significantly impair of empathy for other people in social settings. Whilst the diagnosis of mental retardation includes deficits in both social and academic intelligence, they are considered to be only lowly correlated [1] [4]. Furthermore, some researchers [26] have concluded that there are three different brain systems that are associated with social intelligence (i): a cortical subsystem which relies on long-term memory to make complex social judgments; (ii) a frontal-dominant subsystem to organize and create social behaviours; and (iii) a limbic-dominant subsystem to support emotional responses. If so, different brain lesions will lead to different types of impairment of social intelligence.

From this consideration of social intelligence and disability, it is evident that all the evidence suggests that if social intelligence is correlated with other cognitive functions, any correlations are small but important and not statistically insignificant. If so, social intelligence is an important, semi-autonomous component of human cognition and worthy of consideration along with universal access and augmented cognition based solutions for accessibility problems and cognitive overload when using socially significant systems

10   Social Intelligence and Cognitive User Modelling

There are two relevant groups who will use the notion of social intelligence within the context of universal access. First, there are the researchers who seek to understand the psychology of the intended users, for cognitive user modelling. Second, there are the designers and developers who work on unified user interface design [21]. For the first group, it is recommended that social intelligence can be treated as sub-domains of knowledge and skills within an overall cognitive architecture of the user. For the second group, as suggested below, social intelligence may require a more special treatment if it is not undervalued accidentally in the design process. The theoretical perspective is considered elsewhere [6] and concludes that most, if not all the presently offered components of human cognition can subsume many aspects of social intelligence.

11   Socially Intelligent Interactive Design

From the perspective of the Universal Access interactive system design, social skills must be acknowledged, understood and included by the designers and eventually be supported by the system itself.   This is particularly important to the development of socially based and socially aware systems, for example, the creation of an accessible negotiation system based on remote, visual conferencing.   In that case, we propose that designers and developers should consider social intelligence as a separate factors in addition to the nine cognitive components already provided by Simplex Two [3].

12   Discussion

In this paper we have shown how both universal access and augmented cognition potentially have substantial areas of synergy within the context of the emergence of the Inclusive Information Society [21]. We have also defined a new, five level expansion of the concept of accessibility and introduced the concept of cognitive accessibility to link accessibility and cognitive overload. Furthermore, we have found that social intelligence and social skills are an important development area for both universal access and augmented cognition. Additionally, social intelligence, at the moment, can be subsumed under the current architecture of Simplex [3]. Finally all three concepts of universal access, augmented cognition and social intelligence provide powerful toolboxes for us to meet our objectives, namely (a) the creation of accessible systems that support vocational and social effectiveness for people with special requirements and (b) to build the joint contribution of cognitive and social factors into UA design methodologies for socially relevant systems.

References

1. Adams, R.: Universal access through client-centred cognitive assessment personality profiling. In: Stary, C., Stephanidis, C. (eds.) User-Centered Interaction Paradigms for Universal Access in the Information Society. LNCS, vol. 3196, pp. 3–15. Springer, Heidelberg (2004)

2. Adams, R.G.: Applying advanced concepts of cognitive overload and augmentation in practice: the future of overload. In: Schmorrow, D.D., Stanney, K.M., Reeves, L.M. (eds.) Foundations of Augmented Cognition, 2nd edn. Arlington Virginia: Strategic Analysis (2006)

3. Adams, R.: Decision and Stress: Cognition and e-Accessibility in the Information Workplace. Universal Access in the Information Society (in press) (2007)

4. Adams, R., Langdon, P.: Principles and concepts for information and communication technology design. Journal of Visual Impairment and Blindness 97, 602–611 (2003)

5. Adams, R., Langdon, P.: Assessment, Insight and Awarenes. In: User Centred Design that Includes Users With Special Needs. In: Keates, S., Clarkson, P.J., Langdon, P. and Robinson, P (eds.) London: Springer (2004)

6. Adams, R., Gill, S.P.: User modelling and social intelligence. In: HCII 2007 proceedings (In press) (2007)

7. Baron-Cohen, S.: Mindblindness: An essay on autism and theory of mind. MIT Press, Cambridge (1995)

8. Baron-Cohen, S., Golan, O., Chapman, E., Grander, Y.: Transported to a world of emotion. Psychologist 20, 76–77 (2007)

9. Derks, D., Bos, A.E.R., von Grumbkow, J.: Emoticons and social interaction on the Internet: the importance of social context. Computers in Human Behavior 23, 842–849 (2007)

10. Gardner, H.: Frames of mind: The theory of multiple intelligences. New York: Basic Books (1983)

11. Gardner, H.: Multiple intelligences: The theory in practice. New York: Basic Books (1993)

12. Gill, S.: Designing of inclusivity. HCII proceedings (In press) (2007)

13. Gill, S.P., Borchers, J.: Knowledge in co-action: social intelligence in collaborative design activity. AI & Society 17, 322–339 (2003)

14. Kihlstrom, J.F., Cantor, N.: Social intelligence. In: Sternberg, R.J. (ed.) Handbook of intelligence, 2nd edn. pp. 359–379. Cambridge University Press, Cambridge (2000)

15. Langdon, P., Adams, R., Clarkson, P.J.: Universal Access to Assistive Technology through Client-Centred Cognitive Assessment. In: Carbonell, N., Stephanidis, C. (eds.) Universal Access. Theoretical Perspectives, Practice, and Experience. LNCS, vol. 2615, pp. 555–567. Springer, Heidelberg (2003)

16. Moseley, R.: Developing web applications. Wiley, West Sussex UK (2007)

17. Premack, D., Woodruff, G.: Does the chimpanzee have a theory of mind? Behavioral & Brain Sciences 1, 515–526 (1978)

18. Salvendy, G.: Foreword. In: Stephanidis, C. (ed.) User interfaces for all: concepts, methods and tools, Lawrence Erlbaum Associates, Mahwah (2001)

19. Schmorrow, D.D., Stanney, K.M., Reeves, L.M.: Foundations of Augmented Cognition, 2nd edn. Arlington Virginia: Strategic Analysis (2006)

20. Smith, T.J., Henning, R.A., Adams, R.G.: Social cybernetics of augmented cognition – a control systems analysis. In: Schmorrow, D.D., Stanney, K.M., Reeves, L.M. Foundations of Augmented Cognition, 2nd edn. Arlington Virginia: Strategic Analysis (2006)

21. Stephanidis, C.: User interfaces for all: new perspectives into human-computer interaction. In: Stephanidis, C. (ed.) User interfaces for all: concepts, methods and tools, Lawrence Erlbaum Associates, Mahwah (2001)

22. Sternberg, R.J.: Toward a triarchic theory of human intelligence. Behavioral & Brain Sciences. Behavioral & Brain Sciences 7, 269–315 (1984)

23. Sternberg, R.J.: Beyond IQ: A triarchic theory of human intelligence. Cambridge University Press, New York (1985)
24. Sternberg, R.J.: The triarchic mind: A new theory of intelligence. New York: Viking (1988)
25. Sternberg, R.J. (ed.): Handbook of intelligence, 2nd edn., pp. 359–379. Cambridge University Press, Cambridge
26. Taylor, E.H., Cadet, J.L.: Social intelligence, a neurological system? Psychological Reports 64, 423–444 (1989)

Intent Driven Interfaces to Ubiquitous Computers

Neil G. Scott and Martha E. Crosby

University of Hawaii at Manoa

Abstract. An intent driven interface allows a person to control a computer by stating an intended outcome rather than entering the sequence of tasks required to achieve the same outcome. Techniques that were originally developed as part of a universal access accelerator for individuals with disabilities are now being applied as convenience and productivity tools for accessing any computer based device, appliance or system. An intelligent universal serial bus (USB) Hub, called the iTASK Module, determines user intent independently of the input source or the system that is accessed. iTASK Modules can be interconnected to support multi-user collaboration and sharing of system resources without requiring any hardware or software changes to the accessed system.

Keywords: IDEAL, iTASK Module, NIP, intent, ubiquitous, USB.

1 Introduction

For many people, the term ubiquitous computers conjures up visions of an environment in which there is always some type of personal computer within easy reach. While there are now several billion personal and business computers in use around the world, they are just a small fraction of the total number of computers that have been deployed. Appliances, toys, cell phones, industrial controllers and cars are examples of devices that contain one or more embedded computers. An economy car, contains twenty to forty processors, and a luxury car contains eighty to one-hundred.

Business and personal computers that almost always provide a screen, keyboard and mouse to support user interaction, this is rarely the case with embedded systems where low cost and small size makes conventional human interaction strategies impractical for most applications. When absolutely necessary, dedicated, function-specific buttons and knobs may be provided but most of the embedded systems have no directly accessible human/computer interface.

This paper describes an intent driven user interface that enables an operator to control any computer-based system by simply describing the intended outcome rather than the sequence of commands normally required to reach that outcome. It can be used equally well on conventional business and personal computers or on embedded systems. User input consists of text messages containing one or more words that describe the intent of the user. The interface maintains context information by keeping track of the location, device, application, and control function that was most recently accessed. This context enables the interface to recognize applicable synonyms, such as "tv," "television," and "idiot box;" and to filter out words that don't have meaning

D.D. Schmorrow, L.M. Reeves (Eds.): Augmented Cognition, HCII 2007, LNAI 4565, pp. 241–250, 2007.
© Springer-Verlag Berlin Heidelberg 2007

within the current context. This makes it unnecessary for the operator to adhere to predefined formats or scripts when formulating input messages. For example, "turn on the tv," "turn the tv on," "I want the television turned on," or "turn on the idiot box" all reduce down to "tv on." The operator doesn't need to know the mechanics of how the intended outcome is achieved, in this case, how the tv is actually turned on.

The intent driven interface is implemented as a small standalone device called an iTASK Module that uses universal serial bus (USB) ports for all input and output connections. While similar in appearance to the USB hubs that are used to increase the number of USB host ports on a personal computer, the iTASK Module contains its own processor and an additional USB client port.

The iTASK Module operates independently of the device to which it is connected. It checks every incoming message to determine whether to pass it directly to another port, as in a standard USB hub, or whether to analysis the message to determine user intent and then send out the sequence of commands necessary to achieve the user's intended outcome.

2 Background

The concept of an intent driven interface grew out of research into how individuals with disabilities could use speech recognition and head tracking to simplify and improve their interaction with computers and environmental control systems.

Speech recognition became a practical access tool for individuals with physical disabilities in 1989. The speech recognition software stretched the early PCs to the limits of their capabilities, particularly when used in conjunction with large applications programs, such as MS Word. Speech recognition impacted the computer system in at least three areas: (i) overall performance of the system was often significantly degraded, (ii) the combined user interface was often overwhelming for the user, particularly when he or she had to correct recognition errors, and (iii) software bugs in the applications and operating system were more prevalent when the computer was operating at its upper limit.

Individuals with disabilities who worked with non-IBM personal computers, such as the Macintosh, Sun and SGI were unable to reap the benefits of speech recognition which was only available for the IBM PC.

Under a grant funded by the Fund for Improved Post Secondary Education (FIPSE), one of the authors (Scott) developed a Universal Access System that made it possible to use the speech recognition with any type of computer. It achieved this by splitting the user interface into two separate components: A speech recognizer running in its own dedicated IBM PC, and a Universal Access Port that emulated the keyboard and mouse on whatever type of PC the user was required to work with. The Universal Access System proved to be extremely effective for at least three reasons: the speech recognizer always runs at full speed in a dedicated computer, it connects to any computer that has a Universal Access Port (Universal Access Ports were developed for IBM, Macintosh, and Sun, SGI, and HP workstations) and separating the speech interface from the application reduced the cognitive load on the user.

Conceptually, dictating text into a computer is very simple; you speak, it types. And it really is this simple until the recognizer misrecognizes what you said. Once again, it is conceptually simple to say what is required to make the necessary corrections. It is just a matter of remembering the appropriate commands and speaking them into the computer in the correct order. With practice, you become proficient at making corrections but then, you need to be able to edit what you have written and save your work to a file. Yet again, it is conceptually easy to use predefined spoken commands to access the necessary menu items in your word processor. It is at this point, however, that many people become overwhelmed by the complexity of the system. Remembering which window should have the focus, the correct word or phrase to say, the right time to say it, and the order in which to say each word or phrase rapidly becomes a significant cognitive load.

Prewritten verbal commands, called macros, are used to reduce the number of utterances required to perform a particular task. A macro consists of a short phrase that describes a task linked to the sequence of commands required to perform it. The task is performed automatically each time the phrase is spoken. Properly designed macros significantly increase the productivity of speech recognition in real world working environments but they also introduce significant problems. The first problem is that the user must remember precisely what to say to trigger each macro. This gets increasingly difficult as the number of macros on a system grows. The second problem is part of a good news bad news situation in that the more comprehensive the macros, the more work that can be achieved with each utterance but accidentally triggering one of these macros at the wrong time can be devastating.

When speech recognition first became a viable option for people with disabilities in 1989, it took about two days of intensive training to enable a disabled person to perform non-trivial work tasks. A decade later, when computers were more than fifty times faster and the recognition software was much more advanced, it still took the same amount of time to train a new user. After questioning many disabled users of speech recognition, the author (Scott) concluded that the problem was not caused by the technology but rather, by user uncertainty about what to say to the computer in different scenarios. This uncertainty was exacerbated by a fear of accidentally triggering a macro that would damage or lose what had already been written. Almost without exception, the first utterance a person made when first introduced to speech recognition was "what do I say?"

3 Developing an Intent Driven Interface

The Archimedes Project at Stanford University undertook a project during the summer of 2002 to design a new Universal Access System that would eliminate the "what do I say?" problem. A team of twenty researchers and students worked together to develop a strategy for solving the problem and them broke into small groups to design the hardware and software components. Initial brainstorming sessions led to the development of a scenario in which a user describes the intended outcome to a virtual operator who knows the correct way to perform any required task on the device that is being accessed. In this scenario, users could use cryptic commands like "tv on" or they could be more tentative, using commands such as "I would like to watch the television please." If the user says something that is confusing or unclear, the virtual operator should ask for clarification and remember the response to prevent confusion should the user say the same thing again. A living room was chosen as the primary scenario for the test bed. The goal of the project was to enable a user to turn individual lamps on and off, open and close doors, windows and drapes, control all user functions in an audio visual system and control the operation of a computer.

3.1 The iTASK Module

The overall design of the iTASK, as it became called, is similar to the original Universal Access System except that that all input and output connections are now made through USB ports as shown in Figure 1, and a Natural Interaction Processor (NIP) is incorporated into the internal software to determine user intent based on one or more text messages received from accessors as depicted in Figure 2.

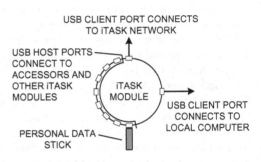

Fig. 1. USB Ports on an iTASK Module

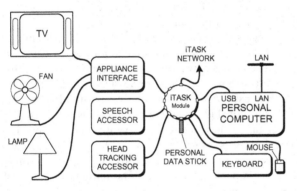

Fig. 2. iTASK module providing access to appliances and a personal computer using speech recognition and head tracking

Note the personal data stick connected to one of the USB host ports in Figure 1. This is a standard flash drive containing vocabulary trees, command definitions and user preferences that personalize the iTASK Module. In some situations, the personal data is stored in an accessor if it is always used by the particular user.

The keyboard and mouse depicted in Figure 2 are the original devices that were attached to the personal computer except that they now pass through the iTASK Module so that their data can be monitored to look for embedded text commands or gestures. The USB standards define devices like the keyboard and mouse as Human Interface Devices (HID) devices. All of the standard operating systems (Windows, Linux, Mac, and so on) incorporate software to automatically recognize and process HID data packets. In most situations, the iTASK Module automatically sends HID packets directly to the local personal computer regardless of the originating USB port. Therefore, sending an HID packet or plugging a USB keyboard or mouse into any port on the iTASK Module will automatically enter keyboard or mouse data into the local personal computer. HID data can also be sent to any computer on the iTASK network by wrapping it in an iTASK packet addressed to the iTASK Module that connects to the target computer. When the iTASK packet is reaches its destination, the iTASK wrapper is removed and the HID packet is delivered to the local computer.

The speech accessor depicted in Figure 2 is a small computer running speech recognition software. It translates spoken messages into plain text that is placed in an iTASK packet and sent to the iTASK Module. The iTASK Module makes all of the decisions about whether the text is to be interpreted as a command or as dictated text, and the destination for the resulting information.

The head tracking accessor translates head movements into 2D direction vectors that mimic the operation of a mouse, 3D direction vectors that point to an object in space, movement dynamics that can be interpreted as gestures, or text messages that specify the name of the object currently being pointed to by the tracker. For example the text message might say "pointing at the tv" or "pointing at the bed lamp." Representing the output of the tracker as text allows the iTASK Module to interpret spoken or typed commands such as "turn that off" that are coincident with the head tracker identifying a particular lamp or appliance.

The Appliance interface depicted in Figure 2 translates generic device commands generated by the iTASK into specific commands and transmission formats expected by the targeted appliance. Much thought went into how the interface to appliances should be handled. The first version of the iTASK Module included infrared (IR) and radio frequency (rf) and X10 power line components that could directly control many different devices. It was later decided to place these components in separate appliance modules because they represent moving targets that are constantly changing as new standards and improved transmission protocols are introduced. For instance, there are more than one-hundred thousand different IR codes currently being used for audio visual equipment. The iTASK Module handles this by generating "iTASK" text commands, such as "volume up," that are translated into specific IR codes by a small natural interaction processor inside the appliance module. The IR codes that match the particular TV, for example, are down loaded from the manufacturer's website and stored in the appliance module when the TV is first installed and set up.

One of the most important characteristics of the iTASK Module is that the personal computer depicted in Figure 2 is absolutely standard and contains no added software or hardware. Applications function exactly as they would if the iTASK Module was not connected, i.e., there is no performance degradation. Furthermore, there is no requirement for the personal computer to be of a particular type; the only stipulation is that it has a USB port. This is particularly liberating for individuals with disabilities who have traditionally had to put up with slow and compromised computer systems containing additional layers of software on top of the operating system and applications.

The arrow at the top of Figure 2 identifies a USB client port that provided for connecting the iTASK Module to a hierarchical network as depicted in Figure 3. Each iTASK Module in the network knows about all devices and other iTASK Modules that are directly connected to it. A discovery mechanism built in to each iTASK Module enables any iTASK Module to automatically locate and interact with devices connected to any other iTASK Module in the network without requiring any stored master lists of available resources. This allows iTASK Modules to be added or removed on the fly without disrupting the network or leaving behind stale data.

3.2 An Example of an Intent Driven Application

The Intent Driven Environment for Active Learning (IDEAL) classroom depicted in Figure 4 shows how iTASK Modules can be configured as an iTASK network to support learning activities in a classroom. The apparent simplicity of the diagram belies the revolutionary features made possible by the iTASK Module.

- The iTASK Modules handle all of the conventional and special user interfaces for each computer. While each keyboard, for example, is normally connected to its local computer, the iTASK Module can easily redirect it to any other computer in the iTASK network. Typing or saying a simple command like "connect my keyboard to the class computer" or "connect my mouse and keyboard to Mary's computer" will automatically redirect the specified peripheral devices.
- Personal data sticks configure each iTASK Module to handle the special needs and personal preferences of individual students.
- The special access requirements of students with disabilities are easily and quickly accommodated by connecting one or more accessors to an iTASK Module, as depicted on the leftmost student computer in Figure 3. If this were a speech accessor, for instance, it could also be used to access any computer in the system simply by saying something like "connect this to the Mary's computer"
- Three different networks are shown in Figure 4. Each network handles a different aspect of the networking requirements.

    o The iTASK network handles all time-dependent communications between the iTASK Modules and the Class Resource Server.
    o A conventional cable or wireless local area network (LAN) delivers bulky material from the class resource server to the other computers.
    o A wide area network (WAN) connects the Class resource server to the school or district server and the internet. The class resource server manages and screens all individual student access to the internet based on lesson requirements and individual permissions.

- The natural interaction capabilities of the iTASK Modules make interaction with the computers more transparent thereby reducing the intimidation of students who are not technically savvy.
- A hands-on activity module is shown connected to each iTASK Module that connects to a student computer. The hands-on activity module operates in conjunction with a set of virtual instruments in the class resource server to incorporate real time measurements into lessons that are managed and delivered by a learning management system also included in the class resource server.
- Apart from the class resource server, every computer in the classroom has minimal performance requirements. Basically, they can be any computer that supports a LAN connection, a USB connection and a standard browser. Disc-less Linux computers are an ideal choice since they eliminate all licensing costs and require almost zero maintenance and technical support. It is not necessary for all of the computers in a class room to be of the same make, type or model, or be running the same operating system, since the only requirement is that they can run a standard browser such as Firefox. Being able to mix and match any

computers in a class set liberates schools from the high costs and major disruptions currently caused by built-in obsolescence. Every purchased or donated computer can be used in a classroom until the hardware actually fails.

- Fewer IT staff will be required to maintain the computers in a school.
- The long term stability of the classroom computer environment will encourage teachers to become more engaged in using computer-based learning because the materials they prepare will continue to run from one year to the next.

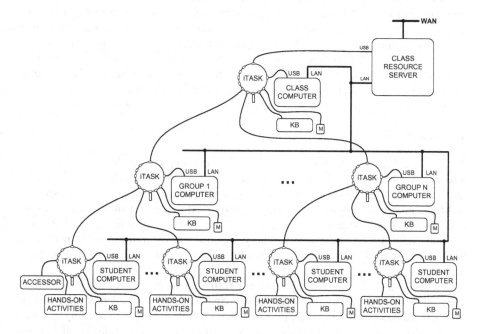

Fig. 3. Example of an iTASK Network supporting computer based learning in a classroom

4 Implementation of the iTASK Module

The proof of concept prototype constructed in 2002 combined conventional linguistics analysis with distributed intelligent agents. The resulting program occupied forty-six Mbytes of memory. A one Gigahertz computer with one Gigabyte of random access memory (RAM) correctly decoded natural language commands for controlling devices in a living room scenario but even with a simple command like "turn on the lamp," there would be a delay of up to five seconds before the lamp would turn on. While the results were functionally correct, the project was considered impractical due to the size and slowness of the software and the cost of the hardware.

Armed with the knowledge that the basic concepts worked, one of the authors (Scott) developed a second prototype based on control engineering algorithms instead of the statistical methods used by linguists. The key to using this more direct approach resulted from continually tracking the context of the interaction between the user and the iTASK Module. Whereas the linguistic approach considers every word in the vocabulary each time a new test word is received, the control engineering approach rejects all words that have no meaning within the current context. For most practical commands, this results in a search space of less than ten words that can be easily handled by a small microprocessor. The second prototype of the iTASK Module was implemented on an eight bit microprocessor that had only four hundred bytes of random access memory (RAM). This system correctly interpreted commands for the living room scenario in less than ten milliseconds.

Two new prototypes are currently being designed. The first system uses a thirty-two bit ARM processor and a recently introduced USB processor chip that performs all of the USB processing in firmware. This system will support multiple, large vocabulary applications with almost imperceptible processing delays. The second system uses an extremely low power sixteen-bit processor. It will handle a medium size vocabulary and make it feasible to incorporate fully functional iTASK Modules into small devices such as infrared remote controls, electronic medical devices, electronic toys, lamp controls, door locks or control panels for smart environments.

4.1 Accessors

As mentioned earlier, an accessor is a portable input/output (I/O) device that provides a personalized bridge between a user and an iTASK Module. Originally developed for individuals with disabilities, accessors translate alternative user inputs such as speech, or Morse code into text messages that are processed by an iTASK Module. Outputs from the accessed system are sent from the iTASK Module to an accessor where they are translated into an alternative modality matched the capabilities of the user, e.g., spoken text or Braille for a blind person or graphically generated sign language for a deaf person.

Accessors and iTASK Modules are not restricted to disability-related scenarios. They provide an ideal way to provide on-demand access to embedded processors that normally function without any direct interaction with a human. Including a small iTASK Module in an embedded industrial control processor, for example, allows any accessor to be used to perform tests, make adjustments or load new software. In this situation, the iTASK Module eliminates the need to use a different proprietary remote terminal for each different controller since a technician can use a single accessor to interact with any type of embedded controller.

4.1.1 Input Accessors

Input accessors fall into two basic categories: Accessors that generate messages to be interpreted as text functions in an iTASK Module, and accessors that generate messages to be interpreted as pointing functions.

Text-related accessors include:

- Keyboards may have larger or smaller dimensions than standard keyboards, specialized keys, customized layouts, and different languages.
- Chordic keyboards that translate combinations of one to seven keys into keystrokes. These can be designed for left or right handed operation, and can support faster text entry than a conventional qwerty keyboard.

- Scanning inputs make it possible to generate full text messages with a single input switch. Statistically organized options are displayed sequentially to the user who operates the switch when the desired option is displayed. Options include: groups of letters, individual letters, icons, spoken words or phrases, musical tones or arbitrary sounds.
- Morse code inputs can be generated with one, two, or three switches, depending on the range of movement and timing/response capabilities of the user. Dash, dot and enter switches are suitable for people who have poor timing control or are subject to spasms. A single two-way bug switch can generate Morse code faster than anyone can type. Morse code characters have been defined for all characters available on a computer keyboard.
- Handwriting recognition on an HP iPAQ PDA is sufficiently fast and accurate for it to be used as a reliable handwriting accessor. Some tablet computers also work well but they are still expensive and clumsy to handle.
- Speech recognition is available with many different vocabulary sizes and processor requirements. The vocabulary of low-cost, chip-based systems ranges from ten words through to a few hundred words. PDA based systems have vocabularies of several thousand words and PC based systems have vocabularies ranging from ten to more that one-hundred thousand words.
- Direct selection accessors use pointing devices such as a mouse, finger, stylus, head trackers or eye gaze trackers to select objects displayed on some type of display screen. The objects can be letters, words, phrases, or icons that are translated to text when selected.

Pointing related accessors translate some form of pointing action into: 2D vectors, 3D vectors, movement dynamics, or messages that specify the object at which the person is pointing. Devices that detect pointing movements include:

- Various types of mouse.
- Tablets or touch pads operated by a finger or stylus
- Gyroscopes for rotational movement
- Accelerometers for linear movement or tilt sensing
- Head tracking using ultrasonics, infrared, gyroscopes, accelerometers, or video cameras
- Eye gaze tracking based on specialized video cameras
- Gestures based on any moving part of the body detected by: video cameras, ultra wideband radar, or electric-field-disturbance detectors,
- EMG, EKG or EOG signals detected by electrodes attached to the skull

4.1.2 Output Accessors

Output accessors were designed to translate information derived from the screen or speaker of the target computer into an alternative modality and/or format that matches the special needs of a person with a disability. They are also useful for non-disabled users who need to access embedded processors that are not normally equipped with a human/computer interface. An output accessor designed specifically to access embedded processors may simply duplicate the functions of a standard computer screen on the screen of a PDA or cellular phone. Examples of output accessors that could be adapted for use with ubiquitous computers include:

- Devices with alternative screen properties optimized particular locations, size constraints, formats and application specific requirements.
- Screens with magnified screen images for visually impaired users.
- Text-to-speech synthesizers are used in screen readers for blind users or communication devices for people with severe speech disorders. Speech output has many uses beyond disability such as talking instruments and interactive controls in smart buildings,
- Text-to-sign language for deaf users. Signing avatars are now supported on PCs, PDAs, and Cellular phones.
- Text-to-flashing lights for telling deaf people to look at a screen message or to inform then that someone is ringing the door bell, etc.
- Braille displays for blind users.
- Graphics-to-haptic displays that represent lines, images, icons and text locations as forces that can be felt by a blind user.
- Graphics-to-sound (sonification) displays for blind users represent screen objects, colors and textures by modifying various sound properties.
- Vibration output devices (tactors) communicate directional information to people who are blind, deaf or performing tasks that heavily load other senses.

5 Summary

While originally designed to provide universal access for individuals with disabilities, the iTASK has the potential to improve and simplify human/computer interaction with any device or system that uses information and computer technology. iTASK Modules will be made available with support for small, medium and large vocabularies. Small vocabulary iTASK Modules will be suitable for embedding into low cost devices that currently use cryptic push button interfaces. Every iTASK Module is compatible with any type of input accessor. At this stage of development, most of the output accessors require special additions to a standard iTASK Module. Examples of specific applications are described in the paper but it is easy to see how these can be extrapolated into almost any area of human/computer interaction.

Foundations for Creating a Distributed Adaptive User Interface

Don Kemper, Larry Davis, Cali Fidopiastis, and Denise Nicholson

Institute for Simulation and Training
3100 Technology Drive
Orlando, FL 32826
USA
407.882.1300
{dkemper, ldavis, cfidopia, dnichols}@ist.ucf.edu

Abstract. Distributed simulation allows multiple users to develop and improve interactions without having to be collocated. To enhance such interaction, we present the foundation for a distributed, multi-modal, adaptive user interface. First, the interface concept is placed within the context of a closed-loop human system. Next, the present prototype implementation is described. Then, the concept of modifying interface elements based upon a combination of actual, physically simulated, and virtual devices is discussed. Finally, we discuss the possibility for self-adaptation, design challenges, and directions for future development.

Keywords: Multi-Modal Adaptive User Interface, Closed-Loop Human Systems.

1 Introduction

"Between stimulus and response, man has the freedom to choose." [1]

The ability of an individual to choose her actions is a fundamental characteristic of humanity. In having the freedom to choose, humans also have the ability to adapt. Humans adapt to internal and external changes on a continual basis, often without conscious awareness.

Another important aspect of humanity is individuality. In identical circumstances, two people may respond differently when presented with the same stimuli. Also, there are known effects of individual personality traits and the emotional and cognitive state of a person on the ability to process information [12].

An ideal computer interface should account for the individuality and adaptability of the human in order to provide optimal human computer interaction. An information system that deals with each user uniquely or treats users displaying certain traits as part of the same group can be considered an adaptive system [3]. A self-adaptive interface is defined as a human-computer interface that changes automatically in response to its experience with users [2].

D.D. Schmorrow, L.M. Reeves (Eds.): Augmented Cognition, HCII 2007, LNAI 4565, pp. 251–257, 2007.
© Springer-Verlag Berlin Heidelberg 2007

Within the context of training, adaptive system designs can accelerate the development of expertise. However, good design remains a challenge; user intent must be translated to the computer in one form or another. A previous survey of adaptive human-computer interfaces [8] states that a major factor of HCI inadequacy is that "the design of effective interfaces is a difficult problem with sparse theoretical foundations." Since the publishing of that research, there have been several theoretical frameworks proposed for static user interface [7] [10] as well as for adaptive user interface [4].

Distributed, multi-user simulation offers a unique opportunity for exploring adaptive user interfaces. In some instances, users participate within the simulation using a heterogeneous mix of simulators. The different simulators require interfaces that must communicate information to one another while providing an optimal experience for the user. In addition, the simulators may possess different interface devices to enable application-specific functionality. For example, a 3D simulator may have a head-mounted display (HMD) interface. The possibility of heterogeneous simulators and/or a range of interface hardware require(s) the application of an adaptive user interface.

The ultimate goal of a distributed simulation is to enable multiple users to share an environment without the requirement of being physically co-located. In this manner, the simulation connects the participants in a form of human-to-human contact. By designing the interface to apply multiple modalities (e.g. sound, motion, touch), the interaction among participants can be closer to that of normal contact and the interaction can be more robust [9]. An adaptive, multi-modal user interface could be used to increase the sense of realism within a simulation. A self-adaptive interface could be used to enhance the situational awareness of the user or mitigate the occurrence of stimuli within the environment so as to not overwhelm or under-task the user.

In remainder of this paper, we present the foundations for the creation of a distributed, adaptive, multi-modal user interface in the context of training within a distributed simulation. We then describe a prototype adaptive interface where the interface elements are modified based upon the combination of actual, simulated, and virtual devices used. The interface adaptation is currently user-driven and will be expanded to include self-adaptive interface elements that mitigate workload requirements within the application environment. Finally, we discuss modifications, improvements, and challenges related to the interface design and implementation.

2 Adaptive User Interfaces

The need for adaptive user interfaces is driven in part by the trend of work environments requiring users to do more with less [6]. In addition, as system complexity increases, system based mitigation efforts on behalf of users can become paramount, the alternative being task overload and possibly task failure. One approach to handling this is via an Augmented Cognition Closed Loop Human System (CLHS), presented by [6]. It is an iterative process which cycles through generating environment and content, presenting stimuli to the user, monitoring the effects and adapting the system according to assessments of the user's state. Interface adaptations may range from simple visual or auditory cues to a combination of multi-modal approaches [11].

2.1 The Cycle of Adaptation

One method of dealing with the cycles of adaptation is presented in the CLHS diagram shown in Figure 1. Initially, application content and environment components are generated and supplied to the UI Adaptation Layer where decisions are made regarding the presentation to the user. This involves selecting visual output and user input options based on system hardware and the presence of supported input devices. The output of the UI Adaptation Layer determines the presentation to the user, which serves as input stimuli to the user. Concurrently, the Operational Neuroscience Sensing Suite (ONSS) actively monitors the user's state and generates user state information parameters which are fed back to the UI Adaptation Layer. The UI Adaptation Layer User State Mitigation component can take actions as needed, which in turn affect the content and environment on the next cycle. The centralized location of the User Interface Adaptation Layer within the cycle is essential to the adaptation process as it dictates output and processes input feedback per iteration.

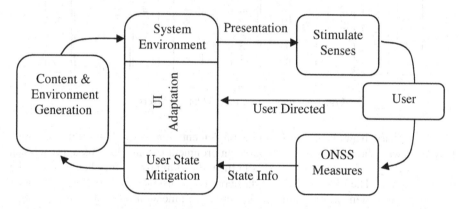

Fig. 1. Closed Loop Human System w/ UI Adaptation Layer

2.2 Our Implementation

The overarching design guidelines for the adaptive interface were to increase the sense of immersion while maintaining compatibility with the original simulation platform. The goal was to have one simulation that adapts to the hardware and the user in order to create the most immersive experience possible with the available components. The baseline simulation uses a typical 2D application style dashboard interface overlaid on a 3D virtual environment. The dashboard includes menu selections and virtual device components used within the system. The user navigates via keyboard and mouse interactions; movement in the virtual environment is accomplished via typical mouse and keyboard actions and the dashboard is point and click to select actions.

Interface Enhancements. We have created enhancements to the interface to increase the fidelity of the simulation to the user. The modifications include support for various visual display configurations, user input and manipulation devices as well as planned support for simulated physical devices. The primary display configurations include single monitor/projector, multi-monitor/multi-projector and head mounted displays. The input options currently include the standard mouse and keyboard, wireless mouse and pointing devices, head tracker, a Nintendo® Wii™ Remote and application specific physically simulated devices such as binoculars, GPS, and compass.

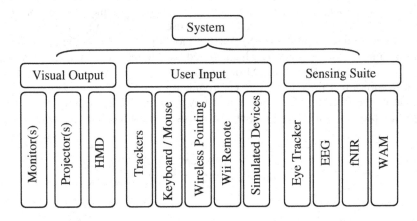

Fig. 2. System Configuration Options Overview

The primary benefit of the baseline implementation is its familiarity to users. However, with the addition of immersive environment extensions, this approach can be completely unacceptable as it significantly diminishes the benefits of the enhancements. The display of a 2D dashboard, for instance, in a multi-projector or HMD display system would diminish the sense of immersion in addition to creating a potentially awkward method of interaction. Therefore, the dashboard was replaced with an on-demand menu system and separate virtual device components. This provides a default view consisting only of the virtual environment, maximizing the immersion for the given hardware configuration.

System Environment UI Adaptation. The system environment adaptation component of the UI Adaptation Layer configures the output display and the user input devices. The process is generally automatic for standard devices such as keyboard, mouse and single displays. The physical hardware configuration for multiple displays, projectors and specialized input devices is separate from this process, with only the knowledge of their presence being of any importance to this component.

This component primarily manages the availability and location of the UI components within the environment. The UI display is adjusted in a manner that is consistent across all supported configurations based on the hardware present. For example, the on-demand menu system is always presented in same relative position with respect to the user's field of view. Additionally, alternative input devices such as the Nintendo Wii Remote perform in similar fashion as those in the baseline system for basic tasks like point and select. However, they add to the experience through the introduction of more natural navigation by virtue of their position and movement sensing capabilities. Finally, three degree-of-freedom (3DOF) tracking devices are used to provide head orientation input for the visual display.

The planned introduction of application-specific physically simulated devices (PSDs) will also be handled within this component. Each PSD will have a virtual analogue in the application and only one should be visible to the user at a time to avoid confusion. For example, the application supports a compass PSD and a virtual analog within the environment. The user will have access to the virtual compass as long as the PSD compass is not detected. The adaptation is dynamic; therefore, if a PSD compass is removed or fails, the system will detect this and make the virtual compass available. There is also conflict resolution built in to handle cases that cannot physically exist or otherwise work. If the display device being used is an immersive HMD, for example, then the user cannot be expected to interact with the PSDs in the normal fashion. Therefore, the virtual analogues will be available.

User State Mitigation UI Adaptation. This component will implement mitigation strategies as intervention techniques in the form of adaptive interactions and performance support techniques to improve human performance [6]. These will include multi-modal adaptations and attention management schemes designed to keep the user from being over or under tasked.

This assessment is made largely based on data provided by the Operational Neuroscience Sensing Suite (ONSS). This suite includes an eye tracker, EEG, functional Near Infrared (fNIR) and Wireless Arousal Meter (WAM). Each component will provide specific user state data that will be integrated by the User State Mitigation component of the UI Adaptation Layer to produce corrective action strategies based on task state knowledge in the system.

The initial mitigation strategies will include selective de-cluttering and UI support mechanisms to manage the user's task level. As ONSS data is fed into the system a decision will be made regarding whether any action is warranted. In the case of a user becoming overloaded, perhaps detected through excessive eye movement and/or increased arousal per the WAM, the system may employ a UI support strategy of highlighting environmental components relevant to the task state. During successive iterations it may be determined that the initial strategy is insufficient and that additional measures are required such as de-cluttering. Once strategies are added into the cycle, they are removed in a step-down manner based on ONSS parameters suggesting reduced workload etc. as well as when the user accomplishes tasks at hand.

3   Discussion

The prototype interface currently allows users to customize the simulator experience through a selection of different input devices and graphical controls. We now expand the discussion to include modifications, improvements, and challenges related to the interface design and implementation. Self-adaptation and current design challenges to direct future development are discussed in the following sections.

3.1 Self-adaptive Interface Elements

The interface adaptation is currently user-driven and will be expanded to include self-adaptive interface elements. These changes will allow the interface to mitigate difficulties the user may have within the application environment or provide additional stimulus if needed. Devices from the ONSS will indicate the need to provide mitigation to the interface. In this way, the interface can be tailored to meet the information processing needs of an individual within the simulation.

The concept of using neurophysiological devices to trigger mitigation is not new. Research in the area of augmented cognition encompasses a wide variety of strategies for applying mitigation based upon user state. Moreover, it is important to note that human-adaptive information research predates augmented cognition. In [5], the authors compare and contrast efforts from associate systems to that of augmented cognition systems. Although the present interface is not involved with the live control of vehicles, the lessons learned expressed in [5] (particularly, keeping the user "in charge" and the importance of co-development and progressive testing) will be leveraged within development of the adaptive interface.

3.2 Design Challenges

The interface design is intended to conform to the requirements given in [9]. In this effort, we attempt to maximize cognitive and physical ability by allowing users multiple modalities to receive information from the simulation. For example, in the case of using binoculars within a simulation, the PSD gives the advantage of physical familiarity. Both the physical and virtual modalities are integrated within the context of simulation and normal usage of the device. Usability consistency across the interface is maintained and the interface is adaptive by design.

The challenges in conforming to the requirements center on feedback and visual consistency in 3D. We are presently researching acceptable, intra-interface feedback methods to mitigate incorrect usage of PSDs. Another challenge is maintaining interface consistency in the case of a 3D simulator. For correct visual stimulus, visual interface elements must be presented at the correct depth with proper cues. Moreover, the perspective of the 3D elements must be correct with regard to the display device

Another design challenge is informing the distributed simulation of interface changes. Any devices used, mitigations, or error conditions must be provided to the distributed network to notify participants of changes in potential interactions. Through the use of the High-Level Architecture (HLA), some of the communication difficulties can be eliminated while others are created. We are presently researching a network communication paradigm using HLA to convey the interface state across the simulation.

Acknowledgements. The authors thank the members of the Applied Cognition and Training in Immersive Virtual Environments (ACTIVE) Laboratory who contributed to the writing and research presented. The results presented were funded by the Office of Naval Research as part of the Virtual Technologies and Environments (VIRTE) program and through a Presidential Equipment Grant from the University of Central Florida. The authors regret the inability to publish pictures of the interface due to export control restrictions.

References

1. Covey, S.R.: Principles of Personal Vision. In: The Seven Habits of Highly Effective People. Simon & Schuster, pp. 66–94, New York, (1990)
2. Edmonds, E.A.: Adaptive Man-Computer Interfaces. In: Coombs, M.J., Alty, J.L. (eds.) Computing Skills and the User Interface, Academic Press, Orlando (1981)
3. Feeney, W., Hood, J.: Adaptive Man/Computer interfaces: information systems which take account of user style. J SIGCPR Comput. Pers. 6, 4–10 (1977)
4. Schneider-Hufschmidt, M., Malinowski, U., Kuhme, T. (eds.): Adaptive User Interfaces: Principles and Practices. Elsiever, New York (1993)
5. Miller, C.A., Dorneich, M.C.: From Associate Systems to Augmented Cognition: 25 Years of User Adaptation in High Criticality Systems. In: Proc Aug Cog, vol. 2, pp. 344–353 (2006)
6. Nicholson, D., Stanney, K., Fiore, S., Davis, L., Fidopiastis, C., Finkelstein, N., Arnold.: An Adaptive System for Improving and Augmenting Human Performance. In: Proc Aug Cog, vol. 2 (2006)
7. Nielsen, J.: Heuristic Evaluation. In: Nielsen, J., Mack, R.L. (eds.) Usability Inspection Methods, John Wiley & Sons, New York (1994)
8. Norico, A.F., Stanley, J.: Adaptive Human-Computer Interfaces: A Literature Survey and Perspective. IEEE Trans. Sys. Man, Cyb. 19, 399–408 (1989)
9. Reeves, L.M., Lai, J., Larson, J.A., Oviatt, S., Balaji, T.S., Buisine, S., Collings, P., Cohen, P., Kraal, B., Martin, J., McTear, M., Raman, T.V., Stanney, K.M., Su, H., Wang, Q.Y.: Guidelines for Multimodal User Interface Design. Commun ACM 47, 57–59 (2004)
10. Shneiderman, B.: Designing the User Interface: Strategies for Effective Human-Computer Interaction, 3rd edn. Addison-Wesley, London (1998)
11. Stanney, K., Samman, S., Reeves, L., Hale, K., Buff, W., Bowers, C., Goldiez, B., Nicholson, D., Lackey, S.: A Paradigm Shift in Interactive Computing: Deriving Multimodal Design Principles from Behavioral and Neurological Foundations. Int J Hum Comp. Inter. 17, 229–257 (2004)
12. Szlama, J.L., Hancock, P.A.: Individual Differences in Information Processing.: In: McBride, D., Schmorrow, D. (eds.) Quantifying Human Information Processing. Lexington Books, pp. 177–193, Oxford, UK (2005)

EMMA: An Adaptive Display for Virtual Therapy

Mariano Alcañiz[1], Cristina Botella[3], Beatriz Rey[1], Rosa Baños[4], Jose A. Lozano[1],
Nuria Lasso de la Vega[3], Diana Castilla[3], Javier Montesa[1], and Antonio Hospitaler[2]

[1] LabHuman, Universidad Politécnica Valencia, Valencia Spain
[2] Dep. Ing. Construcción, Universidad Politécnica Valencia, Valencia Spain
[3] Departamento de Psicología Básica, Clínica y Psicobiología Universitat Jaume
[4] Departament de Personalidad, Evaluación y Tratamientos Psicológicos. Universidad de
Valencia

Abstract. Environments used up to now for therapeutic applications are invariable ones. Their contents can not be changed neither by the therapist nor by the patient. However, this is a technical issue that can be solved with current technology. In this paper, we describe a virtual environment that has been developed taking into account this factor. The main technical feature of the environment is that its aspect can be modified controlled by the therapist that conducts the clinical sessions depending on the emotions that the patient is feeling at each moment, and depending on the purpose of the clinical session. The environment has been applied for the treatment of post traumatic stress disorder, pathological bereavement, and adjustment disorder in adult population. In the paper we present some data showing its utility for the treatment of a phobia in a 9-year-old child.

Keywords: Virtual Reality, Adaptive display, Virtual therapy.

1 Introduction

The concept of "adaptative displays" has being considered for many years. It is a request to obtain technical devices that adapt to the requirements of the user, instead of having the users to adapt to the device. The term "adaptative display" has been used in some places to refer to displays that change their contents depending only on situational content rather than on any awareness of the user [1]. These adaptative displays can be used in many different applications: medicine, industry, architecture, psychology...

In the field of clinical psychology, virtual reality has been used in the latest years for the treatment of different psychological disorders. The idea was first thought in November 1992 in the Human-Computer Interaction Group of the Clark Atlanta University. The first experiment was a pilot study with a 32-years-old woman that suffered flying phobia. She was treated using a virtual environment [2] in which she followed eight thirty-minute sessions. At the beginning of each session, the subject had a high level of anxiety, which was decreasing in a gradual way after remaining in the situation during several minutes. This effect also was transferred from the virtual to the real world.

D.D. Schmorrow, L.M. Reeves (Eds.): Augmented Cognition, HCII 2007, LNAI 4565, pp. 258–265, 2007.
© Springer-Verlag Berlin Heidelberg 2007

Since that moment, this technique has been used for the treatment of different phobias. We can point out the environments designed for acrophobia treatment [3], [4], agoraphobia [5] or flying phobia [6], [7]. It has also been analyzed its effectiveness for fighting against other psychological problems: obsessive-compulsive disorders, attention deficit disorders, post-traumatic stress and eating disorders [8],[9].

However, environments used up to now for therapeutic applications are invariable ones. The contents cannot be changed, or only minor changes can be made, so no modification can be made in the contents of the virtual environment even when high emotional responses can be obtained from the user. Nevertheless, from a clinical point of view, it could be very useful for the psychologist to have a greater control over the aspect of the virtual environment that is shown to the user. In the environment that we are presenting in this paper, the psychologist can make changes in the aspect of the environment depending on the reactions of the patient to the different parts of the therapy session, and depending also on the purpose of the clinical session. This work has been conducted inside the EMMA Project (IST-2001-39192). The environment has been applied for the treatment of post traumatic stress disorder, pathological bereavement, and adjustment disorder in adult populations [10], [11]. In this paper we present some data showing its utility for the treatment of a phobia in a 9-year-old child.

2 Technical Description of the System

The purpose of the virtual environment is to be used in the context of a psychological treatment. The user is a person who suffers from psychological problems, such as affective disorders, anxiety disorders or adjustment disorders. All the sessions of the treatment are conducted by a therapist and, in some of them, the virtual environment is used as a help for this treatment. Both the therapist and the patient are physically present in the room during the evolution of the session. The patient visualizes the virtual environment in a retro-projected screen, and the interaction is made by means of a wireless joystick.

The application has been developed using Brainstorm eStudio software. This is an advanced, multiplatform real time 3D graphics development tool. It incorporates features such as: the inclusion of 3D objects in a very easy way, they can be imported from files, erased or animated; generation of 3D texts, whose colors can be changed; adding videos to surfaces; generation of new interfaces and timers; addition of actions to objects when they are selected; addition of sounds; loading or saving configurations. All these possibilities are controlled using the mouse, pop-up menus or drag and drop actions. The interpreted language that is used to program is python. Brainstorm eStudio can be defined as an interface that the programmer can use to create 3D complex visualizations using only tool options

2.1 Description of the Environment

The environment can be modified dynamically by the therapist taking into account the state of the patient at each moment during the treatment, so different aspects have

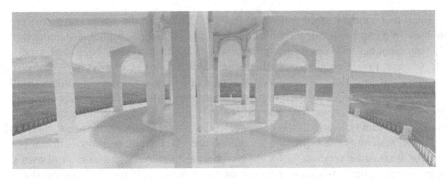

Fig. 1. Aspect of the room

been developed. The environment is not a static one. Initially, the user appears inside a big hall with circular shape and no walls.

The user can visualize the outer part of the environment, which initially is an open area of meadows. The user can navigate freely along the entire environment, even going out from the big hall and going though the meadows.

However, the meadows constitute only one of the five possible aspects of the outer part of the environment. The other pre-defined aspects are: a desert, an island, a forest with many trees and branches, and a snowed city. These five environments can be related to different emotions. For example, the forest with braches can be related to anxiety. On the other hand, if the purpose of the therapist is to induce relaxation in the patient, the island can be used. The desert can be related to rage, and the snowed city with sad situations, so it can be used during the session when the patient is remembering a situation that induces sadness in him or her. However, the real use that is given to each aspect of the environment depends on the context of the session and can be selected by the therapist in real time.

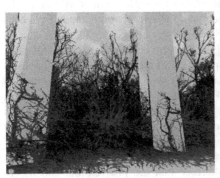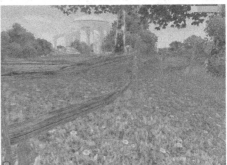

Fig. 2. Virtual environments corresponding to anxiety and joy

In order to control the appearance of the different aspects that have been developed, a special interface has been prepared. The application is running on a different computer from the one where the virtual environment has been launched. The therapist can select in an easy way (pressing different buttons) the aspect of the environment that has to be shown at each moment, and the needed command will be sent using TCP/IP to the computer where the environment is running. As soon as this computer receives the command, the appearance of the environment will change depending on the concrete order that it has received.

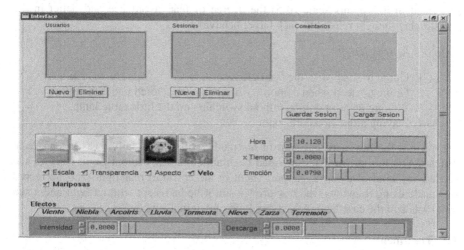

Fig. 3. Interface for the therapist

2.2 Application of Special Effects

Besides the big-scale control that we have described in the previous point, the therapist can also control small-scale changes. Different effects can be applied to the environment: a rainbow can appear, it can start raining, snowing, an earthquake can be generated, and the illumination can change to the one corresponding to different hours of the day and the night. All these effects are also launched from the same interface that controls the big-scale changes. The therapist can control by means of a slider the moment when the effect is launched and its intensity.

3   Method

3.1 Participant

The participant was a 9-year-old boy who presented a severe fear of darkness. His mother informed that he always has had sleeping problems. When he slept with his older brother he needed a light on, so his family changed him to sleep alone in another bedroom because the light molested his brother.

At the moment they seek help, the parents had to leave a light on in the corridor so the boy could fall asleep. After a while, they switched off this light but they left a little table lamp on in the bedroom. The boy belonged to a *"boy scouts"* group but when he went camping he only slept with a torch. When we was asked about his fear he informed that he was afraid of the "monsters" he could see in the darkness. The parents had tried to solve the problem using several strategies (reinforcements, persuasion…), obtaining poor and no lasting results.

3.2 Measures

Fear and Avoidance Scale: Before completing this instrument, four target behaviours or situations he avoided in relation to his darkness phobia were established. Then the boy rated in a 5 points scale (0-5) the degree of fear, avoidance and belief in the catastrophic thought related to each target behaviour.

TARGET BEHAVIOURS

1. Going to sleep with the light off
2. Going to sleep when camping without having a torch under the pillow
3. Waking up at midnight without switching on the little table lamp.
4. Staying alone in a dark room.

Self-record: the boy with the help of his mother filled in a daily basis a register in which they wrote down if the boy had been able to sleep without Light or if he had needed any kind of external support (light in the corridor, rear light...). The record was made using drawings (the boy drew a sun if he had slept without light and a sun with clouds in the case he had used any kind of external support).

3.3 Treatment

The treatment program is an adaptation of the emotive imaging procedure designed by [12] but applied using a VR program "EMMA's world". The application procedure of the emotive imaging procedure is described in several works [13], [14]. In the adaptation we have made of this procedure we use as treatment components, like Méndez, the exposure to the feared situation using narratives, the modelling of courage behaviours on the part of the therapist and the material and social reinforcement (by means of a token economy program) of the behaviours approaching the phobic situation. The novelty of the application of the emotive imaging procedure in this case study is that the in vivo exposure component is applied with the support of the virtual environment "EMMA's world".

3.4 Procedure

After being informed about the treatment program using VR that his child was going to receive, the mother signed an informed consent accepting his participation of the in the study.

The treatment program consisted of 11 weekly sessions with a duration of approximately 60 minutes.

Considering the anxiety levels informed by the boy in the different "EMMA's World" environments, the beach environment was chosen and the following VR exposure hierarchy was elaborated:

1. Beach environment at sunset (lantern lamp on)
2. Beach environment at night (lantern lamp on)
3. Beach environment at night (lantern lamp off)
4. Forest environment at night.

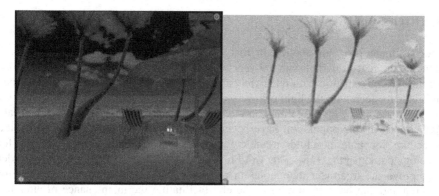

Fig. 4. Virtual environments used for the treatment

Once the hierarchy was defined the child was exposed to the first item (beach environment at subset with a lantern lamp on) and then he was progressing along the hierarchy. Furthermore, some multimedia elements were introduced in the VR *software* with the aim of constructing the emotive imaging. In "EMMA's room" a photo of the child and his favourite hero (Spiderman) were introduced. Besides, an audio was also prepared in which Spiderman introduces himself and asks the child for help to develop a "mission" in the beach at night, including in the narrative one of the anxiety provoking stimulus (thieves).

After the VR sessions were finished e in vivo exposure sessions were carried out, with the aim of testing to which extent the gains obtained with VR helped the child to confront the feared situations and to guarantee the generalization to real situations.

4   Results

In Table 1 the scores for fear and avoidance before and after treatment are presented. All scores for fear and avoidance related to the target behaviours are reduced.

On the other hand, the levels of anxiety and avoidance recorded by the child during the VR exposure sessions show that at the beginning of the session the levels of anxiety and avoidance are high diminishing progressively along the exposure session, thereby following the traditional exposure rules. This seems to indicate that the used environments are clinically significant for the child, that is, able to generate anxiety levels similar to those the child experiences in real feared situations.

Table 1.

Behaviour	PRE		POST	
	Fear	Avoidance	Fear	Avoidance
1	5	5	0	0
2	4	5	2	2
3	4	4	0	0
4	4	3	0	0

5 Discussion

The treatment program applied in this case study has shown to be effective in reducing the fear of darkness in a 9-year-old. After treatment the child is able to cope with the feared situation with no anxiety and this is generalised to real situations since he is able to sleep with the light off every day.

There are a few investigations on the use of VR in children. The most important applications in this population have been centred on the use of VR as a distraction procedure for pain in children undergoing medical treatment [15], [16], or for oncology patients [17], [18]. This work reveals that VR can be highly useful in order to improve the treatment of phobias in children. It is a less aversive treatment for children and can be very attractive, thereby facilitating the maintenance of attention during more time and they can also feel more

References

1. Schmeisser, E.T.: Dream of a Display that Pays Attention to the Viewer. CyberPsychology & Behavior 7(6), 607–609 (2004)
2. North, M.M., North, S.M., Coble, J.R.: Virtual environment psychotherapy: a case study of fear of flying disorder. Presence: Teleoperators and Virtual Environments 6(1), 127–132 (1997)
3. North, M., North, S.: Virtual reality psychotherapy. The Journal of Medicine and Virtual Reality 1, 28–32 (1996)
4. Rothbaum, B., Hodges, L., Kooper, R., Opdyke, D., Williford, M., North, M.: Effectiveness of computer-generated (virtual reality) graded exposure in the treatment of acrophobia. American Journal of Psychiatry 152, 626–628 (1995)
5. North, M., North, S., Coble, J.R.: Effectiveness of virtual environment desensitization in the treatment of agoraphobia. Presence 5(3), 346–352 (1996)
6. Rothbaum, B., Hodges, L., North, M., Weghorst, S.: Overcoming phobias by virtual exposure. Communications of the ACM 40, 34–39 (1997)
7. Baños R., Botella C., Perpiñá C.: El abordaje de la fobia a volar mediante realidad virtual (Approach to flying phobia by virtual reality). Communication presented at the IX Meeting of the Psychiatric Association of the Comunidad Valenciana, Castellón, Spain (2000)
8. Riva, G., Baccheta, M., Cesa, G., Conti, S., Molinari, E.: Virtual Reality and Telemedicine Based Experiential Cognitive Therapy: Rationale and Clinical Protocol. In: Fiva, G., Galimberti, C. (eds.) Towards CyberPsychology: Mind, Cognitions and Society in the Internet Age, IOS Press, Amsterdam (2001)
9. Perpiñá, C., Botella, C., Baños, R., Marco, J.H., Alcañiz, M., Quero, S.: Body Image and virtual reality in eating disorders: Is exposure by virtual reality more effective than the classical body image treatment? Cyberpsychology and Behavior 2, 149–159 (1999)
10. Botella, C., Quero, S., Lasso de la vega, N., Baños, R., Guillén, V., García-palacios, A., Castilla, D.: Clinical Issues in the application of Virtual reality to treatment of PTSD. In: Roy, M. (ed.) Novel approaches to the diagnosis and treatment of posttraumatic stress disorder. NATO Security Through Science Series, vol. 6, IOS Press, Amsterdam (2006)
11. Botella, B.: Baños, R., Rey, B., Alcañiz, M., Guillen, V., Quero, S., Garcia-Palacios.: Using an Adaptative Display for the Treatment of Emotional Disorders: A preliminary analysis of effectiveness. CHI 2006, pp. 586–591 (2006)

12. Méndez, F.X., García, M.J.: Emotive performances: A treatment package for children's phobias. Child and Family Behavior Therapy 18, 19–34 (1996)
13. Bados, A.: Fobias específicas. In: Vallejo Pareja, M. A. (ed.) Manual de terapia de conducta, vol. 1, pp. 169–218. Dykinson, Madrid (1998)
14. Bragado, C.: Terapia de conducta en la infancia: trastornos de ansiedad. Fundación Universidad Empresa, Madrid (1994)
15. Hoffman, H.G., Garcia-Palacios, Kapa, V., Beecher, J., Sharar, S.: Virtual Reality for reducing experimental ischemic pain. International Journal of Human Computer Interaction 15, 469–486 (2003)
16. Das, D., Grimmer, K., Sparnon, A., McRae, S., Thomas, B.: The efficacy of playing a virtual reality game in modulating pain for children with acute burn injuries: a randomized controlled trial [ISRCTN87413556]. BMC Pediatrics [Electronic Resource] (Electronic), vol. 5(1), pp. 1–1 (2005)
17. Gershon, Zimand, Pickering, Rothbaum, Hodges.: A Pilot and Feasibility Study of Virtual Reality as a Distraction for Children With Cancer. Journal of the American Academy of Child & Adolescent Psychiatry 43(10), 1243–1249 (2004)
18. Wolitzky, Fivush, Zimand, Hodges, Rothbaum.: Effectiveness of virtual reality distraction during a painful medical procedure in pediatric oncology patients. Psychology & Health 20(6), 817–824 (2005)

Closed-Loop Adaptive Decision Support Based on Automated Trust Assessment

Peter-Paul van Maanen[1,2], Tomas Klos[3], and Kees van Dongen[1]

[1] TNO Human Factors, P.O. Box 23, 3769 ZG Soesterberg, The Netherlands
{peter-paul.vanmaanen, kees.vandongen}@tno.nl
[2] Department of Artificial Intelligence, Vrije Universiteit Amsterdam,
De Boelelaan 1081a, 1081 HV Amsterdam, The Netherlands
[3] Dutch National Research Institute for Mathematics and Computer Science (CWI),
P.O. Box 94079, 1090 GB Amsterdam, The Netherlands
tomas.klos@cwi.nl

Abstract. This paper argues that it is important to study issues concerning trust and reliance when developing systems that are intended to augment cognition. Operators often under-rely on the help of a support system that provides advice or that performs certain cognitive tasks autonomously. The decision to rely on support seems to be largely determined by the notion of relative trust. However, this decision to rely on support is not always appropriate, especially when support systems are not perfectly reliable. Because the operator's reliability estimations are typically imperfectly aligned or calibrated with the support system's true capabilities, we propose that the aid makes an estimation of the extent of this calibration (under different circumstances) and intervenes accordingly. This system is intended to improve overall performance of the operator-support system as a whole. The possibilities in terms of application of these ideas are explored and an implementation of this concept in an abstract task environment has been used as a case study.

1 Introduction

One of the main challenges of the Augmented Cognition Community is to explore and identify the limitations of human cognitive capabilities and try to let technology seemlessly adapt to them. This paper focuses on augmenting human cognitive capabilities concerning reliance decision making.

Operators often under-rely on the help of a support system that provides advice or that performs certain cognitive tasks autonomously. The decision to rely on support seems to be largely determined by the notion of relative trust. It is commonly believed that when trust in the support system is higher than trust in own performance, operators tend to rely on the system. However, this decision to rely on help is not always appropriate, especially when support systems are not perfectly reliable. One problem is that the reliability of support systems is often under-estimated, increasing the probability that support is rejected. Because the operator's reliability estimations are typically imperfectly aligned or calibrated with true capabilities, we propose that the aid makes an estimation of the extent of this calibration (under different circumstances) and intervenes accordingly. In other words, we study a system that assesses whether human

D.D. Schmorrow, L.M. Reeves (Eds.): Augmented Cognition, HCII 2007, LNAI 4565, pp. 266–275, 2007.

decisions to rely on support are made appropriately. This system is intended to improve overall performance of the operator-support system as a whole.

We study a system in which there is an operator charged with making decisions, while being supported by an automated decision support system. As mentioned above, the aim is to make the operator-support system as a whole operate as effectively as possible. This is done by letting the system automatically assess its trust in the operator and in itself, and adapt or adjust aspects of the support based on this trust. This requires models of trust, including a way of updating trust based on interaction data, as well as a means for adapting the type of support.

In this study, trust is defined as the attitude that an agent will help achieve an individual's goals, possibly the agent itself, in a situation characterized by uncertainty and vulnerability [1]. Trust can refer to the advice of another agent or to one's own judgment. Trust, like the feelings and perceptions on which it is based, is a covert or psychological state that can be assessed through subjective ratings. To assess trust, some studies have used scales of trust (e.g., [2]) and some studies have used scales of perceived reliability (e.g., [3]). The latter is used because no operator intervention is needed. We distinguish trust from the decision to depend on advice, the act of relying on advice, and the appropriateness of relying on advice [4,5].

As a first implementation of this closed-loop adaptive decision support system, the operator-system task described in [6] has been extended.[1] This architecture instantiation leads to an overview of the lessons learned and new insights for further development of adaptive systems based on automated trust assessment. The present paper discusses some key concepts for improving the development of systems that are intended to augment cognition. The focus is on improving reliance on support.

In Section 2 an overview is given of the theoretical background of reliance decision making support systems and its relevance to the Augmented Cognition Community. In Section 3 the conceptual design of a reliance decision making support system is given. In Section 4 an instantiation of this design is described and evaluated. We end with some conclusions and future research.

2   Theoretical Background

The goal of augmented cognition is to extend the performance of human-machine systems via development and usage of computational technologies. Adaptive automation may be used to augment cognition. Adaptive automation refers to a machine capable of dynamic reallocation of task responsibility between human and machine. Reallocation can be triggered by changes in task performance, task demands, or assessments of workload. The goal of adaptive automation is to make human-machine systems more resilient by dynamically engaging humans and machines in cognitive tasks. Engaging humans more in tasks may solve out-of-the-loop performance problems, such as problems with complacency, situation awareness, and skills-degradation. This may be useful in situations of underload. Engaging machines more in tasks may solve performance degradation when the demand for speed or attention exceeds the human ability. This may be useful in situations of overload.

---

[1] A description and analysis of this system will be published in another paper in preparation.

It should be noted that the potential benefits of adaptive automation turn into risks when the system wrongly concludes that support is or is not needed, or when the timing or kind of support is wrong [7]. For the adaptive system there may be problems with the real-time acquisition of data about the subject's cognition, with determining whether actual or anticipated performance degradations are problematic, and with deciding whether, when, and in what way activities need to be reallocated between human and machine. When the adaptive system is not reliable we create rather than solve problems: unwanted interruptions and automation surprises may disrupt performance and may lead to frustration, distrust, and disuse of the adaptive system [8]. In this paper we focus on computational methods that can be used to adjust the degree in which the machine intervenes.

When machine decisions about task reallocation are not reliable under all conditions the human operator should somehow be involved. One way is to make the reasoning of adaptive automation observable and adjustable for the operator. Understanding the machine's reasoning would enable her to give the system more or less room for intervention. Another and more ambitious way to cope with unreliable adaptive automation is by having a machine adjust its level of support based on a real-time model of trust in human reliance decision making capabilities. In this case it is the machine which adjusts the level of support it provides. The idea is adjusting the level of support to a level that is sufficiently reliable for the user, that problems with frustration, distrust and disuse of the adaptive system are reduced.

A rational decision maker accepts support of an adaptive system when this would increase the probability of goal achievement and reject this support when it would decrease goal achievement. We rely more on support when we believe that it is thought to be highly accurate or when we are not confident about our own performance. People seem to use a notion of relative trust to decide whether to seek or accept support [9,10,11]. We also rely more on support when the decision of the system to provide support corresponds to our own assessment. The performance of an adaptive support system has to be trusted more than our own performance as well as be appropriately timed. In making a decision to accept support, users are thought to take the reliability of past performance into account. This decision to accept support is not based on a perception of actual reliability, but on how this is perceived and interpreted. Unfortunately, research has shown that trust and perceptions of reliability may be imperfectly calibrated: the reliability of decision support is under-estimated [3,6]. This could lead to under-reliance on systems that provide adaptive support. In this paper we argue that, because of this human bias to under-rely on support, reliance decision support designs are needed that have the following properties:

Feedback. They should provide feedback about the reliability of past human and machine performance. This would allow humans to better calibrate their trust in their own performance and that of the machine, and support them to appropriately adjust the level of autonomy of adaptive support.

Reliance. They should generate a machine's decision whom to rely on. Humans could use this recommendation to make a better reliance decision. This decision could also be used by the machine itself to adjust its level of autonomy.

Meta-reliance. They should generate a machine's decision whom to rely on concerning reliance decisions. This decision could combine and integrate the best reliance decision making capabilities of both human and machine. This could also be used by the machine itself to adjust its level of autonomy.

In the following sections we show how the above three functions could be realized by a system that automatically assesses trust in real-time.

3 Conceptual Design of Reliance Decision Support

In this section the three properties mentioned above are described in more detail, in terms of three increasingly elaborate conceptual designs of reliance decision support. First we abstract away from possible application domains in order to come to a generic solution. The designs presented in this section are applicable if the following conditions are satisfied:

- The application involves a human-machine cooperative setting concerning a complex task, where it is not trivial to determine whether the machine or the human has better performance. In other words, in order to perform the task at hand, it is important to take both the human's and the machine's opinion into account.
- Both the human operator and the automated aid are able to generate solutions to the problems in the application at hand. In other words, both are in principle able to do the job and both solutions are substitutable, but not necessarily generated in a similar way and of the same quality.
- Some sort of feedback is available in order for both machine and human to be able to estimate their respective performances and generate trust accordingly. In other words, there is enough information for reliance decision making.

In many cases, if for a certain task the above conditions do not hold (e.g., the operator's solution to a problem is not directly comparable to the aid's solution, or no immediate feedback is available), then for important subtasks of the task they generally still hold.

One could say that for all automated support systems the aid supports the operator on a scale from a mere advice being asked by the user, to complete autonomous actions performed and initiated by the aid itself. More specifically, for reliance decision making support, this scale runs from receiving advice about a reliance decision, to the reliance decision being made by the aid itself. In a human-machine cooperative setting, a *reliance decision* is made when either the aid or the operator decides to rely on either self or other. In the designs presented below the terms *human advice* and *machine advice* refer to the decision made for a specific task. The terms *human reliance* and *machine reliance* refer to the reliance decisions made by the human and the machine, respectively, i.e., the advice (task decision) by the agent relied upon. Finally, the term *machine meta-reliance* refers to the decision of the machine whether to rely on the human or the machine with respect to their reliance capabilities.

3.1 Feedback

Agreement or disagreement between human and machine concerning their advice can be used as a cue for the reliability of a decision. In case of agreement it is likely that (the decision based on) the corresponding advice is correct. In case of disagreement, on the other hand, at least one of the advices is incorrect. To decide which advice to rely on in this case, the operator has to have an accurate perception of her own and the aid's reliability in giving advice. The machine could provide feedback about these reliabilities, for instance by communicating past human and machine advice performance. This would allow humans to better calibrate their trust in their own performance and that of the machine, and support them to adjust the machine's level of autonomy. In Figure 1 the conceptual design of machine feedback is shown.

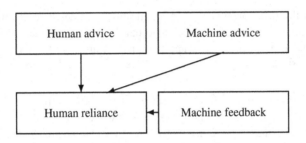

Fig. 1. Both human and machine generate an advice on which the human's reliance decision is based. The machine provides feedback, for instance about the reliability of past human and machine performance. This allows humans to better calibrate their trust.

3.2 Reliance

Unfortunately, by comparing advice, one introduces an extra cognitive task: making a reliance decision. In this particular design the machine augments the cognitive function of reliance decision making, resulting in a decrease of the operator's workload. This can be in the form of a recommendation, or the reliance decision can be made autonomously by the machine, without any intervention by the human operator. The machine or human could adjust the machine's level of autonomy in that sense. Additionally, the human could provide feedback in order to improve the machine's decision. For instance, the human can monitor the machine in its reliance decision making process and possibly veto in certain unacceptable situations. In Figure 2 the conceptual design of such machine reliance is shown.

3.3 Meta-reliance

Since in some situations humans make better reliance decisions, and in others machines do, reliance decision making completely done by the machine does not result in an optimal effect. Therefore, it may be desirable to let the machine decide whom to rely on concerning making reliance decisions. We called this process *meta-reliance decision making* and it combines the best reliance decision making capabilities of both human and machine. If the machine's meta-reliance decision determines that the machine itself should be relied upon, the machine would have a high level of autonomy, and otherwise a lower one. Hence the machine is capable of adapting its own autonomy. In Figure 3 the conceptual design of machine meta-reliance is shown.

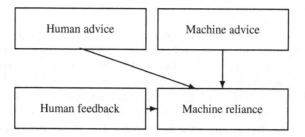

Fig. 2. The machine generates a reliance decision. In this particular design the machine augments the cognitive function of reliance decision making. Both human and machine generate an advice on which the machine's reliance decision is based. It is possible that the human gives additional feedback.

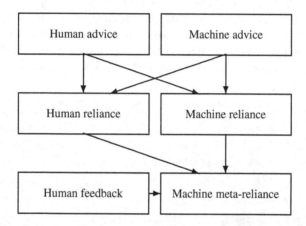

Fig. 3. The machine generates a meta-reliance decision. It combines the best reliance decision making capabilities of both human and machine. Both the human and the machine generate advices and reliance decisions, on the latter of which the machine's meta-reliance decision is based.

4 Implementation and Evaluation

In this section we describe a proof-of-concept for the ideas presented above. In previous work [6], a collaborative operator-aid system was used in laboratory experiments to study human operators' reliance decision making. None of the additions described in Sec. 3 were employed, the setting was essentially that described in Sec. 3.1, without the aid's feedback. We have now extended the aid's design to provide the reliance and meta-reliance properties, and simulated the extended system's performance, compared to the results from the laboratory experiments. Below, we first describe the original and the extended task, and then the corresponding extensions in the aid's design. Finally, we present the improvements in system performance resulting from these additions.

4.1 The Task

For the experiment described in [6], participants read a story about a software company interested in evaluating the performance of their adaptive software before applying it to more complex tasks on naval ships. The story pointed out that the level of reliability between software and human performance was comparable and around 70%. Participants were asked to perform a pattern recognition task with advice of a decision aid and were instructed to maximize the number of correct answers by relying on their own predictions as well as the advice of the decision aid. The interface the participants were presented with is presented in the first 3 and the 6th rows of Figure 4. The task consitutes making a choice between 3 alternatives, as shown in each of the rows in the interface. In phase 1 the operator chooses, based on her own personal estimation of the pattern to be recognized. Then in phase 2 the machine chooses, with a pre-fixed average accuracy of 70%. Finally, in phase 3, the operator makes a reliance decision, by selecting the answer given in the first 2 phases by the agent she chooses to rely on. (The operator is free to choose a different answer altogether, but this happened only rarely in the experiments.) The last action of each trial consists of the feedback given by the system about which action was the correct one (phase 6), the corresponding button colored green if the operator's reliance decision was correct, and red if it was incorrect.

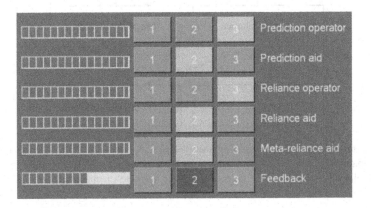

Fig. 4. An example interaction between the operator and the automated decision aid. The rows represent the different phases of the operator-aid task. For the current research, phases 4 and 5 were added to the task environment described in [6].

In order to support the operator in making reliance decisions the above operator-aid task was extended by adding 2 phases representing the aid's reliance (Sec. 3.2) and meta-reliance (Sec. 3.3) decisions. The next section details the aid's design in this respect.

4.2 Design of the Aid

In the original experiments, the aid did nothing more than provide an advice to the human operator. The enhancements to the aid's design were intended to provide the properties Reliance and Meta-reliance discussed in Section 3, to allow improvement upon the operator's Reliance Decision Making (RDM) in the form of Reliance Decision Making of the Machine (RDMM) and Meta-Reliance Decision Making of the Machine (Meta-RDMM).

Both RDMM and Meta-RDMM are based on a generic trust model [4] that allows the aid to estimate the operator's and the aid's abilities to make advice (task-related, prediction) and reliance decisions. The RDMM module makes the decision in phase 4 in Figure 4 ('Reliance Aid'), based on a comparison of the aid's trust in the operator's and the aid's own prediction abilities (phases 1 and 2). Like the operator in phase 3, the aid proposes in phase 4 the answer given in phases 1 and 2 by the agent it trusts most hightly, where trust refers to *prediction* capability. In case of disagreeing reliance decisions in phases 3 and 4, the aid chooses among the operator and the aid in phase 5, this time based on a comparison of its trust in the two agents' *reliance decision making* capabilities.

As mentioned above, the same basic trust model is used for both estimates (prediction and reliance decision making capabilities). Essentially, the respective abilities are modeled as random variables $0 \leq \theta_a^x \leq 1$, which are interpreted as the probabilities of each of the agents $a \in \{\text{operator}, \text{aid}\}$ making the correct decision $x \in \{\text{prediction}, \text{reliance}\}$. The aid uses Beta probability density functions (pdfs) over each of these 4 random variables to model its belief in each of the values of $\theta \in [0, 1]$ being the correct one. Based on the feedback obtained in phase 6, each of the answers given in phases 1 through 4 can be classified as 'success' or 'failure' depending on whether the operator and the aid, respectively, were correct or incorrect in their prediction and reliance decisions, respectively. At the end of each trial, the aid uses Bayes' rule to update each of its estimates given the newly obtained information from phase 6. The advantage of using a Beta pdf as a prior in Bayesian inference about a binomial likelihood (such as that of θ), is that the resulting posterior distribution is again a Beta pdf [12,13].

In the next trial, the aid uses the new estimates about the agents' prediction abilities for RDMM in phase 4, and the estimates about the agents' reliance decision making abilities for Meta-RDMM in phase 5.

4.3   Experimental Results

The original experimental design and results are discussed in [6]. Here, we show to what extent the elaborations of the aid's design were able to enhance the system's overall performance. Table 1 shows these results. Each participant played two experiments of 101 trials each. For each row, the improvements from operator reliance decision making (Operator-RDM) to RDMM, and from Operator-RDM to Meta-RDMM are significant. No significant difference in performance is found between RDMM and Meta-RDMM. There are no significant differences between experiment 1, 2, and both, for RDMM and Meta-RDMM. However, the differences between experiment 1, 2, and both, for Operator-RDM are significant. This means that, in our experiments, there was no measurable effect on performance of (Meta-)RDMM due to operator learning effects.

Our results indicate that the quality of the decision to rely on the prediction of either the operator or the aid is higher when it is made by RDMM than when it is made by

Table 1. Performance (percentage correct) of operator reliance decision making (Operator-RDM), RDMM, and Meta-RDMM. Per row, the differences between Operator-RDM and RDMM, and Operator-RDM and Meta-RDMM, are significant.

	Operator-RDM	RDMM	Meta-RDMM
exp. 1	0.65	0.70	0.70
exp. 2	0.67	0.70	0.69
both	0.66	0.70	0.69

human participants. When a computer would make reliance decisions based on RDMM it would outperform most human participants. However, it also became clear that in some situations humans make better reliance decisions than aids, and in others aids do. This means that reliance decision making completely done by the aid does not necessarily result in optimal performance. Meta-RDMM tries to take advantage of this and is based on the idea that the aid itself decides when to rely on RDMM and when to rely on the operator for reliance decision making (meta-reliance). Our results show that Meta-RDMM also outperforms human participants in reliance decision making, but (surprisingly) significant differences between RDMM and Meta-RDMM were not found.

5   Conclusion

The goal of augmented cognition is to extend the performance of human-machine systems via development and use of computational technology. In the context of the current work, performance can be improved when, like in human-human teams, both human and machine are able to assess and reach agreement on who should be trusted more and who should be relied on in what situation.

In this paper we showed that human reliance decisions are not perfect and reliance decision making can be augmented by computational technology. Our machine reliance decision making model outperforms human reliance decision making.

Now that we have our proof-of-concept in an abstract task, we intend to investigate how human-machine cooperation can be augmented in more complex and more realistic situations. We intend to focus on how models of trust and reliance can be practically used to adjust the level of autonomy of adaptive systems. We want to investigate in what domains this kind of support has an impact on the effectiveness of task performance, and how the magnitude of the impact depends on the task's and the domain's characteristics. How serious are the conditions mentioned in section 3, both in terms of limiting the scope of application domains, and in terms of determining the effectiveness of our solutions. An important question is whether the properties of our abstract task environment are paralleled in real-world settings.

Acknowledgments

This research was partly funded by the Royal Netherlands Navy under program number V206 and by the Dutch government (SENTER) under project number TSIT2021.

References

1. Lee, J.D., See, K.A.: Trust in automation: Designing for appropriate reliance. Human Factors 46, 50–80 (2004)
2. Lee, J.D., Moray, N.: Trust, control strategies and allocation of function in human machine systems. Ergonomics 22, 671–691 (1992)
3. Wiegmann, D.A., Rich, A., Zhang, H.: Automated diagnostic aids: the effects of aid reliability on user's trust and reliance. Theoretical Issues in Ergonomics Science 2, 352–367 (2001)
4. Klos, T.B., La Poutré, H.: A versatile approach to combining trust values for making binary decisions. In: Stølen, K., Winsborough, W.H., Martinelli, F., Massacci, F. (eds.) iTrust 2006. LNCS, vol. 3986, pp. 206–220. Springer, Heidelberg (2006)
5. van Maanen, P.-P., van Dongen, K.: Towards task allocation decision support by means of cognitive modeling of trust. In: Proceedings of the Eighth International Workshop on Trust in Agent Societies (Trust 2005), pp. 168–77. Utrecht, The Netherlands (July 2005)
6. van Dongen, K., van Maanen, P.-P.: Under-reliance on the decision aid: A difference in calibration and attribution between self and aid. In: Proceedings of the Human Factors and Ergonomics Society's 50th Annual Meeting, San Francisco, USA (2006)
7. Parasuraman, R., Mouloua, M., Hilburn, B.: Adaptive aiding and adaptive task allocation enhance human-machine interaction. Automation Technology and Human Performance: Current Research and Trends 22, 119–123 (1999)
8. Parasuraman, R., Riley, V.A.: Humans and automation: Use, misuse, disuse, abuse. Human Factors 39, 230–253 (1997)
9. Moray, N., Inagaki, T., Itoh, M.: Adaptive automation, trust, and self-confidence in fault management of time-critical tasks. Journal of Experimental Psychology: Applied 6, 44–58 (2000)
10. Dzindolet, M.T., Peterson, S.A., Pomranky, R.A., Pierce, L.G., Beck, H.P.: The role of trust in automation reliance. International Journal of Human-Computer Studies 58, 697–718 (2003)
11. van Dongen, K., van Maanen, P.-P.: Designing for dynamic task allocation. In: Proceedings of the Seventh International Naturalistic Decision Making Conference (NDM7), Amsterdam, The Netherlands (2005)
12. D'Agostini, G.: Bayesian inference in processing experimental data: Principles and basic applications. Reports on Progress in Physics 66, 1383–1419 (2003)
13. Gelman, A., Carlin, J.B., Stern, H.S., Rubin, D.B.: Bayesian Data Analysis. 2nd edn. Chapman & Hall/CRC (2004)

A Closed-Loop Adaptive System for Command and Control

Tjerk de Greef[1] and Henryk Arciszewski[2]

[1] Department of Human in Control, TNO Human Factors,
PO BOX 23, 3769 ZG Soesterberg, The Netherlands
[2] Department of C2 and Information, TNO Information & Operations,
PO BOX 23, 3769 ZG Soesterberg, The Netherlands
{Tjerk.deGreef,Henryk.Arciszewski}@tno.nl

Abstract. On Navy ships, technological developments enable crews to work more efficiently and effectively. However, in such complex, autonomous, and information-rich environments a competition for the users' attention is going on between different information items, possibly leading to a cognitive overload. This overload originates in the limitations of human attention and constitutes a well-known and well-studied bottleneck in human information processing. The concept of adaptive automation promises a solution to the overwhelmed operator by shifting the amount of work between the human and the system in time, while maintaining a high level of situation awareness. One of the most critical challenges in developing adaptive human-machine collaboration concerns the design of a trigger mechanism. This paper discusses and evaluates a number of possible triggers for the usage in closed-loop adaptive automation from the perspective of command and control.

1 Introduction

On navy ships, technological developments enable crews to work more efficiently and effectively. However, in such complex, autonomous, and information-rich environments, task demands may exceed the users' limited cognitive resources, possibly leading to a state of overload. This constitutes a well-known and well-studied bottleneck in human information processing. Besides the technical developments, the manning reduction initiatives of many navies cause a further increase of the workload of crew.

It is suggested that the adaptive automation paradigm may present a good equilibrium between task demands and the available cognitive resources. Adaptive automation (AA) takes as its starting point that the division of labor between man and machine should not be static but dynamic in nature. It is based on the conception of actively supporting the operator only at those moments in time when human performance in a system needs support to meet operational requirements [1]. Some argue that the appliance of adaptive automation enhances performance, reduce workload, and improve situation awareness [2]. Since 1988 various empirical studies have proven beneficial effects of the concept of adaptive automation [3] [4] [5] [6] [7] [8].

D.D. Schmorrow, L.M. Reeves (Eds.): Augmented Cognition, HCII 2007, LNAI 4565, pp. 276–285, 2007.

One of the challenging factors in the development of a successful adaptive automation concept concerns the question of *when* changes in level of automation must be effectuated. With respect to methods of invocation, one of the most critical challenges facing designers of adaptive systems is how to effectively switch between the levels and/or modes of operation. The definition of augmented cognition extends the AA paradigm by explicitly stating the symbolic integration of man and machines in a closed-loop system whereby the operator's cognitive state and the operational context are to be detected by the system [9].

Workload generally is the key concept to invoke such a change but this concept is used in the broadest sense only. The measurement of workload is again much debated and we would like to elucidate the relationship between workload, task demands, and performance. Fig 1 shows the relationship between these three variables.

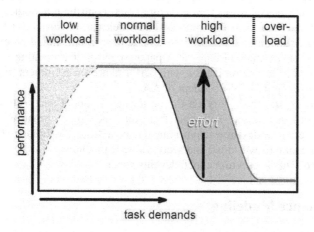

Fig. 1. The relation between task demands, performance, and workload (taken from [10])

It shows that an operator can experience different levels of workload dependent on the demands of a task. It also shows that the performance does not necessarily decline as the operator experiences a high workload. We can cope with changing conditions without decreasing our performance or getting into a state of overload by putting more energy into it thereby making ourselves an adaptive system. The difference between maintaining the level of performance and an increased workload is referred to as the *effort* of the operator.

The majority of the studies have facilitated allocations based on critical events, performance models, or physiological measurements, all with their benefits and pitfalls. The critical-event method uses specific tactical events as triggers and suffers from the fact that this method is insensitive to the operator's available resources. Performance models have been argued as being totally reactive and unlikely to craft a comprehensive database [11]. The psychophysical approach uses deviations in EEG power bands, heart rate variability, respiration, galvanic skin response, and brain activity as trigger mechanisms. These studies suggest that it is indeed possible to obtain indices of one's brain activity and use that information to drive an adaptive automation system to improve performance and moderate workload. There are, however, still many critical conceptual and technical issues that must be overcome before systems such as these can move from the laboratory to the field [12].

None of the studies have reported on the application of AC in the actual operational field such as command and control (C2), although a number of studies have generalized a number of tasks from C2 for experimental purposes. These studies demonstrate enhanced performance, a reduction of workload, and improved situation awareness, though none report on the utilization of AA in an operational settings. Manning reduction initiatives and technological developments confront warfare officers with more information and the risk of overload and underload seems eminent. This study centralizes on the application of AA in the field of C2, particularly on the question which triggers are useful in this area of operation. This study abstains from the usage of psychophysical triggers since research by Veltman & Jansen [10] report on the difficulties of such measure in the field of C2. This study centralizes on the operational field and the question which factors could contribute as indicators of overload. We gathered data from the same as study Veltman & Jansen [10] and demonstrate that performance modeling provides one indicator, but should be extended with clever usage of environmental data. This paper suggests that creating triggers based on environmental data in combination with performance measurement might deliver a reliable trigger for applying the concept of AA.

Section two reports the theory on the performance model and section three validates the performance model with data from the study by Veltman & Jansen [10]. Chapter four demonstrates how environmental data from the field of C2 might be used as an indication of workload and section five learns how *pro-active* behavior can be incorporated. The last section concludes this paper.

2   Performance Modeling

As stated previously, we focus on a performance measure and state that the measure of operator performance provides an indication of the cognitive state. Specifically, the acknowledgement time (AT) of the operator on signals from the combat management system (CMS) is the primary base of the performance measure. Accordingly, a performance-decrease is regarded as a situation where the operator fails to cope with the situation and the operation requires assistance of the system. These situations arise due to temporal limited human information processing capacity.

The chosen feedback approach works only under the premise that the system signals the operator intelligently. Hence, the operator is prompted only when *true* information is available and *true* information should be regarded according to the definition of Shannon & Weaver [13] as the *reduction of uncertainty*. This premise is achieved through the separation of the user and system understanding of the surrounding world (see fig. 2). Both user and system use its own particular reasoning mechanisms to create such an understanding. The system reasons through artificial intelligence mechanisms using sensory information while the human applies cognitive resources to craft such an understanding. The information elements (e.g. track) are present in each view though their attributes (e.g. speed, height) may differ. Each element can be compared for differences. For instance, the identities assigned by system and user may not be the same. Accordingly, the CMS signals information to the operator only when the system finds *new* evidence that adjusts the current understanding. The operator on the other hand, can acknowledge signaled information by explicitly stating its understanding of the situation and the CMS stores this opinion in the user world view (see fig. 2).

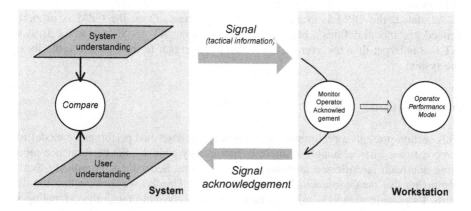

Fig. 2. The workstation receives information from the system and communicates the operator's understanding of the situation opinion to the system for storage in the user understanding space. The operator performance is calculated real-time and is based on the acknowledgement of the operator responses to signals.

The workstation has two responsibilities. First, the workstation ought to keep the information element within the system synchronized with the user's state of mind. Secondly the workstation must measure the user's cognitive state. The first responsibility is achieved through the passing of the user's understanding, and the second responsibility is accomplished by comparing the acknowledgement times against an operator performance model (OPM). A significant increase in the AT corresponds with a drop in performance and with a state of overload, which on its turn leads to increased assertiveness of the workstation.

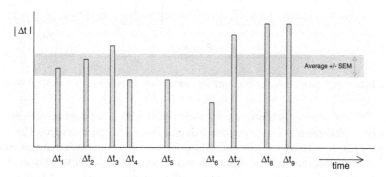

Fig. 3. Detecting an increase in acknowledgement time means a decrease in performance

The OPM is crafted in a learning phase from the average AT of the user to signals of the CMS regarding elements that are signaled. The OPM determines the average response (AVG) time and the standard error of means (SEM). Standard errors of means are important because they reflect how much sampling fluctuation, that is the extent to which a statistic takes on different values with different samples, a statistic will show.

As stated, the OPM is crafted in a learning phase. Once the OPM is properly trained, the model defines a bandwidth of the average AT +/- SEM (see fig 3). Any AT that is larger than the average AT + SEM is a trigger to increase the authority of the system.

3 Validation

This section presents a preliminary validation of the described performance model for three reasons. First, although sensitive to momentary changes, the performance modeling approach is criticized as being totally reactive. Secondly it is unlikely that a comprehensive database could be established [11]. Thirdly, we surmise that the described signaling paradigm might demonstrate a low sample rate, since signaling is only done in those cases where reduction of uncertainty is achieved. Prior to running an experiment with the performance model, we applied the model using data from another experiment and looked into these issues.

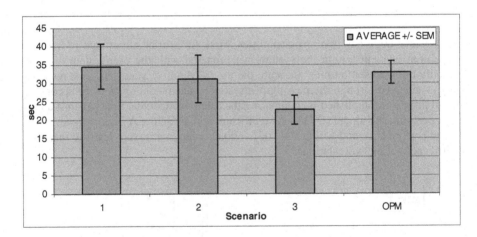

Fig. 4. The average acknowledge time and standard error of means per scenario for one WO

During the evaluation of a novel workstation [14] with eight warfare officers (WO) of the Royal Netherlands Navy, acknowledgement-times were recorded. The evaluation was arranged to prove the power of the workstation. Mitigation strategies were not available. The workstation was designed around a simulation environment that fed environmental and entity data to a ship model containing sensors, weapons and a highly automated combat management system (CMS). The information flow from the CMS communicates information in the form of tracks that include position, velocity, identity, and threat-level. The CMS is able to build and retrieve track information thanks to its range of sensors and reasoning functionality. When new information regarding a track becomes available, the CMS signals this information to the workstation only when the user has a different understanding of the situation. Said differ ently, no signaling is undertaken when the operator already identified a track as hostile. After an acquaintance period of one day, the WO performed three scenarios. Fig. 4 and table 1 summarize the average AT and the standard error of means for each scenario for one WO. These three scenarios served in the learning phase and the last column describes the outcome of the operator performance model by combining all three AT for the three scenarios. Accordingly, the OPM states that the operator should be aided by the CMS when the average response time reaches the threshold of 35.9 seconds (=32.9 + 3 seconds).

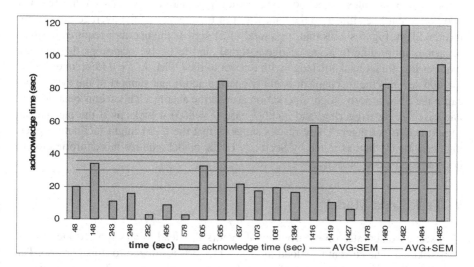

Fig. 5. The acknowledgement time and the OPM as a function of the second scenario

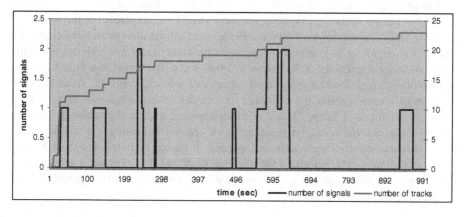

Fig. 6. The number of signals for the second scenario displays quiet areas

Table 1. The expected level of information of an important feature of a track

Identity	Presumable intention	Expected LIP
Pending	System is gathering information	Skill-based
Unknown	Unknown	Knowledge-based
Friendly	Track of own nation	Skill-based
Assumed Friendly	Presumably own nation track	Knowledge-based
Neutral	Track is commercial	Skill-based
Suspect	Track might attack	Knowledge-based
Hostile	Track might attack	Rule-based

Fig. 5 demonstrates the acknowledgement times as a function of scenario two. The two horizontal lines illustrate the bandwidth of the model, i.e. the average plus or minus the SEM. Fig. 5 shows that for a total of 21 signals the operator requires in seven occasions more time to acknowledge a signal, and in twelve occasions the operator requires less time to acknowledge with respect to the OPM. At $t = 148$ seconds and at $t = 605$ seconds the mechanism is not triggering additional support of the system because the SEM absorbs slight fluctuation around the average. This seems beneficial in one case for not triggering, and another case $(t = 605)$ it looks as if the mechanism should lead to a trigger. These results suggests that the OPM might facilitate triggering occasionally but, as stated by Scerbo [11], the model requires more information to become useful, and proactive.

4 Task Load Model

This section elaborates on environmental factors that lead to an expected increase of the workload. The current task load model (CTL) [15] is utilized for this purpose. The (CTL) model distinguishes three factors that have a substantial effect on the workload. The first factor, percentage time occupied (TO), has been used to assess workload in practice for time-line assessments. Such assessments are often based on the notion that people should not be occupied more than 70 to 80 percent of the total time available [16]. The second load factor is the level of information processing (LIP). To address the cognitive task demands, the cognitive load model incorporates the skill-rule-knowledge framework of Rasmussen (1986) where the knowledge based component involves a high load on the limited capacity of working memory. To address the demands of attention shifts, the cognitive load model distinguishes task-set switching (TSS) as a third load factor. The tree factors present a three-dimensional space in which human activities can be projected with regions indicating the cognitive demands that the activity imposes on the operator. It should be noted that these factors represent task demands that affect the operator workload (i.e., it is not a definition of the operator cognitive state). Fig 7 shows from the perspective of the operational demands a number of expected cognitive states.

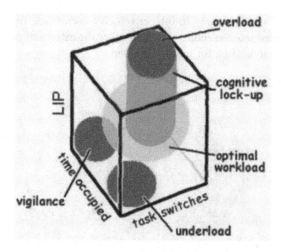

Fig. 7. The three dimensions of the task load model. Neerincx [14] distinguished several critical regions.

The workload cube may inspire us to find more workload indicators. First of all the number of information element, i.e. the tracks, may lead to an increase in the number of TS (switching between information elements for monitoring purposes) and TO. Fig 6 provides a nice example of this case in the timeframe $t = 496$ untill $t = 694$. The LIP, sometimes referred to as complexity, of the information element in C2 depends mainly on the identity (friend or foe) of a track. The identity often provides an intention, but sometimes the identity involves a lot of uncertainty. We state that uncertain elements lead to a higher LIP and table 1 provides an overview of the identities and expected LIP. For example, an increase in unknown tracks results in an increase in complexity since the operator has to put effort in the process to ascertain the identity of a track of which relatively little is known. The cognitive burden will be less when the same increase of track is labeled friendly.

5 Workload Predictors

Scerbo [11] mentions that a mitigation strategy should not be entirely reactive but preferably demonstrate a kind of pro-active behavior. This section describes an approach where such pro-activeness is achieved.

In C2, tracks are the predominant information elements and it is common that a number of operators split the surrounding world into sectors. Usually these sectors are divided geometrically (e.g. range), but not necessarily and the sectors could easily consist other attributes (e.g. speed, identity). Each operator is responsible for information elements in that sector, and the amount and identity of tracks provide an indicator of workload. The amount of information elements that is likely to enter the operator's sector in the following few minutes could therefore be an indicator of future workload, so pro-active adaptation could be based on estimates of this variable. The CMS uses the trajectories of the tracks to infer a velocity vector (see fig 8). This velocity vector is extrapolated into the future which provides the estimated number of tracks in the future hence an indication for future workload.

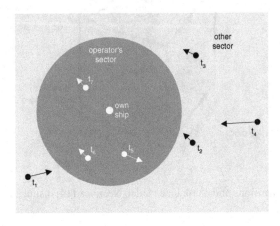

Fig. 8. Information elements that are not in the operational space may eventually enter

6   Conclusion

Technological developments enable crews of navy frigates to work more efficiently and effectively. These complex, autonomous, and information-rich environments creates a competition for the operator's attention between different information items, possibly leading to a cognitive overload. Limitations in human cognition are due to intrinsic restrictions and these may fluctuate from moment to moment depending on a host of factors including mental fatigue, novelty, boredom, and stress. The concept of adaptive automation promises a solution to the overwhelmed operator by shifting the amount of work between the human and the system in time, while maintaining a high level of situation awareness. One of the most critical challenges in developing adaptive human-machine collaboration concerns the design of a trigger mechanism. This paper discusses a performance model in the field of C2 and the proposed model hints towards a description of cognitive state. The evaluation shows that additional factors should be incorporated in the model. These are found by applying the cognitive task load model [15] to the field of C2 and a number of workload factors are identified. Also, it is suggested that triggering could be improved by a predictive measure.

This study demonstrates that the design of a trigger mechanism is difficult and that a number of factors need to be incorporated. We will continue research and evaluation along this path, and combine critical workload factors to an operator model.

Acknowledgements. CAMS-Force Vision, a software development company associated with the Royal Netherlands Navy, funded this research.

References

1. Rouse, W.B.: Adaptive aiding for Human/Computer Control. Human factors, 431–443 (1988)
2. Bailey, N.B., Scerbo, M.W., Freeman, F.G., Mikulka, P.J., Scott, A.S.: Comparison of a Brain-Based Adaptive System and a Manual Adaptable System for Invoking Automation. Human factors, 693–709 (2006)
3. Parasuraman, R., Mouloua, M., Molloy, R.: Effects of adaptive task allocation on monitoring of automated systems. Human factors, 665–679 (1996)
4. Kaber, D., Endlsey, M.: The effects of level of automation and adaptive automation on human performance, situation awareness and workload in a dynamic control task. Theroretical Issues in Ergonomics Science (2004)
5. Hilburn, B., Jorna, P., Byrne, E., Parasuraman, R.: The effect of adaptive air traffic control (ATC) decision aiding on controller mental workload. In: Mouloua, M., Koonce, J.M. (eds.) Human-automation interaction: research and practice, pp. 84–91. Lawrence Erlbaum Associates, Mahwah (1997)
6. Scallen, S., Hancock, P., Duley, J.: Pilot performance and preference for short cycles of automation in adaptive function allocation. Applied ergonomics, 397–404 (1995)
7. Inagaki, T.: Situation-adaptive Autonomy for Time-critical Takeoff Decisions. International journal of modelling and simulation, 175–180 (2000)
8. Moray, N., Inagaki, T., Itoh, M.: Adaptive Automation, Trust, and Self-Confidence in Fault Management of Time-Critical Tasks. Journal of experimental psychology 6(1), 44–58 (2000)
9. Kruse, A.A., Schmorrow, D.D.: Session overview: Foundations of augmented cognition. In: Schmorrow, D.D. (ed.) Foundations of Augmented Cognition, pp. 441–445. Lawrence Erlbaum Associates, Mahwah (2005)
10. Veltman, J.A., Jansen, C.: The role of operator state assessment in adaptive automation, TNO Human Factors Research Institute (2006)
11. Scerbo, M.: Theoretical perspectives on adaptive automation. In: Parasuraman, R., Mouloua, M. (eds.) Automation and human performance: theory and applications, pp. 37–63. Lawrence Erlbaum Associates, Mahwah (1996)
12. Scerbo, M.W., Freeman, F.G., Mikulka, P.J., Parasuraman, R., Nocero, F.D., Prinzel, L.J.: The Efficacy of Psychophysiological. NASA/TP-2001-211018 (2001)
13. Shannon, C., Weaver, W.: The mathematical theory of communications. University of Illinois Press, Urbana (1949)
14. van Delft, J.H., Arciszewski, H.F.R.: The evaluation of automation and support tools in the naval command & control environment. TM-04-A067, Soesterberg, The Netherlands, TNO Human Factors (2004)
15. Neerincx, M.A.: Cognitive task load design: model, methods and examples. In: Hollnagel, E. (ed.) Handbook of Cognitive Task Design, pp. 283–305. Lawrence Erlbaum Associates, Mahwah (2003)
16. Beevis, D.: Analysis techniques for man-machine systems design, vol. 1 & 2. NATO/Panel 8-RSG.14, Technical Report AC/243(Panel 8)TR/7, Brussels: North Atlantic treaty organization (1992)

Attuning In-Car User Interfaces to the Momentary Cognitive Load

Marika Hoedemaeker[1] and Mark Neerincx[1,2]

[1] TNO Human Factors, P.O. Box 23, 3769 ZG, Soesterberg, The Netherlands,
[2] Delft University of Technology, 4, Mekelweg, 2628 CD, The Netherlands

Abstract. Cars, trucks and busses are more and more equipped with functions and services that drivers are supposed to operate and understand. The most important developments in this area are the Advanced Driver Assistance Systems (ADAS) and In Vehicle Information Systems (IVIS). In order to make sure that the driver understands and appreciates (comfort) these services and traffic safety is not at risk (distraction, workload), the HMI's (Human Machine Interfaces) of all these functions should be attuned to each other, to the driver, and to the context. For attuning the functions to each other, a HMI platform is needed on which these functions are integrated. For attuning the functions to the driver it is necessary to have knowledge about the momentary state of the driver and of the intentions of the driver at a certain moment. For attuning the functions to the context, it is required to sense the relevant environmental conditions or states. This paper shows that a recent cognitive task load model from process control domain can be applied for the design of adaptive in-car user interfaces. Furthermore, current developments of such interfaces are being discussed.

Keywords: In-car services, workload, adaptive user interface, central management.

1 Introduction

A car driver is sitting in a relatively fixed position, performing his or her tasks in a closed environment that can be relatively easily enriched with driver-state sensing technology. The driver's tasks can be tracked rather well, and context factors can be easily assessed via both current sensor technology (e.g., slippery road) and data acquisition via wireless networks (e.g., traffic density and weather). So, the automotive domain seems very well suited to further develop and implement the first results of augmented cognition technology.

And there is a real need for such technology. Drivers can access more and more services in the car, for example for navigation, traffic information, news and communication. Furthermore, the car itself provides more and more information that should support drivers' tasks, such as speed limit warnings and parking guidance "beeps". The consequences of providing in-car traffic management information (like route information) in combination with infotainment services (like news headlines) can be negative; distraction or high workload could adversely affect the interaction

D.D. Schmorrow, L.M. Reeves (Eds.): Augmented Cognition, HCII 2007, LNAI 4565, pp. 286–293, 2007.

between the driver and the in-car system (e.g. [1]). Increases in workload can result from numerous sources inside and outside the car. Recently interactions of the driver with in-vehicle systems while driving have received considerable interest in the literature because of their potential impacts on road traffic safety. The additional workload imposed on the driver by an in-vehicle system easily results in overload of the driver. Overload means that the driver is unable to process all relevant information necessary to perform the primary driving task. This may lead to increased error rates and delayed detection of other traffic participants and, hence, to reduced safety [2]. This paper presents a practical theory of cognitive task load and current approaches to attune the in-car user interfaces to the momentary task load of the driver.

2 Cognitive Task Load

For process control tasks, Neerincx [3] developed a practical theory on cognitive task load (CTL) and applied it for the design of adaptive interfaces. This theory can be a good starting point for such interfaces in the car, distinguishing three types of cognitive load factors.

First, the *percentage time occupied*, has often been used to assess workload in practice for time-line assessments. Driver's cognitive processing speed determines this time for an important part, that is, the speed of executing relatively over-learned or automated elementary cognitive processes, especially when high mental efficiency (i.e., attention and focused concentration) is required (cf. [4]). Cognitive processing speed is usually measured by tasks that require rapid cognitive processing, but little thinking. It contains elements such as perceptual speed (the ability to rapidly search for and compare known visual symbols or patterns), rate-of-test-taking (the ability to rapidly perform tests which are relatively easy or that require very simple decisions) and number facility (the ability to rapidly and accurately manipulate and deal with numbers). The processing speed of older adults is relatively slow and can result in decreased driver performances [5].

Second, the *level of information processing*, affects the cognitive task load. At the skill-based level, information is processed automatically resulting into actions that are hardly cognitively demanding. At the rule-based level, input information triggers routine solutions, resulting into relatively efficient problem solving. At the knowledge-based level, based on input information the problem is analysed and solution(s) are planned, in particular to deal with new situations. This type of information processing can involve a heavy load on the limited capacity of working memory. Driver's expertise and experience with the tasks have substantial effect on their performance and the amount of cognitive resources required for this performance. Higher expertise and experience result in more efficient, less-demanding deployment of the resources. New situations, such as driving at the other side of the road in England by a Dutch driver, or complex traffic situations will raise the cognitive load substantially.

Third, the CTL theory distinguishes *task-set switching or sharing* as a third load factor to address the demands of attention shifts or divergences. Complex task situations consist of several different tasks, with different goals. These tasks appeal to different sources of human knowledge and capacities and refer to different objects in the environment. We use the term task set to denote the human resources and environmental objects with the momentary states, which are involved in the task performance. Switching entails a change of applicable task knowledge. The capacity to switch between, or share task-sets affects driver's mental load. Older adults seem to have generally less capacity for switching [6]. Kramer et al. [7] found large age-related differences in switch-costs early in practice (i.e., the costs in reaction time and errors due to switching between two tasks). After relatively modest amounts of practice the switch costs for old and young adults became equivalent and maintained equivalent across a two-month retention period. However, under high memory loads older adults were unable to capitalize on practice and the switch costs remained higher for them. In case of increased diverse information supply, drivers cannot compensate by directing more attention to the task and avoiding other tasks such as thinking or talking. Perceiving and processing of simultaneous information from in-vehicle systems can lead to a situation of overload where safe driving performance is very likely to suffer. Keeping the level of driver workload below some critical level, i.e. avoiding overload, can also in the long run be considered as an important contribution to road traffic safety (c.f. [8]).

It should be noted that the effects of cognitive task load depend on the concerning task duration. In general, the negative effects of under- and overload increase over time. Under-load will only appear after a certain work period, whereas (momentary) overload can appear at every moment. When task load remains high for a longer period, carry-over effects can appear reducing the available resources or capacities for the required human information processing [9]. Vigilance is a well-known problematic task for operators in which the problems increase in time. Performance decrease can already occur after 10 minutes when an operator has to monitor a process continuously but does not have to act [10, 11]. Vigilance can result in stress due to the specific task demands (i.e. the requirement to continuously pay attention on the task) and boredom that appears with highly repetitive, homogeneous stimuli. Consequently, the only viable strategy to reduce stress in vigilance, at present, appears to advise to stop when people become bored (cf. [12]). With respect to safety of car driving, on one hand vigilance, boredom and fatigue are of special concern, and

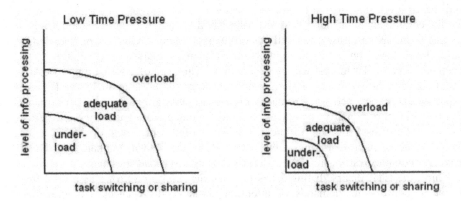

Fig. 1. Cognitive Task Load (CTL) under low and high time pressure (cf. the practical CTL theory of Neerincx, [3])

at the other side short-lasting peaks in workload are potentially dangerous. These peaks appear when the complexity of the situation increases suddenly and/or the driver is involved in several tasks. An adaptive interface should take care that the driver remains in the "safe task load area". Figure 1 shows how the three cognitive load factors determine the adequate load area, and the regions of under- and overload.

3 Adaptation and Central Management

Currently, the difficulty of adding new applications and services to an existing in-vehicle system often means that stand-alone solutions are introduced, each with its own Human Machine Interface (HMI). As the number of new intelligent services increases, therefore, so does the number of human-machine interfaces. This may lead to potentially dangerous situations given that each application competes for the driver's attention and that the driver may be distracted by the HMI's blinking, beeping or speech [13]. In current practice, services provide information to the driver automatically. In other words, the driver cannot decide whether information comes in at the appropriate moment. That is, at a moment which will not cause distraction and when the primary driving task has a sufficiently low workload. Secondly, not all information is equally essential at the same time.

To guarantee that driver's workload is kept low enough to allow a safe driving, there is the need to design and develop an on-vehicle multimedia HMI, able to harmonize the huge volume of messages coming from the new and traditional functions for the driving support. At the same time the HMI should be able to control and manage all the different input and output devices of the vehicle in order to provide an optimised interaction between the driver and the vehicle.

A central management system like this should manage the information data flow coming from the different in-car tasks, according to the current traffic and environment assessment and to the driver's state in terms of distraction, fatigue and alertness. Driving workload managers continually assess the difficulty of driving and regulate the flow of information to drivers that could interfere with driving, such as automatically diverting an incoming phone call to an answering machine when a driver is turning at an intersection. Therefore Green [14] defined a workload manager as a device that attempts to determine if a driver is overloaded or distracted, and if they are, alters the availability of telematics and the operation of warning systems .

The final goal of a central management system is to let the in-vehicle communication to adapt to:

- the state of the driver,
- the vehicle and the surrounding environment
- the different in-car tasks

Workload managers often use a look-up table to determine the workload from the rules. Real workload managers depend primarily on sensors that are already installed in a vehicle.

It still is a real challenge to measure in real time the state of the driver. Eye-tracking systems can measure the time and frequency of the driver's eyes off the road (i.e. not looking at the road ahead) and the amount of visual time sharing, in which the driver is continuously sharing his visual focus between the road ahead and something else (like an in-vehicle display). Cognitive distraction, in which the driver thinking, daydreaming or taking part in a conversation, is much more difficult to measure.

Measuring eye fixations is extremely difficult under any situation and particularly difficult to accomplish at low cost in a moving vehicle. Direction of gaze can be determined by measuring the electrical potentials around the orbit or shining an infrared beam off of the cornea and measuring its angle of reflection. Now various video based systems track the face, find the eye, and then by judging the amount of white on either side of the iris, determine the direction of gaze.

Technologies designed to detect declines in driver alertness due to drowsiness or fatigue have involved monitoring the driver's physiological state (heart rate, brain activity etc) as well as bio behaviour (head movements, eye movements etc) or performance (lane deviations, speed variability etc). In simulator studies there has been a high correlation between physiological and behavioural deterioration in the fatigued or drowsy driver. However, analyses of on-the-road performance data from commercial vehicle drivers have shown much lower correlations between bio behavioural and performance measures, because deliberate or strategic driving in the real world is a large component in the variability seen in the performance measures such as lane keeping. In addition to monitoring the driver to detect drowsy driving, a second option is to monitor the vehicle that is being controlled by the driver. Vehicle measures have several advantages over driver measurements. They have greater face validity and are less obtrusive. Steering wheel movements for example have shown promise as an early indicator of impaired performance as well as lateral lane variance.

In general it is believed that a combination of bio behaviour and performance measures are important components of an overall drowsy driver monitoring and detection system. However, a performance measure alone is not sufficient to predict drowsiness.

Measurement of the surrounding environment can be done by taking into account the current road type and the speed that the vehicle is driving on that road type from vehicle sensors. By combining these two, one can get an indication of the traffic flow and the workload the environment imposes on the driver (see Table 1 for an example).

Table 1. Simple lookup table with information from the environment and the effect on driver workload

Road Type	Velocity [km/hr]	Driver Workload
Highway	0-30	Low
	30-50	Medium
	50-80	Medium
	80-100	Low
	100-120	Low
	>120	High
Roundabout	0-30	Medium
	30-40	High
	>40	High

4 Adaptive Interface Examples

4.1 CoDrive

Recently, the Dutch Co-drive project developed a demonstrator to show how an in-car system can attune the provision of applications and services to the current driving context [13]. The proposed CoDrive system consists of three components. First, a common Human-Machine Interface (HMI) for different applications and services aims at improved road safety while maintaining optimal freedom and flexibility with regard to the content. Second, a distributed in-vehicle ICT platform enables information sharing, while guaranteeing undisturbed, real-time behaviour of each and every application and service. Third, additional support for the driver focuses on enhanced effectiveness and safety of his or her journey.

The HMI framework, or management system contains: an auctioneer (prioritising mechanism), a workload estimator, a set of design rules, and a basic display lay-out. Essential to the framework is that each service is responsible for and generates its own HMI. This HMI, however, has to comply with the design rules and with the framework interaction mechanisms. In this way safety is increased while application developers are constrained to a minimum.

Every service that wants to use the shared HMI sends a Request to the auctioneer accompanied by three variables: "Identity", "Priority" and "Workload". The auctioneer determines which service is granted access to the screen. It separates requests that have a higher workload than allowed – information delivered by the workload estimator – from the ones that comply with the allowable workload. If requests comply with the allowable workload the auctioneer selects the ones with the highest priority and then gives the request that came in first access to the HMI. At any time, the user may request a service to show its information by pushing the corresponding service button on the touch screen display. The auctioneer once again handles the request and passes the request to the corresponding service. The service then activates an HMI compliant with the allowable workload. The auctioneer disables the user buttons when the allowable workload is lower than the minimum workload of the corresponding service.

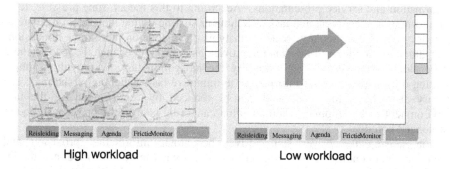

High workload   Low workload

Fig. 2. Example of a high and low workload HMI

4.2 AIDE

The main objective of the ongoing EU project AIDE is to improve driver system interaction in terms of distraction and usability to increase driving safety and improve user comfort [15]. In order to reach this goal the AIDE project, in contrast to usual approaches, is focused on:

- considering the effects of HMI interdependences, i.e. for example preventing interference between different messages presented at the same time to the driver;
- taking into account the driving situation, driver state and driver preferences to adapt the HMI according to these conditions, i.e. the interaction may be changed in critical conditions or according to the preferences to reduce driver's distraction and to draw drivers attention to the driving task;
- including nomad devices in a common in-vehicle HMI in a way that they do not differ in terms of the HMI strategy from integrated applications.

In AIDE the communication between the driver and the in-vehicle system is managed by a central intelligence to avoid critical effects of interdependences. This intelligence, named "Interaction and Communication Assistant" (ICA) ensures that the information is given to the driver at the right time and in the right way and that only functions that are relevant in the present driving context are active. ICA is responsible for managing all the interaction and communication between the driver and the vehicle, based on the assessment of the driver-vehicle-environment (DVE) state/situation. This includes the selection of modality for presentation, the message prioritisation and scheduling and the general adaptability of the driver-vehicle interface (e.g. display configuration and function allocation).

Within AIDE three different demonstrators are being built that cover different vehicle types; a luxury car demonstrator, a city car demonstrator as well as a system applicable for trucks. At this moment the three demonstrators are being evaluated in in-road studies.

5 Conclusions

This paper presented theory, the design space and some examples of adaptive in-car information and service presentations. According to this theory, time pressure, level of information processing and task switching or sharing define the critical load areas. Adaptive interfaces should provide estimations of the load on these three dimensions and attune the service and information provisions in order to change the load on these dimensions when needed (e.g., simplify the navigation task by providing simple routing information or filter information to minimize task switching or sharing). The theory also shows that underload can be reduced by "enrichment" of the task environment or by stopping when attention cannot be paid to the driver task due to prolonged boredom.

Via sensing the driver state, driver behaviour, information provision and environmental conditions, the actual critical load areas can be quantified, and the in-car interfaces can be changed to establish adequate load levels. The most important developments in this area are the Advanced Driver Assistance Systems (ADAS) and In Vehicle Information Systems (IVIS). For attuning the different functions and services to each other, these developments provide a HMI platform on which these functions are integrated. For attuning the functions to the driver, they provide estimations of the momentary state of the driver and of the intentions of the driver at a certain moment. In this way, these systems try to ensure that the information from the different services is presented to the driver without causing driver overload and endangering traffic safety.

Acknowledgments. Part of this research on adaptive interfaces has been supported by the Dutch MultimediaN project (http://www.multimedian.nl).

References

1. McKnight, J., McKnight, S.: The effect of cellular phone use upon driver attention. Accidents Analysis and Prevention 25, 259–265 (1991)
2. Verwey, W.B.: Evaluating safety effects of traffic congestion information systems. In: Hancock, P.A., Desmond, P. (eds.) Stress, workload and fatigue, pp. 409–425. Erlbaum, Mahwah (2001)
3. Neerincx, M.A.: Cognitive task load design: model, methods and examples. In: Hollnagel, E. (ed.) Handbook of Cognitive Task Design (Chapter 13), pp. 283–305. Mahwah, NJ: Lawrence Erlbaum Associates (2003)
4. Carroll, J.B.: Human Cognitive Abilities: A Survey of Factor Analytic Studies. Cambridge University Press, New York (1993)
5. Korteling, J.E.: Multiple-task Performance and Aging. Doctoral Thesis, University of Groningen, The Netherlands (1994)
6. Sit, R.A., Fisk, A.D.: Age-related performance in a multiple task environment. Human Factors 41(1), 26–34 (1999)
7. Kramer, A.F., Hahn, S., Gopher, D.: Task coordination and ageing: explorations of executive control processes in the task switching paradigm. Acta. Psychologica 101, 339–378 (1999)
8. Verwey, W.B.: On-line driver workload estimation. Effects of road situation and age on secondary task measures. Ergonomics 43, 187–209 (2000)
9. Rouse, W.B.: Adaptive aiding for human computer control. Human Factors 30, 431–443 (1988)
10. Levine, J.M., Romashko, T., Fleishman, E.A.: Evaluation of an abilities classification system for integrating and generalizing human performance research findings: an application to vigilance tasks. Journal of Applied Psychology 58(2), 149–157 (1973)
11. Parasuraman, R.: Vigilance, monitoring, and search. In: Boff, K.R., Kaufman, L., Thomas, J.P. (eds.) Handbook of perception and human performance, volume 2: cognitive processes and performance, chapter 43, Wiley, New York (1986)
12. Scerbo, M.W.: Stress, workload and boredom in vigilance: a problem and an answer. In: Hancock, P.A., Desmond, P.A. (eds.) Stress, Workload and Fatigue, Lawrence Erlbaum Associates, Mahwah, New Jersey (2001)
13. Zoutendijk, A., Hoedemaeker, M., Vonk, T., Schuring, O., Willemsen, D., Nelisse, M., van Katwijk, R.: Implementing Multiple Intelligent Services in an Intelligent Vehicle with a Safe Workload Aware HMI. In: Proceedings ITS Madrid (2003)
14. Green, P.: Driver distraction, telematics design, and workload managers: Safety issues and solutions. SAE Paper Number 2004-21-0022 (2004)
15. Amditis, A., Andreone, L., Polychronopoulos, A., Engstrom, J.: Design and development of an adaptive integrated driver-vehicle interface: overview of the AIDE project. In: Proceedings of the IFAQ conference, Prague (2005)

EEG-Based Drivers' Drowsiness Monitoring Using a Hierarchical Gaussian Mixture Model

Roman Rosipal[1], Björn Peters[2], Göran Kecklund[3], Torbjörn Åkerstedt[3],
Georg Gruber[4], Michael Woertz[1], Peter Anderer[4,5], and Georg Dorffner[1,4,6]

[1] Austrian Research Institute for Artificial Intelligence, Vienna, Austria
[2] Swedish National Road and Transport Research Institute, Linköping, Sweden
[3] Karolinska Institutet, Stockholm, Sweden
[4] The Siesta Group Schlafanalyse GmbH, Vienna, Austria
[5] Department of Psychiatry and Psychotherapy, Medical University of Vienna,
Vienna, Austria
[6] Institute of Medical Cybernetics and Artificial Intelligence, Center for Brain Research,
Medical University of Vienna, Vienna, Austria
roman.rosipal@ofai.at,bjorn.peters@vti.se,
goran.kecklund@ki.se,torbjorn.akerstedt@ipm.ki.se,
georg.gruber@thesiestagroup.com,michael.woertz@ofai.at,
peter.anderer@meduniwien.ac.at,georg.dorffner@meduniwien.ac.at

Abstract. We developed an EEG-based probabilistic model, which effectively predicts drowsiness levels of thirty-two subjects involved in a moving base driving simulator experiment. A hierarchical Gaussian mixture model (hGMM) with two mixture components at the lower hierarchical level is used. Each mixture models data density distribution of one of the two drowsiness cornerstones/classes represented by 4-second long EEG segments with low and high drowsiness levels. We transfer spectral contents of each EEG segment into a compact form of autoregressive model coefficients. The Karolinska drowsiness scoring method is used to initially label data belonging to individual classes. We demonstrate good agreement between Karolinska drowsiness scores and the predicted drowsiness, when the hGMM is applied to continuously monitor drowsiness over the time-course of driving sessions. The computations associated with the approach are fast enough to build up a practical real-time drowsiness monitoring system.

1 Introduction

Drowsiness from combination of sleep loss, high workload prior to driving, and long driving under difficult conditions (night driving, rain, fog, dense traffic) is a significant risk factor that substantially contributes to the number of motor vehicle accidents. For this reason, the drivers' drowsiness has been the subject of intensive research studies followed by the development of the efficient drowsiness monitoring systems. These systems were designed using behavioral (for example, frequency of body movements–actigraph data, steering wheel control), visual (for example, facial

D.D. Schmorrow, L.M. Reeves (Eds.): Augmented Cognition, HCII 2007, LNAI 4565, pp. 294–303, 2007.
© Springer-Verlag Berlin Heidelberg 2007

expression, eyelid movement and closure, head movement, gaze) or physiological (electroencephalogram (EEG), electrooculogram (EOG), electromyogram (EMG)) measures. It has been observed that changes in the human EEG and EOG are very sensitive physiological indicators of drowsiness [11]. The advantage of the EEG-based systems is their high-temporal resolution allowing to track second-to-second drowsiness fluctuations.

However, there is no gold-standard drowsiness scoring system available for scoring EEG/EOG on alert subjects. In this study, the Karolinska drowsiness scoring method [3] was used to visually assign drowsiness levels of 20-second data epochs recorded from subjects participating in a driving simulator experiment.

An EEG-based hierarchical Gaussian mixture model (hGMM) with high-temporal resolution is designed and trained to continuously and automatically monitor/predict drowsiness. The measure of different drowsiness states of subjects participating in a driving experiment are the visually assigned Karolinska drowsiness score (KDS) values. Instead of the strict following of the KDS values, the hGMM is initialized using the information about the extreme drowsiness states–low and high drowsiness cornerstones–only. An output of the model is the continuous curve of the posterior probabilities reflecting a belief about class-membership of the particular data input to the one of the drowsiness cornerstones. Such an output representation may become advantageous in the process of building a practical real-time drowsiness monitor with an adaptable threshold triggering a warning system. Finally, a probabilistic framework of the hGMM can be extended in a principled way by considering different sensor modalities and by the inclusion of the contextual/prior information influencing subjects' drowsiness, such as information about the expected physiological state of subjects while driving or about the driving environment itself.

2 Materials and Methods

2.1 Driving Simulator Study

Procedure: The study was carried out at the Swedish National Road and Transport Research Institute in Linköping (VTI) using the third generation moving base driving simulator, which consists of

- Cut-off passenger car cab
- Computerized vehicle model
- Large moving base system
- Vibration table
- PC-based visual system
- PC-based audio system

The driving simulator is shown in Fig. 1, left. The simulator provides a realistic experimental driving condition that is fully controllable and with a high internal validity (same conditions for all subjects). Furthermore, the simulator makes it possible to carry out safety critical experiments that might be very difficult to do in field studies. The external validity has been found to be very good in previous experiments carried out at VTI [12]. The simulated passenger car had a manual gearbox with 5 gears. The time delay introduced in the simulator is very short (max. 40 ms), which is important when focusing on the control and maneuvering aspects of driving. The noise, infra-sound and vibration levels inside the cabin corresponded to those of a modern vehicle.

The simulated road had the dimensions and geometry according to a real rural road (Fig. 1, right). The road was 9 m wide with moderate curves and with a speed limit of 90 km/h. The driving condition was daylight clear view and full fiction.

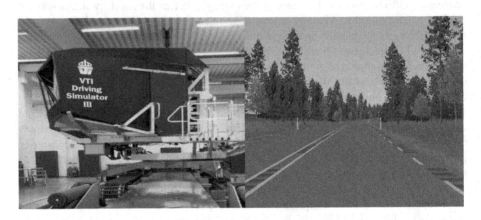

Fig. 1. *Left*: The moving base driving simulator at VTI. *Right*: A simulated road example.

Subjects: Forty-four shift workers, all non-professional drivers, participated in the experiment. All drove during morning hours directly after a full night-shift with no sleep. Prior to the experiment the subjects received information on how to prepare and they were instructed not to i) drink alcohol for 72 hours before the experiment, ii) drink coffee, tea or other drinks that have an alerting effect for 3 hours before arriving at VTI, iii) eat for 3 hours before arriving at VTI, iv) take a nap during the night shift before the experiment, v) wear make-up when arriving at VTI. All drivers drove at least 45 minutes with a maximum of 90 minutes.

Physiological data: A wide range of data was collected including pre- and post-questionnaires, sleep diary, subjective sleepiness ratings, driving behavior, pupillometry, eye gaze and eye-lid opening, etc. However, in the current work only EEG, EOG, and EMG physiological data were used. Vitaport 2 from Temec Instruments BV was used for all electrophysiological measurements. Vitaport 2 is a portable digital recorder with a hardware-configurable number of channels for physiological measurements. EEG was measured with two monopolar derivations positioned at Fz-A1, Cz-A2 and a bipolar derivation Oz-Pz. Horizontal and vertical EOG movements on both eyes were recorded with three channels. The single EMG electrode was placed under the jaw. The sampling frequency was 256 Hz for EEG and EMG and 512 Hz for EOG. Silver cup electrodes were used for all signals. The input data were stored on a flash memory card and were downloaded to a personal computer hard drive for off-line analysis.

2.2 Karolinska Drowsiness Scoring Method

The collected physiological data were used to visually score the drivers' drowsiness level using the Karolinska drowsiness scoring method [3]. The method was developed for quantification of drowsiness in "active" situations (situations when the subject should be awake) and uses EEG and EOG recordings. EMG may be a valuable indicator of arousals and artifacts but is not included among the criteria for drowsiness. The scoring method is based on the Rechtschaffen & Kales (R&K) sleep scoring rules [9]. Single channel EEG data from a bipolar Oz-Pz montage were used in the present analysis.

First, the recorded data were divided into 20-second long epochs. The entire epoch was separated into 2-second bins. The outcome KDS measure described the number of bins in the epoch that contains slow eye movements, alpha activity and/or theta activity; that is, signs of sleepiness. If no sleepiness signs were found, the entire epoch was assigned the KDS value equal to 0. If one 2-second bin showed signs of sleepiness KDS = 10 was assigned to the epoch and so on. The maximum KDS level could be 100, which means that the sleepiness signs occur in all 2-second long bins. The epochs with KDS > 50 were considered to represent "sleep onset". However, according to most definitions of sleepiness, a sleep onset should include theta activity and slow eye movements. The visual scoring was done using the Somnologica® software (Embla). Spectral analysis is an optional step of the scoring method. However, in this study, an advantage of the Fast Fourier transform to examine the temporal patterns and the dynamics of drowsiness on a detailed level was exploited.

2.3 Hierarchical Gaussian Mixture Model

The hGMM was used to automatically discriminate and monitor drowsiness. The basic principle of the proposed model architecture is to approximate class-conditional densities of individual drowsiness classes arbitrarily closely. This is achieved with one Gaussian mixture model (GMM) fitted to each class. By defining prior class probabilities, Bayes' theorem can be applied to arrive at posterior probabilities. Thus, the proposed approach can be seen as the extension of Mixture Discriminant Analysis [5] and to be similar to the model called MclustDA [4] (see also [7], [1]). In the current study, the lower hierarchical level of the hGMM consists of two GMMs approximating densities of the low and high drowsiness cornerstones/classes. The upper hierarchical level of the model is then the mixture of these two GMM elements.

The class-conditional distributions at the lower hierarchical level were approximated by GMMs with density function parameters and a number of components being class-specific,

$$p\left(x \mid C_i\right) = \sum_{k \in |Ci|} \alpha_k \, p(x \mid \theta_k) \text{ with } \sum_{k \in |Ci|} \alpha_k = 1, \quad \alpha_k \geq 0 \qquad (1)$$

where $x \in R^d$ represents a d-dimensional observation vector (it this study a vector of the autoregressive coefficients), α_k are mixing coefficients, $C_{i,(i=1,2)}$ is the class membership index and $|C_i|$ denotes the total number of Gaussian components in each mixture. The Gaussian density function for a given component k has the form

$$p\left(x \mid \theta_k\right) = \left(2\pi\right)^{-d/2} \left|\Omega_k\right|^{-1/2} e^{-\left(x-\mu_k\right)^T \Omega_k^{-1}\left(x-\mu_k\right)/2} \tag{2}$$

where the parameter θ_k consists of a mean vector μ_k and a covariance matrix Ω_k.

By applying Bayes' theorem, the posterior probability for a class C_i can be calculated as

$$p(C_i \mid x) = \frac{p(x \mid C_i)\, p(C_i)}{p(x)} \propto p(x \mid C_i)\, p(C_i) \tag{3}$$

where $p(C_i)$ is the non-negative prior class probability. The unconditional density $p(x)$ is not necessarily needed for calculation of the class posteriors, but can be obtained by integrating out the unknown class membership

$$p(x) = \sum_{i=1,2} p(x, C_i) = \sum_{i=1,2} p(x \mid C_i) p(C_i) \tag{4}$$

The prior probability $p(C_i)$ has to be non-negative and sum to one considering both classes. In the current study the prior probabilities were not estimated and were set to be equal; that is, $p(C_1) = p(C_2) = 1/2$.

By fixing the prior probabilities and by training the hGMM on class labeled data, the set of unknown parameters $\Theta_i = \{\theta_k = (\mu_k, \Omega_k), \alpha_k ; k \in C_i\}$ can be estimated independently for each Gaussian mixture. This can be done by maximizing the log of the likelihood function

$$L(\Theta_i \mid x_1, ..., x_{N_i}) = \log \prod_{n=1}^{N_i} p(x_n \mid C_i) = \sum_{i=1}^{N_i} \log \sum_{k \in |Ci|} \alpha_k\, p(x_n \mid \theta_k) \tag{5}$$

where N_i represents a number of samples from the ith class used to estimate the parameters of the corresponding Gaussian mixture. A powerful, well-known framework called *expectation maximization* (EM) was used to maximize the likelihood function with respect to the unknown parameters $\{\mu_k, \Omega_k, \alpha_k\}$ [2]. Detailed description of the closed form formulas for estimating the individual parameters can by found in [7], [1]. The GMM routines from the Netlab toolbox[1] (Matlab toolbox for data analysis, [8]) were used to train and test the hGMM.

2.4 Experiments

EEG data pre-processing: Prior to building the actual drowsiness models the raw EEG data were pre-processed using the following four steps i) re-sampling the original data to 100Hz by using a method that applies an anti-aliasing filter and

---

[1] http://www.ncrg.aston.ac.uk/netlab/

compensates for the filter's delay, ii) band-pass filtering of the re-sampled data into the range of 0.5 – 40Hz by using the 4th order Butterworth filter with zero-phase distortion, iii) windowing of the filtered data into 4-second long non-overlapping segments[2], iv) computation of the autoregressive (AR) coefficients for each segment. The AR model order was set to 10. If more than one EEG channel was used the AR coefficients were concatenated into a single input vector. These pre-processing steps were found to be useful in previous sleep process modeling studies [10]. A KDS value was assigned to each 4-second segment based on its membership to the corresponding 20-second segment. Finally, segments containing artifacts visually observed during the Karolinska drowsiness scoring process were removed.

Study A: The performance of the hGMM to classify the EEG epochs with KDS = 0 and KDS $\geq$ 50 was investigated. The purpose of this classification exercise was to demonstrate separability of the two drowsiness cornerstones. Available 4-second data segments of each subject were randomly split into training and testing parts. Ten percent of the segments from each class were kept in the testing part. This procedure was repeated 100 times. The first 20 training partitions were used to determine the number of Gaussian components for each mixture. This was achieved by using the 20-fold cross-validation method with the validation part representing randomly selected 20% of each training set. The number of Gaussian components varied in the range 2 to 16 and the final selection was done based on the minimum of the mean classification error computed over 20 validation runs. The hGMM was then trained on all 100 training partitions and the performance was tested on the corresponding testing sets. Using the described validation and testing procedures, all possible combinations of the three EEG electrodes were compared. The aim of this comparison was to determine the influence of different EEG combinations to discriminate between low and high drowsiness.

Study B: In the second step, the hGMM reflecting continuous changes in drowsiness levels was developed. This was achieved using the following strategy. First, 30% percent of 4-second segments representing the two drowsiness cornerstones were randomly selected from each subject. The hGMM was trained using the selected segments. Next, the posterior values for all data segments arranged in the time-course of the driving experiment were computed. Note that in contrast to the previous classification experiment, also the segments with the KDS values in the range 10 - 40 were used and their posterior values were computed. These segments were not used during the training step. For visual purposes the posterior values were re-scaled from their 0 - 1 range into KDS range of 0 - 100. The scaled values were smoothed using a moving average filter. The same smoothing was applied to the KDS values and both smoothed curves were visually compared. The agreement between the smoothed curves was also numerically compared using the nonparametric Spearman rank correlation method [6].

---

[2] This windowing was done in synchrony with 20-second long epochs used for the KDS values assignment. This allows to uniquely determine a KDS value to each 4-second segment based on its membership to the corresponding 20-second epoch.

3 Results

Out of the forty-four participants, thirty-two subjects (16 females and 16 males) were considered useful for the current study. Based on visually observed artifacts 18% of the all 4-second EEG segments were removed resulting in 35295 segments left for the analysis. The histogram of the KDS values of these segments is depicted in Fig. 2. It can be observed that the KDS value equal to 100 was not reached. The number of segments with KDS = 0 represented 16.8%. Similarly, there were 16.7% segments with KDS ≥ 50 meaning that 66.5% of the KDS values fell into the range 0 - 50.

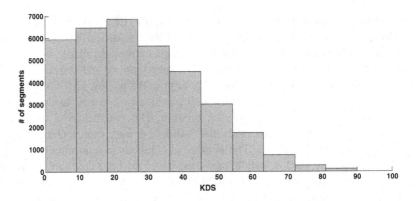

Fig. 2. Histogram of the KDS values for the 4-second segments used in the analysis

Study A: Table 1 summarizes the resulting hGMM test set correct classification rates. The values represent averages over 100 different runs. For each combination of the EEG electrodes, the number of mixture components was found by applying the previously described cross-validation method. Reasonable high correct classification rates can be observed. It is important to note that the KDS values were assigned to 20-second long segments while the current hGMM operates on 4-second segments. Furthermore, in contrast to the Karolinska scoring procedure, broadband spectral information from more than one EEG electrode was used in the case of the hGMM.

Table 1. Comparison of the mean and standard deviation of the test set correct classification rates. Values are averaged over 100 runs. The last column represents the number of Gaussian mixture components found by the cross-validation method applied to the first 20 training sets.

EEG electrodes set	Correct classification rates Mean (Standard deviation)	Number of Gaussian components Mixture1 / Mixture2
Fz-A1, Cz-A2, Oz-Pz	77.27 (1.65)	4 / 8
Cz-A2, Oz-Pz	72.90 (1.47)	4 / 8
Fz-A1, Oz-Pz	76.28 (1.21)	6 / 12
Fz-A1, Cz-A2	73.46 (1.30)	2 / 6
Oz-Pz	67.21 (1.30)	8 / 16
Cz-A2	67.80 (1.37)	8 / 10
Fz-A1	71.45 (1.27)	4 / 12

The degradation of the performance in comparison to the full–three EEG electrodes–set can be observed when dropping the Cz-A2 electrode. The results also suggest the importance of the Fz-A1 electrode inclusion. In Table 2, the confusion tables comparing the performance of the full EEG montage for three different sets of Gaussian mixture components are depicted. In general, very small variability in performance can be observed. Slightly preferable can be the case of using 10 components in each mixture when the most balanced error rates between two classes are observed. Following the results of Tables 1 and 2, the hGMM with 10 Gaussian components in each mixture and using all three EEG electrodes was used in Study B.

Table 2. Confusion tables comparing the performance of the full EEG (Fz-A1,Cz-A2,Oz-Pz) montage for three different sets of mixture components. Results are averages of 100 test sets.

Mixture1 / Mixture2 4 / 8		Mixture1 / Mixture2 8 / 8		Mixture1 / Mixture2 10 / 10	
76.13	23.87	77.97	22.03	77.45	22.55
21.57	78.43	22.97	77.03	22.69	77.31

Study B: After training the hGMM on 30% of the segments from the two drowsiness cornerstones (KDS = 0 and KDS ≥ 50), the model was applied to all subjects' data following the time-course of the driving experiment. In general, good visual agreement was observed between the posterior curves representing the predicted drowsiness and the actual KDS values. In Fig. 3 (top plots) the curves of two subjects with the highest Spearman rank correlation coefficient between the smoothed posterior and KDS curves are plotted (0.81 – subject 5 and 0.85 – subject 11). The 40-second long moving averaged filter was applied for smoothing the both curves. In three subjects the correlation coefficient values were smaller than 0.2. It is interesting to point out that in these cases the subjects show predominately lower values of KDS with small variability over the whole driving session. An example is plotted in Fig. 3 (bottom left plots, 0.15 - subject 19; note shorter, about 46 min driving in this case). The small posterior values of the prediction model, which are in good agreement with the assigned low drowsiness of the subject (KDS ≤ 30), can be seen. The curves of the subject with the value of the correlation coefficient closest to the median correlation equal to 0.53 are plotted in Fig. 3, bottom right plots (0.53 – subject 34). Again, good agreement can be observed between the predicted and actual KDS values.

Finally, the sensitivity of the hGMM to a random selection of the training set and to the EM method convergence was studied. The same training procedure, using 30% of the two drowsiness cornerstones segments, was repeated 20 times. In the top plot of Fig. 4 an example of 20 curves of the predicted drowsiness of the subject 5 are plotted. Consistent drowsiness prediction can be observed with a low variability among different runs. This is also confirmed with a narrow boxplot representing the distribution of the Spearman rank correlation coefficients computed over 20 runs (bottom plot of Fig. 4). The median value of the correlation coefficients is 0.81, which is in good agreement with a single run case used in Fig. 3. Similarly, the reasonably narrow boxplots for the other three subjects, used in Fig. 3, can be observed in the bottom plot of Fig. 4.

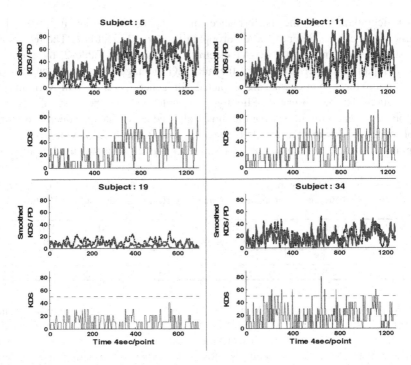

Fig. 3. *Top plots*: The KDS (dash-dotted) and predicted drowsiness (PD) (solid line) curves. A moving average filter 40 sec long was used. *Bottom plots*: The non-smoothed KDS values.

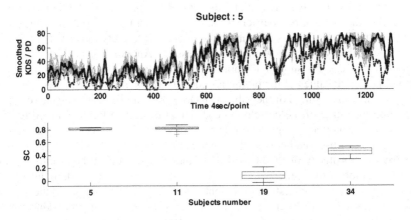

Fig. 4. Top: The KDS (dash-dotted) and twenty predicted drowsiness (PD) (solid lines) curves. The thicker line is the mean value of the PD curves. A moving average filter 40 sec long was used. Bottom: The boxplot of the Spearman rank coefficients (SC) for subjects 5, 11, 19 and 34.

4   Conclusions

The study has shown promising results in applying the presented probabilistic approach to the drivers' drowsiness monitoring task. A reasonably high level of correlation was observed between predicted drowsiness levels and the KDS values. This was despite the fact that the hGMM was applied to shorter data segments, no EOG information was used and, in contrast to the Karolinska scoring protocol, broadband spectral information from multi-electrode EEG setting was considered. The computations associated with the approach are fast enough to build up a practical real-time system. Moreover, such system can be applied and tested in different human drowsiness, vigilance, or fatigue monitoring tasks. Future steps will involve the principled probabilistic inclusion of other physiological signals, visual measures of drowsiness and contextual information into the system. Moreover, implementation of an automatic artifact processing scheme would be a necessary step to build a real-time drowsiness monitoring system.

Acknowledgments. Research supported by the EU project SENSATION/IST 507231. The Austrian Research Institute for Artificial Intelligence is supported by the Austrian Federal Ministry of Education, Science and Culture and the Austrian Federal Ministry of Transport, Innovation and Technology.

References

1. Bishop, C.: Pattern Recognition and Machine Learning. Springer, Heidelberg (2006)
2. Dempster, A.P., Laird, N.M., Rubin, D.B.: Maximum likelihood from incomplete data via the EM algorithm. J. Royal Stat. Soc. B 39, 1–38 (1977)
3. Gillberg, M., Kecklund, G., Åkerstedt, T.: Sleep and performance of professional drivers in a truck simulator - comparison between day and night driving. J. of Sleep Res. 5, 12–15 (1996)
4. Fraley, C., Raftery, A.E.: Model-Based Clustering, Discriminant Analysis, and Density Estimation. J. Am. Stat. Assoc. 97, 611–631 (2002)
5. Hastie, T., Tibshirani, R.: Discriminant Analysis by Gaussian Mixtures. J. Royal Stat. Soc. B 58, 155–176 (1996)
6. Heckman, N., Zamar, R.: Comparing the shapes of regression functions. Biometrika 87, 135–144 (2000)
7. McLachlan, G.L., Peel, D.: Finite Mixture Models. John Wiley & Sons, New York (2000)
8. Nabney, I.T.: NETLAB: Algorithms for Pattern Recognition. Springer, Heidelberg (2004)
9. Rechtschaffen, A., Kales, A.: A manual of Standardized Technology, Techniques, and Scoring Systems for Sleep Stages of Human Subjects. Technical Report, Brain Research Institute UCLA, Los Angeles (1968)
10. Rosipal, R., Neubauer, S., Anderer, P., Gruber, G., Parapatics, S., Woertz, M., Dorffner, G.: A continuous probabilistic approach to sleep and daytime sleepiness modeling. ESRS2006, P299, Innsbruck (September 2006)
11. Santamaria, J., Chiappa, K.H.: The EEG of Drowsiness. Demos Medical Publishing (1987)
12. Törnros, J.: Driving behaviour in a real and simulated road tunnel — a validation study. Accident Analysis & Prevent. 4, 497–503 (1998)

The Effect of Fatigue on Cognitive and Psychomotor Skills of Surgical Residents

Kanav Kahol[1,2], Mark Smith[1], Stephanie Mayes[1], Mary Deka[1], Vikram Deka[1], John Ferrara[1], and Sethuraman Panchanathan[2]

[1] Phoenix Integrated Surgical Residency Program, SimET Center
Banner Good Samaritan Medical Center, Phoenix Arizona
[2] Arizona State University

Abstract. Surgical residents are exposed to a significant amount of cognitive load during call. While various efforts have been made to quantify the effect of fatigue and sleep deprivation on the psychomotor skills of surgical residents, there is very little investigations into the effect of these factors on cognitive skills. However, this is an important issue in medical curriculum design, as much of the medical errors are procedural in nature and are not psychomotor. In this paper, we present a study that aimed to quantify the effect of fatigue on cognitive skills. We employed hand movement data for developing a proficiency measure of surgical skill. The difference in proficiencies measured through hand movement post call and pre call was determined. The simulation tasks were designed to challenge working memory, attention of the user. The results showed a significant difference in hand movement proficiencies as well as behavioral errors pre and post-call. EEG Data was also gathered during simulation tasks pre and post call through the B-Alert® Bluetooth EEG technology. The B-Alert® software was analyzed to reveal ratings of alertness/drowsiness, engagement, mental workload and distraction. The results showed statistically significant difference in EEG ratings in pre call and post call condition.

1 Introduction

In 1999 the Institute of Medicine published the now famous study "To Err is Human" on the unacceptably high rate of errors in medicine, and that has generated even more demand for changes in the status quo in healthcare. As a result, many of the prevalent approaches in medical field are being questioned. One of the burning questions is the effect of fatigue and sleep deprivation on the skills of residents. Residency programs require medical residents to perform various kinds of medical duties over extended periods of 16-24 hours. These extended hours of operation can significantly influence a doctor's ability to perform. This factor can be even more critical in surgical procedures that require both cognitive and motor skills. Two decades ago minimally invasive surgery was introduced, and along with it came a more extensive and lengthy learning curve. More complex procedures are being continually developed and introduced, accompanied by more serious risks and complications. These procedures require a

D.D. Schmorrow, L.M. Reeves (Eds.): Augmented Cognition, HCII 2007, LNAI 4565, pp. 304–313, 2007.
© Springer-Verlag Berlin Heidelberg 2007

significant amount of cognitive as well as psychomotor acuity. It is important to measure the effect of fatigue on these skills. This will provide guidelines on development of residency programs and how to handle fatigue and sleep deprivation.

Many systems have been proposed to study the effect of fatigue, sleepiness, noise and interruptions on surgical proficiency. These systems rely on existing measures of surgical proficiency to measure the effect of operating conditions on skill. Eastridge et al. (Tendulkar et al., 2005) used the MIST VR system for analyzing the effect of sleep deprivation due to calls on the technical dexterity of residents. Thirty-five surgical residents were prospectively evaluated pre-call (rested), on-call (rested), and post-call (acutely sleep deprived). Participants completed questionnaires regarding sleep hours and level of fatigue. Technical skill was assessed using the MIST VR. Speed, errors, and economy of motion were automatically recorded by the MIST VR system. Data were analyzed by pairing Student t-test and analysis of variance. They showed that Call-associated sleep deprivation and fatigue are associated with increased technical errors in the performance of simulated laparoscopic surgical skills. While studies on fatigue, sleep deprivation have been performed, these studies have relied on existing measures of surgical proficiency. Existing measure of surgical proficiencies include simple measure of proficiency such as time, tool movement smoothness etc. These measures are not sufficient to quantify effect of fatigue comprehensively. In the first section of the paper we define a system for measuring hand movement based proficiency. We then describe an experiment with the developed apparatus to quantify the effect of fatigue.

2 Hand Movement Based Proficiency System

Surgical movements such as suturing, knot tying, etc are composed of a few basic movements herein referred to as gestures or basic gestures. These gestures form the building block of most complex surgical procedures. The advantage of deconstructing a complex motion into simplex units lies in facilitating understanding of the complex movements and ease of communication while training. It also allows for detailed evaluation of surgical procedures and pinpointing where the resident is making errors and the type of errors. The overall approach of proficiency analysis relied on recognizing the accuracy of individual basic movements and combining the proficiency measures of individual basic gestures that form a complex movement pattern like suturing.

In order to develop proficiency system, simulation tasks were chosen. The complex surgical procedure that was chosen for analysis involved picking up a linear object with a probe, passing the object through an opening, grasping it with the probe with the other hand, and then passing it back through a vertical opening. The procedure was simulated on a Simuvision® Simulator. Simuvision is a portable laparoscopic video trainer that has a camera and two surgical probes plugged into a laptop. The view of the surgical pad was provided on the laptop and it simulates the work environment in minimally invasive surgery. We chose to de-construct complex movements into 9 basic gestures: (i) In movement (ii) Out movement (iii) Left movement (iv) Right movement (v) Up movement (vi) Down movement (vii) Clockwise Rotation (viii) Counter-clockwise Rotation (ix) Grasping (closing and opening both). These elemental movements were chosen based on data from the literature that suggests that complex gestures in minimally invasive surgery is a combination of these basic movements (Rosen, J.D. Brown, L. Chang, M. Sinanan, & Hannaford, 2006). The complex movement selected spans the entire range of the 9 gestures.

In addition to this complex motion, a simulation was designed for virtual ring transfer task. In the virtual ring transfer task, residents were tasked with grasping a series of a "virtual" rings and placing each on randomly highlighted pegs on a board. The simulation was implemented using the Sensable® haptic joystick. The Sensable haptic joystick allows for generation of 3 degrees of force feedback in response to events in the virtual environment. OpenHL® programming API was used to design the simulation. The simulation allows for measurement of tool tip in the virtual environment. Additionally the sessions could be played back in the software with traces of tool tip movement being shown at various speeds. This allowed for visual analysis of movement.

The basic task involved 10 rings. After the participant places a ring on a highlighted peg, another peg is randomly chosen for participant to the put the ring on. This is repeated till all the 10 rings are correctly placed. The time taken for completing the task is displaced on the bottom middle part of the screen for the participant to follow.

In addition to the basic ring transfer task three variations of the task were designed. In the basic version, the ring is stationary and can be grasped by picking it from a fixed location. To include more manipulations and greater range of motion, a variation of the basic simulation was designed where the ring moved slowly in the environment. This variation required the participants to track the ring movement and pick it while it is in motion. In this variation, the ring moved in the plane of the peg board. In a second variation, the ring was allowed to move anywhere in a 3D environment. In the third variation, the entire peg board moves slowly, creating different orientations in which the surgeons need to accomplish the task. These tasks trained the user to accomplish the tasks in different orientations, a common requirement in actual surgical environments. In addition it also allowed for capture of rotation movements of the wrist. Overall there were 4 different types of ring transfer tasks.

2.1 Participants

Table 1 shows the participant groups included in the initial study.

Table 1. Participants Groups in the initial study

	Senior Surgeons	*1st year residents*	*2nd Year Residents*	*3rd Year Residents*
OBGYN: Male	1	1	4	2
OBGYN: Female	0	5	5	2
General Surgery: Male	2	3	4	2
General Surgery: Female	1	2	4	2
Total	**4**	**11**	**17**	**8**

2.2 Data Capture Methodology

There were 2 different types of capture sessions. The first type of sessions involved basic movements with no specific simulation task. The participants initially filled in a demographic questionnaire which documented their age group, sex, ethnicity and handedness. In addition a laparoscopic experience questionnaire was employed to gauge the overall experience of the participant. Both the questionnaires were filled by the user before the task. In this type of capture sessions, participants performed the 9 basic gestures and the complex surgical procedure using the Simuvision® Simulator. The collection of data was randomized across subjects in a counter-balanced fashion. While performing surgical gestures, the participants were requested to wear CyberTouch® Gloves with a Flock of Bird® Tracker attached to the back of the gloves. The glove required to be calibrated to a users' hand. This was done by the procedure highlighted in the Cyberglove software that requires users to mimic certain poses shown on the computer screen while wearing the gloves. These poses are employed by the software to calibrate the position of joints and measurement points on the glove as suited to a user's hand. The software allowed for saving the calibration and for subsequent sessions the saved calibration for every user was loaded.

CyberTouch datagloves are capable of measuring hand movement (angles at various joints). The gloves use bend sensing technology to measure angles. We measured both wrist and digit kinematics. For wrist kinematics, we recorded flexion/extension and adduction/abduction angles. Digit kinematics consisted of: angles at the metacarpal–phalangeal (mcp), proximal and distal interphalangeal (pip and dip, respectively), joints of the four fingers and the angle of abduction (abd) between adjacent fingers. For the thumb, the mcp, abd, and interphalangeal (ip) angles were measured together with the angle of thumb rotation (rot) about an axis passing through the trapeziometacarpal joint of the thumb and index mcp joint.

We also measured palm arch, minimum and maximum values being associated with the thumb and little finger either touching or being maximally separated. Flexion and abduction were defined as positive; the mcp and pip angles were defined as $0°$ when the finger are straight and in the plane of the palm. At the thumb, positive values of thumb rotation denoted internal rotation. The spatial resolution of the CyberGlove is ~$0.1°$. Fingertip and hand 3-D position and orientation are measured by magnetic trackers (Flock of Birds). The sampling rate of the CyberTouch and magnetic trackers was 120 Hz each. The gloves were open at the fingertips and hence they did not interfere with tactile perception.

In addition to the 3D data, video data was gathered for documentation. Three video cameras were employed. The first video camera stream was obtained from the camera on the Simuvision® simulator. This camera captured the tool movements. Two cameras focused on the two hands for capturing the movements. These video streams were synchronized with the 3D data streams. Each surgeon performed the entire set of gestures. Twenty trials for each basic gesture were performed. Ten trials for each complex gesture were captured as it contained enough repetitions of basic gestures for analysis.

In the second type of data capture, the ring transfer task was performed. In general the ring transfer task covered all the 9 basic gestures and the task served as an appropriate procedure to evaluate proficiency of users in accomplishing the task. The software designed for ring transfer recorded time taken to complete simulations and hand movements from the Cybergloves® and Flock of birds.

The following was the data capture methodology for the ring transfer tasks. The participants initially filled in a demographic questionnaire which documented their age group, sex, ethnicity and handedness. Then the participants were requested to fill a questionnaire that assessed their fatigue level. The questionnaire designed by Behrenz et al. (Behrenz & Monga, 1999) was used for this purpose. This questionnaire allowed for gauging the beginning stress levels and fatigue levels of the residents when doing the task. In addition a laparoscopic experience questionnaire was employed to gauge the overall experience of the participant. All the questionnaires were filled by the user before the task. The user was then requested to wear the Cyberglove®. In the first capture session for each user, the Cyberglove had to be calibrated to a user's hand. Cyberglove was calibrated and the calibration was saved for each user as per the procedure documented above. For subsequent sections, the saved calibration was loaded and employed for measurements.

After wearing the gloves, the participants were randomly assigned a ring transfer task to perform. Data was collected randomized across subjects in a counter balanced fashion. As mentioned above, there were 4 different types of task. In each capture session, the participants performed 2 repetitions of each of the 4 ring transfer tasks. The repetitions allowed for compensation of lack of familiarization with the simulations within a session. For 4 weeks, subjects were requested to perform the tasks before their call and then return and perform the tasks after call. Hence overall, there were overall 8 capture sessions for each user with 4 capture sessions being pre-call and 4 capture sessions being post-call. This methodology enabled gathering data on the effect of fatigue and sleep loss on surgical skills. Additionally, capturing 4 sessions enabled analysis of learning on surgical skill development.

2.3 Data Capture Methodology

The basic movement capture sessions on the Simuvision simulator were recorded through three video cameras. The senior surgeons involved in the experiments viewed the three video streams. The complex movement was divided into basic gestures by senior surgeons. The senior surgeons viewed all the data capture sessions. The corresponding basic gestures in the 3D data stream were identified (the streams were synchronized in capture). The senior surgeons then rated each individual gesture for their subjective measure of proficiency. Each basic movement was rated on a scale of 0 through 10, 0 being the least proficient and 10 being the most proficient. Fractional values were not permitted. The identity of the participant as well as time of capture was not revealed to the senior surgeon preventing any bias in the ratings. Each senior surgeon rated all the performed data sessions except the sessions performed by the senior surgeon themselves. Both the hand movements were rated for proficiency separately as each gesture in the approach was not bimanual in nature. In analysis, left hand and right hand were treated equally as the investigators deemed ambidexterity to be a desirable feature of surgical training. Surgeons were requested to rate proficiency based on visual appearance of the basic gesture as well as the behavioral effect it would produce if conducted in a real surgical environment. For example, a very fast in movement may be detrimental and should get low proficiency rating. The ring transfer data capture sessions were segmented into individual gestures and rated for their proficiency by viewing playback of the virtual simulation in the software. The hand movements were also played back synchronously through visualization software. The same rating system and scale was employed as detailed above.

The next step in data analysis was to find kinematic features for each gesture that depicted high correlation with the subjective measures of proficiency. For each gesture, a set of kinematic features was determined that showed a significant correlation ($p<0.05$) with the subjective proficiency ratings of gestures performed by all the groups. The combination of kinematic features that revealed statistically significant correlation with subjective proficiency measures of all samples of gestures (each gesture class is presented separately) performed by senior surgeons is shown in Table 2. For example, Table 2 shows that the thumb MCP angle value, wrist flexion and the wrist pitch had statistically high correlation with subjective measures. Similarly the thumb MCP angle, x and y component of the wrist, and the wrist flexion and wrist pitch together showed high correlation with rotation gesture. These measures showed high correlation with subjective ratings of the senior surgeon group. These kinematic features were employed as the basis to develop a model that could predict subjective ratings based on the set of kinematic features. Hence for example as shown in table 2, the thumb MCP angle, wrist flexion and wrist pitch were employed for developing predictive model for Grasping subjective proficiency ratings while for in gesture x,y,z component of wrist velocity was employed for development of the model.

Multiple regression analysis was employed to determine a linear model that predicted subjective proficiency ratings for a gesture based on kinematic features identified for the gesture as shown in Table 2. The subjective proficiency measures and the associated feature values were divided into a training set and testing set. The ratings were normalized to fit between a range of ($0 - 1$). The training set employed 70% of all the data capture sessions and the remaining 30% of the data capture sessions were testing set. Parameters were determined for a regression model for the confidence interval of 95% based on the training set between normalized proficiency ratings and predicted ratings. These parameters are shown in Table 2. The test data feature values were fed to the linear model determined by the regression analysis to determine the predicted values of subjective measures. The predicted values were multiplied by 10 to fit in a range of 0 through 10 and then rounded to determine the predicted subjective measure. Correlation coefficient between predicted measures and actual subjective measures was determined. In all the gestures, the correlation between predicted measures and actual subjective measure was above 0.89.

The developed regression models showed high construct validity and predictive validity. In addition, the developed computational measures of proficiency were sensitive to fluctuations in proficiency due to fatigue. This was established by the following methodology. Surgical proficiency of gestures as assigned by the senior surgeons was correlated with normalized fatigue ratings. The questionnaire included tasks in which participants had to rate their present level of fatigue and the maximum and minimum fatigue level during the past 24 hours on a scale of 0 through 10. The normalized rating was obtained taking the weighted average of the three ratings in the questionnaire with the current fatigue level given twice the weight of the minimum and maximum fatigue ratings. The normalized fatigue ratings showed statistically significant correlations ($p<0.1$) with predicted proficiency ratings and the subjective proficiency ratings obtained through senior surgeons. The developed proficiency measures served as a robust computational method to automatically judge proficiency of the performed movements by surgeons. They are based on de-constructing a complex motion sequence into simple gestures and analyzing the gesture for their proficiency through hand movements. This approach offers an easy to understand rating which surgical residents can employ to gauge their skill levels and improve their skills.

Table 2. Set of kinematic features that showed high correlation with subjective proficiency measures for each gesture. The regression coefficients for the linear model are also shown.

Movement	Thumb MCP Angle	Wrist Component Velocity			Aggregate Palm Angle	Wrist Adduction	Wrist Flexion	Wrist Pitch
		X	Y	Z				
Grasp	0.9	-	-	-	-	-	-0.9	-0.8
Rotation(CW)	0.9	0.3	0.2	-	-	-	-0.67	0.23
Rotation(CCW)	0.8	0.4	0.23	-	-	-	-0.23	-0.78
In	-	0.2	0.67	-0.11	-	-	-	-
Out	-	-0.2	-0.56	0.12	-	-	-	-
Up	-	0.8	0.1	0.1	0.1	-0.23	-0.34	-0.12
Down	-	0.21	0.56	0.11	0.23	0.67	-0.23	-0.17
Left	-	0.45	0.56	0.11	-	-0.23	0.36	0.79
Right	-	-0.45	0.56	-0.11	-	-0.45	0.23	0.67

This simple system showed that it is possible to predict deterioration of psychomotor skill. We then further developed a system to predict cognitive skill deterioration. In order to do so, we developed some more variations of the ring transfer tasks.

3 Cognitive Skill Deterioration

For psychomotor skill evaluation, residents were tasked with grasping a series of a "virtual" rings and placing each on randomly highlighted pegs on a board. This task was modified to evaluate attention and memory. The attention task primed the user by highlighting a peg for 1 second with the user tasked to place the ring on the peg. The software does not permit placement of the ring on an incorrect peg. The memory task consisted of 3 sessions in which 4 pegs are highlighted in a sequence. The user is tasked with remembering the sequence and place the ring in that sequence on the pegs. An error is recorded every time the user did not correctly identify the peg for both tasks. Time taken to complete the task was measured in all the three tasks.

In addition to the cited above, we also included EEG based analysis. Research conducted over the past 40 years has established that electroencephalogram (EEG) reliably and accurately reflects subtle shifts in alertness, attention and workload that can be identified and quantified on a millisecond time-frame. We tested the hypothesis that EEG based analysis would predict effect of fatigue on surgical residents.

Advanced Brain Monitoring (ABM) Inc. implemented an integrated hardware and software solution for acquisition and real-time analysis of the EEG and demonstrated feasibility of operational monitoring of EEG indices of alertness, attention, task engagement and mental workload. The system includes an easily-applied wireless EEG system designed to be used in a mobile environment. A novel analytical approach was developed that employs linear and quadratic discriminant function analyses (DFA) to identify and quantify cognitive state changes using model-selected variables that may include combinations of the power in each of the 1-Hz bins from 1-40 Hz, ratios of power bins, event-related power and/or wavelet transform calculations. This unique modeling technique allows simultaneous selection of multiple EEG characteristics across brain regions and spectral frequencies of the EEG, providing a highly sensitive and specific method for monitoring neural signatures of cognition in both real-time and off-line analysis.

Participants wore the wireless EEG sensor headset configured to include the following bi-polar sensor sites: F3-F4, C3-C4, Cz-PO, F3-Cz, Fz-C3, Fz-PO while conducting the ring transfer task. The wireless sensor headset combines battery-powered hardware with a sensor placement system to provide a lightweight, easy-to-apply method to acquire and analyze six channels of high-quality EEG. The headset requires no scalp preparation and provides a comfortable and secure sensor-scalp interface for 12 to 24 hours of continuous use. The headset was designed with fixed sensor locations for three sizes (e.g., small, medium and large). Sensor placement was determined using a database of over 225 subjects so that each sensor is no more than one centimeter from the Residentational 10 – 20 system coordinates. The headset has been evaluated in over 800 healthy participants (fully-rested and sleep-deprived) and more than 200 patients with obstructive sleep apnea. Bi-polar recordings were selected in order to reduce the potential for movement artifacts that can be caused by linked mastoid or ear references during applications that require ambulatory recordings. The seven sensor site locations were selected to optimize the cognitive state classifications while ensuring the sensor headset could be easily applied in less than 10 minutes. Amplification, digitization and radio frequency (RF) transmission of the signals are accomplished with miniaturized electronics in a portable unit worn on the head. The combination of amplification and digitization of the EEG close to the sensors and wireless transmission of the data facilitates the acquisition of high quality signals even in high electromagnetic interference environments. Data are sampled at 256 samples/second with a bandpass from 0.5 Hz and 65Hz (at 3dB attenuation) obtained digitally with Sigma-Delta A/D converters. When utilized in the bi-directional mode, the firmware allows the host computer to initiate impedance monitoring of the sensors, select the transmission channel (so two or more headsets can be used in the same room), and monitor battery power of the headset.

Quantification of the EEG in real-time, referred to as the B-Alert^{TM} system, is achieved using signal analysis techniques to identify and decontaminate fast and slow eye blinks, and identify and reject data points contaminated with excessive muscle activity, amplifier saturation, and/or excursions due to movement artifacts. Decontaminated EEG is then segmented into overlapping 256 data-point windows called overlays. An epoch consists of three consecutive overlays. Fast-Fourier transform is applied to each overlay of the decontaminated EEG signal multiplied by the Kaiser window ($\alpha = 6.0$) to compute the power spectral densities (PSD). The PSD values are adjusted to take into account zero values inserted for artifact contaminated data points.

Wavelet analyses are applied to detect excessive muscle activity (EMG) and to identify and decontaminate eye blinks. Once the artifacts are identified in the time-domain data, the EEG signal is decomposed using a wavelets transformation. Thresholds are developed for application to the wavelet power in the 64 – 128 Hz bin to identify epochs that should be rejected for EMG. The wavelets eye blink identification routine uses a two-step discriminant function analysis. The DFA classifies each data point as a control, eye blink or theta activity. Multiple data points that are classified as eye blinks are then linked and the eye blink detection region is established. Decontamination of eye blinks is accomplished by computing mean wavelet coefficients for the 0-2, 2-4 and 4-8 Hz bins from nearby non-contaminated regions and replacing the contaminated data points. The EEG signal is then reconstructed from the wavelets bins ranging from 0.5 to 64 Hz. Zero values are inserted into the reconstructed EEG signal at zero crossing before and after spikes, excursions and saturations. EEG absolute and relative power spectral density (PSD) variables for each 1-second epoch using a 50% overlapping window are then computed. The PSD values are scaled to accommodate the insertion of zero values as replacements for the artifact.

A single 30-minute baseline EEG test session is required for each participant to adjust the software to accommodate individual differences in the EEG. The output of the B-Alert software includes EEG metrics (values ranging from 0.1-1.0) for alertness/drowsiness, engagement, mental workload and distraction calculated for each 1-second epoch of EEG using quadratic and linear discriminant function analyses of model-selected EEG variables derived from power spectral analysis of the 1-Hz bins from 1-40Hz. These metrics have proven utility in tracking both phasic and tonic changes in cognitive states, in predicting errors that result from either fatigue or overload and in identifying the transition from novice to expert during skill acquisition. We employed these measures for analysis of fatigue on sleep deprivation.

Before and after taking in-hospital call, 32 obstetrical and surgical residents performed a predefined order of ring transfer tasks while wearing datagloves to measure hand movements. They also answered survey's assessing fatigue levels and, activities during call. Acceleration of the hand wrist was measured as smoothness of hand movement. This was calculated through Cyberglove system. Errors in attentional and memory task and time lags in each trial were evaluated. Data was collected over a period of 1 month with 4 pre call and post call trials for each resident. Average number of errors per trial per person and time lag in the pre-call and post call condition was used to perform t-test. A statistically significant decrement ($p<0.01$) in the smoothness of hand movements was observed post-call (Fig 1(b))and in errors in attentional and memory task (Fig (1(c) and 1(d)). Average time lags in post call conditions are also shown in Fig (1b,c,d).

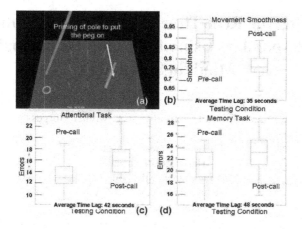

Fig. 1.

In addition, the EEG signals based ratings showed a statistically significant difference between post call and pre call ratings. All the measured metrics were averaged across a task. It was determined that averaged alertness/drowsiness, engagement, mental workload and distraction ratings across tasks were significantly different across call. Further the ratings showed high correlation with subjective fatigue ratings (0.91).

Call-associated fatigue is associated with increased error rates in psychomotor and cognitive skills. Cognitive skill as measured through the task and EEG analysis showed a significant decline. These results need to be accounted for in the design of resident curriculum.

References

1. Behrenz, K., Monga, M.: Fatigue in Pregnancy: A comparative study. American Journal of Perinatology 16(4), 185–188 (1999)
2. Rosen, J., Brown, J.D., Chang, L., Sinanan, M., Hannaford, B.: Generalized Approach for Modeling Minimally Invasive Surgery as a Stochastic Process Using a Discrete Markov Model. IEEE Transactions on Biomedical Engineering 53, 399–413 (2006)
3. Tendulkar, A., Victorino, G., Chong, T., Bullard, M., Liu, T., Harken, A.: Quantification of Surgical Resident Stress "On Call". Journal of the American College of Surgeons 201(4), 560 (2005)

Assessing the Real-Time Cognitive Capabilities of First Responders Using Emerging Technologies in Manikin Simulators

Kathleen Kihmm Connolly and Lawrence Burgess

Telehealth Research Institute
University of Hawaii
651 Ilalo Street, MEB, Suite 212
Honolulu HI, 96813, USA
{kihmm,lburgess}@hawaii.edu

Abstract. Medical triage can be a highly stressful situation in which decisions and task performance may have life or death consequences. Individual responses in stressful situations may affect task performance. Increased injury or casualties may occur without proper training and competency of the first-responder. The emerging technologies of advanced manikin simulators have afforded anatomic, physiological, and pharmacologic realism, which can be dynamically programmed in real-time. This has increased the capabilities and realism of manikin simulations, thus allowing advanced learning techniques that were not previously possible. By employing physiological measures of the learner to determine areas of overwhelming task complexity, which may degrade performance, a method such that the training can be adjusted to the real-time cognitive needs/load of the learner (*adaptive scaffolding*) can be applied. This has the potential to enhance learning and human data processing in medical triage training.

Keywords: Triage, manikin simulators, first-responder, physiological sensors, adaptive scaffolding.

1 Introduction

Medical triage is the act of prioritizing patients according to severity of injury in order to prevent further injury or death. In mass casualty situations, the nature and pace of the workload may vary depending on the scale of the event. First-responders must be able to process information and act accordingly in order to optimize medical and logistical outcomes. The leading challenge of medical triage is the ability to identify those that need immediate care from those that are less critically injured in a timely manner [1]. Performance may suffer when first responders are overwhelmed by multiple demanding tasks in stressful and volatile situations. Hence training is necessary for first-responders to be able to cognitively act in the most optimal way, minimizing casualties and maximizing outcomes.

D.D. Schmorrow, L.M. Reeves (Eds.): Augmented Cognition, HCII 2007, LNAI 4565, pp. 314–322, 2007.
© Springer-Verlag Berlin Heidelberg 2007

Instructional theories suggest that learning based on real-life tasks helps the learner to integrate the knowledge and skills necessary to be able to perform the task in real life [2]. Emerging technologies of advanced manikin simulators with anatomic, physiological, and pharmacologic realism have increased the capabilities and realism of trauma simulations. Now more widely available and accessible, these advanced technologies in manikin simulators are facilitating the ability to provide advanced cognitive training in areas of acute care medicine, including medical triage, which was not previously possible.

Currently available technology in manikin simulations allows the modeling of complex physiological functions that have the ability to be dynamically programmed on-the-fly. By employing physiological sensors to monitor the human trainee, medical triage learning tasks which cause cognitive overload or overwhelming task complexity can be detected in real-time [3]. Cognitive overload or overwhelming task complexity can cause stress and may degrade performance and learning effectiveness. Using this information, a training methodology, referred to as adaptive scaffolding, can then be applied to adjust the state of the manikin to achieve optimal levels of performance and learning. This mitigation strategy has the potential to improve learning and enhance real-life performance, which may not be achieved by traditional didactic or scenario-based training alone.

2 Background

In mass casualty or trauma events, triage is an area where decision-making is vital for achieving positive outcomes; the larger the number of victims on the scene, the more difficult it becomes to determine the order of those that need to be treated. To add to the complexity, in a mass casualty situation, there must be a balance between treatment of the population versus treatment of the individual. Decisions that determine the outcomes of the greater good must be analyzed and carefully weighed, which may result in degrading the medical needs of particular individuals. This is largely based on the number and types of casualities and the available resources. Consequently some victims may not be treated despite the possibility of preventing death or further injury. This decision-making process is atypical from normal trauma management, where each individual victim is treated. Hence, mass casualty trauma situations must require advanced training and planning which are crucial in saving lives and reducing further injury [1].

2.1 The Need to Train First-Responders

Despite that it is vital that first responders and medical personnel are thoroughly trained and prepared for action, there are few opportunities to obtain the training and experience necessary for optimal performance specifically in mass casualty emergency situations. In particular, surgical residents, who are critical in emergency medical situations, lack the training necessary for mass casualty, triage and emergency medicine. Medical training must be expanded to include triage training, especially for surgeons since they are often expected to take lead roles in mass casualty events [4]. The vast number of civilian emergency personnel (150,000 emergency medical technicians and 1.7 million fire fighters) that can benefit from such training must also be underscored. The Federation of American Scientists (FAS) report in 2003, *Training Technology Against Terror: Using Advanced Technology to Prepare America's Emergency Medical Personnel and First Responders for a Weapon of Mass Destruction Attack* [5], found that the U.S.' need for first responder training was dramatically larger than previously recognized. There are over 150,000 emergency medical technicians and 1.7 million firefighters in the U.S. who would be expected to use complex critical thinking skills, such as triage, as part of incident management teams

In light of potential terrorist attacks, civilian populations of first responders and local trauma centers may not be equipped to handle the emotional, logistical and medical load that such an event may present. The military is probably the most trained for mass casualty situations, however, performance and health care of the fighting force has become increasingly challenging. A high operational pace with frequent deployments shortens training time even more. On the battlefield, in command and control situations, it is essential to assess, triage, and treat medical emergencies accurately, proficiently and in a timely manner. This task is made more difficult in stressful battlefield environments where victims may be scattered over distances in foreign, austere terrain with active gunfire.

Physicians have traditionally depended on bedside teaching to impart knowledge to trainees. This concept has become less popular because of concern over patient safety, as well as it being difficult to have a representative patient available for each diagnosis. The desire to use simulation in training whenever possible is important, as patients are protected instead of being commodities in training [6]. As such, simulation training provides an important and well-recognized bridge between the textbook and the bedside, and should be utilized whenever possible.

2.2 Overview of Manikin Technology

Simulation technology can provide a solution for the need to train triage by providing readily available cognitive and procedural training platforms that can supplement a didactic triage curriculum. In addition to skills training, simulation exercises can help lower psychological barriers in stressful emergency situations by providing a safe and controlled environment for practice [7].

Manikin based simulations have been mainstays in medical education for many years [8]. Less advanced manikins are utilized in certification courses such as Cardio-Pulmonary Resuscitation (CPR) and Basic Life Support (BLS). Advanced manikin simulation technologies, which are computer driven, can simulate a multitude of real-life medical scenarios. These advanced manikins are currently being used to train Acute Trauma Life Support (ATLS), Pediatric Advanced Life Support (PALS), as well as, other acute medical emergences, such as hemmorhagic shock or tension pneumothorax. Manikin simulation technology provides the opportunity for students to practice routine, complex or unusual medical procedures in a controlled environment without risk to patients. The software that drives the simulations is interactive and offers real-time feedback to interventions, allowing students to be immediately assessed. A debriefing session allows students to repeat scenarios to enforce learning.

Advances in manikin technology have enabled the ability to simulate human physiology realistically, interactively and with the ability to preprogram or dynamically program the scenerios. The SimMan™ manikin simulator physiological features include breathing, talking, heart, breath and bowel sounds. In addition, haptic feedback features include palpable bilateral Dorsalis Pedis, Posterior Tibialis and carotid pulses. Radial and brachial pulses are available on the left arm, while the right arm may be cannulated for IV and blood work procedures. Airway management procedures include bag-valve-mask ventilation, supraglottic airway adjuncts, endotracheal intubation and cricothyrotomy. Pupils may be modified for assessment. The trauma module for SimMan™ includes interchangeable parts to simulate fractures, burns, impaled objects, and projectile entry/exit wounds [9].

Another advanced feature of manikin simulators is the ability to be dynamically programmed, in real-time, via a wireless laptop computer. An instructor can manipulate the manikin physiology and initiate physiological trends, while students are simultaneously assessing and treating the manikin. This includes vital signs parameters, such heart rate, O2 saturation, arterial blood pressure, pulmonary artery pressure, end tidal CO2, respiratory rate and blood pressure. Trends that occur over time can also be preprogrammed and dynamically initiated. This includes the aforementioned vital signs and central line monitoring such as central venous, pulmonary artery and wedge pressures, and cardiac output.

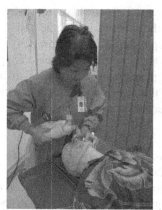 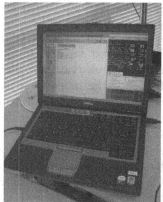

Fig. 1. SimMan™ manikin simulator and laptop computer, which controls the manikin via wireless technology

These advanced emerging manikin capabilities afford the ability for dynamic and interactive simulations of real-life physiological states, changes in states and complex medical scenarios, which can be used to train first-responder, medical and allied health students and health professionals. The realism and ability to conduct complex cognitive tasks on a virtual patient has the potential to be a valuable learning platform.

3   Mitigating Augmented Cognitive Strategy

Medical triage can be a highly stressful situation in which decisions and task performance may have life or death consequences. Individuals may vary in their cognitive capabilities depending on factors the may include expertise, experience, stress, fatigue, distractions, or other internal psychological states. Cognitive overload and stress caused by individual responses may negatively affect and degrade task performance. An intervention of using physiological sensors can be used to determine areas of overwhelming task complexity which may affect performance [3]. Using this information, an individual mitigation strategy of scaffolding can be used to manage and recognize areas of difficulty in order to enhance learning and human data processing by adjusting learning to the individual cognitive needs of the learner [10].

3.1   Assessment of Cognitive State Using Physiological Measures

Cognitive Load Theory (CLT) assumes that the human working memory has a limited capacity. When humans are tasked to the maximum, overload occurs in which learning and performance is degraded. Accordingly reducing cognitive load to accommodate better learning can be more effective in the transfer of performance to real world tasks. Research has also confirmed that emotional influences play a vital role in cognitive processing, such as relationships between anxiety and attention, or emotional state and memory [11].

In addition to the existing cognitive state, learners have difficulty integrating knowledge due to cognitive overload by the complexity of the task. In a study conducted by Crosby and Ikehara (2006) physiological measures of eye tracking, heart rate, electrodermal activity, finger temperature and pressure applied to a computer mouse was used to determine physiological responses to a task with increasing difficulty. The results showed that anomalous individual physiological responses to tasks can be detected, which may affect performance in critical situations [3]. This information can then be used to individually adjust training to allow for improved task proficiency.

In managing cognitive load, to achieve optimal learning, the presentation of learning material cannot alone determine that the learner is assimilating information optimally. It is desireable that cognitive resources be balanced between two type of cognitive states. These are external cognitive load, which may be adequate instructional materials, and on the individual learners internal cognitive load or strategies in dealing with the task [12]. Non-invasive physiological sensors can measure and help detect the cognitive state of the learner in real-time during task performance. The advantages to using physiological measures, versus measurements of speech, facial expressions, body language, or self-reporting, are that they are functions of the human autonomic system that are difficult to falsely generate and can be detected in real-time. With the availability of commercially available wearable sensors, emotions, such as stress can be detected. Table 1 describes some of the non-evasive physiological measures that can be used to determine stress related emotions while training triage.

Table 1. Biosensor Measures that can Determine Cognitive State [13]

Biosensor Measure	Cognitive State
Skin Conductivity	Arousal
Peripheral Temperature	Relaxation
Heart Rate	Stress
Pupil size	Fatigue
Eye Tracking	Difficulty or stress

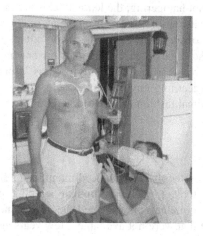

Fig. 2. Example of noninvasive physiological sensors (Nexan Ltd.), which can transmit data wirelessly via an attached PDA. Measures 2-lead electrocardiogram, pulse oximetry, heart rate, respiration rate and temperature.

3.2 Scaffolding as a Mitigation Strategy

Once cognitive overload is detected, a mitigation strategy of scaffolding can be used in enhancing triage training. The concept of scaffolding is based on the developmental theories of Vygotsky (1978) [14]. The concept is based on the theory that with controlled guidance of an expert or teacher, higher levels of thinking can be achieved. Scaffolding can supplement affective (emotional) strategies and create a context in which active exploration of ideas is encouraged [15]. Studies using scaffolding in hypermedia have shown significant increases in student's learning as indicated by performance, understanding, the ability to process data. Results showed higher conceptual understanding than those learning without scaffolding [16]. In a study using computer based scaffolding to design and simulate clinical trials, students were able to demonstrate a 34% increase in the number of elements they included in their research proposals. Also, the students were able to improve their critiques of flawed proposals by 48% [17].

Based on the concept of scaffolding, *adaptive scaffolding* is the idea that task difficulty can be adjusted based on the individual learners level of ability. In other words, simulated tasks can be restructured dynamically to improve understanding in particular topics [18]. This can facilitate the student's success in the task beyond their current capability, similar to the idea of adaptive learning. It is important to note that, in accordance with CLT, learners should be exposed fully to the task at hand. Breaking up a task may cause increased cognitive load due to the need to piece together and reintegrate the information [19].

Applying scaffolding to training triage has the potential to improve cognitive skills. It is critical to be able to determine the when and how much to adjust the cognitive load, thus helping, and not hampering, the learner. This is can be accomplished by the feed back of physiological sensors to detect moments of cognitive overload or stress. When the learner is overwhelmed by the task situation, the instructors can dynamically program the manikin to either maintain or change physiological state, giving the user time to reassess and internally process information. This mitigating strategy may provide a learning environment where information may be processed and stored in a more optimal fashion than traditional training.

4 Conclusion

This paper has focused on the use of advanced manikin simulators and physiological sensors as a potential tools to enhance human learning performance. Emerging technologies in manikin simulators has opened the door to new methods of training, learning and assessment that were not available a few years ago. Advances in human-computer interaction are evolving in such a way that learning activities are no longer constrained by the limitation of technology. Employing methods such as adaptive scaffolding in conjunction with physiological measures of learner stress has the potential to optimize learning. The student can be given "just-in-time" training assistance (learners are able to access information when they need it) so that they can learn and integrate knowledge more effectively than previously possible.

In accordance with the Defense Advanced Research Projects Agency (DARPA) Augmented Cognition Program, employing the emerging technologies of manikin simulation and physiological sensors to detect and augment the training of medical triage has the potential to increase the effectiveness and improve the transfer of knowledge to real-life situations. This is facilitated by the ability to manipulate training based on the individual's cognitive capacity and in turn, improve the mental processes and performance of the trainee. At a disaster site, triage may be the most important medical task performed [20]. The ability to optimally train first-responders in a realistic and safe environment in conjunction with adaptive scaffolding optimized for the individual student's cognitive processing can be of great value.

References

1. Frykberg, E.R.: Medical management of disasters and mass casualties from terrorist bombings: how can we cope? The Journal Of Trauma 53(2), 201–212 (2002)
2. van Merrienboer, J.J.G., Kirschner, P.A., Kester, L.: Taking the Load Off a Learner's Mind: Instructional Design for Complex Learning. Educational Psychologist 38(1), 5–13 (2003)
3. Crosby, M.E., Ikehara, C.S.: Using Physiological Measures to Identify Individual Differences in Response to Task Attributes. In: Schmorrow, D.D., Stanney, K.M., Reeves, L.M. (eds.) Foundations of Augmented Cognition, 2nd edn. San Ramon: Strategic Analysis, Inc. (2006)
4. Galante, J.M., Jacoby, R.C., Anderson, J.T.: Are Surgical Residents Prepared for Mass Casualty Incidents? J. Surg. Res. (2005)
5. Kelly, H., Blackwood, V., Roper, M., Higgins, G., Klein, G., Tyler, J., Fletcher, D., Jenkins, H., Chisolm, A., Squire, K.: Training Technology against Terror: Using Advanced Technolgy to Prepare America's Emergency Medical Personnel and First Responders for a Weapon of Mass Destruction Attack, The Learning Federation, Washinton, DC (September 2002)
6. Ziv, A., Wolpe, P.R., Small, S.D., Glick, S.: Simulation-based medical education: an ethical imperative. Academic Medicine 78(8), 783–788 (2003)
7. Hendrickse, A.D., Ellis, A.M., Morris, R.W.: Use of simulation technology in Australian Defence Force resuscitation training. J. R. Army Med. Corps 147(2), 173–178 (2001)
8. American College of Surgeons, Advanced Trauma Life Support for Doctors Instuctor Manual, 6th edn. Chicago: Fisrt Impressions (1997)
9. Laerdal Medical [Website]. Last Accessed 11 February 2007 (2006) http://www.laerdal.com/.
10. Ikehara, C., Chin, D.N., Crosby, M.E.: A Model for Integrating an Adaptive Information Filter Utilizing biosensor Data to Assess Cognitive Load. In: 9th International Conference on User Modeling (2003)
11. Hudlicka, E.: To feel or not to feel: The role of affect in human-computer interaction. International Journal of Human-Computer Studies 59, 1–32 (2003)
12. Bannert, M.: Managing cognitive Load–Recent trends in cognitive load theory. Learning & Instruction 12(1), 139–146 (2002)
13. Andreassi, J.L.: Psychophysiology Human Behavior and Physiological Response, 4th edn. Lawrence Erlbaum Associates, Publishers, Mahwah (2000)
14. Vygotsky, L.S.: Mind in society: the development of higher psychological processes. Harvard University Press, Cambridge (1978)
15. Yelland, N., Masters, J.: Rethinking scaffolding in the information age. Computers & Education 48(3), 362–382 (2007)
16. Azevedo, R., Cromley, J.G., Seibert, D.: Does adaptive scaffolding facilitate students' ability to regulate their learning with hypermedia? Contemporary Educational Psychology 29(3), 344–370 (2004)
17. Hmelo, C.E., Ramakrishnan, S., Day, R.S., Shirey, W.E., Brufsky, A., Johnson, C., Baar, J., Huang, Q.: Oncology thinking cap: scaffolded use of a simulation to learn clinical trial design. Teaching And Learning In Medicine 13(3), 183–191 (2001)

18. Component Roadmap: Instructional Design in Technology-Enabled Learning Systems: Using Simulations and Games in Learning, The Learning Federation Project, Washington, DC (2003)
19. Kalyuga, S., Chandler, P., Sweller, J.: Managing split-attention and redundancy in multimedia instruction. Applied Cognitive Psychology 13(4), 351–371 (1999)
20. Waeckerle, J.F.: Disaster planning and response. New England Journal of Medicine 324(12), 815 (1991)

Physiologic System Interfaces Using fNIR with Tactile Feedback for Improving Operator Effectiveness

Erin M. Nishimura[1], Evan D. Rapoport[1], Benjamin A. Darling[2], Dennis R. Proffitt[2], Traci H. Downs[1], and J. Hunter Downs III[1]

[1] Archinoetics, LLC, 700 Bishop St, Ste 2000, Honolulu, HI 96813
[2] Dept. of Psych., University of Virginia, P.O. Box 400400, Charlottesville, VA 22904

Abstract. This paper explores the validation of tactile mechanisms as an effective means of communications for integration into a physiologic system interface (PSI). Tactile communications can offer a channel that only minimally interferes with a primary or concurrent task. The PSI will use functional brain imaging techniques, specifically functional near-infrared imaging (fNIR), to determine cognitive workload in language and visual processing areas of the brain. The resulting closed-loop system will thus have the capability of providing the operator with necessary information by using the modality most available to the user, thus enabling effective multi-tasking and minimal task interference.

Keywords: physiologic system interfaces, functional near-infrared (fNIR), tactile, tactile communications.

1 Background

The data presented to humans on a daily basis by interactive electronic systems is ever-increasing. Physiologic system interfaces (PSIs) have been developed in response to this increasing demand on the user and utilize signals from the heart, brain, and skin to provide information to the control systems of these interactive platforms. Additionally, the increasing use of multi-modal communications systems allow for hands-free interaction between the user and the system. As a result, critical information can be conveyed in a two-way stream between the user and the system with minimal interference with the primary task at hand.

By integrating physiologic state data about the operator into a closed-loop system, human performance can be improved by augmenting the computer environment. This is accomplished through providing the operator with feedback through sensory channels that are not required, or minimally required, for working on the primary task. For example, if the subject is focused on a phone conversation, incoming auditory messages may not be heard or processed appropriately. In some scenarios, the new messages could even distract the subject, causing him or her to miss parts of the phone conversation. Because the relative importance or urgency of the new

D.D. Schmorrow, L.M. Reeves (Eds.): Augmented Cognition, HCII 2007, LNAI 4565, pp. 323–328, 2007.

messages compared to the primary task would not always be known, the operator must be given all the information without significant decreases in comprehension.

1.1 Functional Brain Imaging with fNIR

One type of physiologic sensor that helps characterize a user's state is functional brain imaging, which can provide real-time data about the cognitive processes at work, such as working memory. Numerous technologies exist, but only a few would be appropriate for use in real world environments. For example, functional magnetic resonance imaging (fMRI) is widely used in studying the brain's activity, but is the size of a room and requires the subject lie motionless on a table. For this PSI to be widely usable, all component parts must be wearable and minimally intrusive on the subject.

Functional near-infrared imaging (fNIR) technology is a non-invasive technique that is an ideal choice for this PSI. Available systems can be small, comfortable, and easily placed on the user's head over the cortical areas of interest. Additionally, fNIR is relatively affordable, less constraining to the user, and easier to setup than other technologies.

The functionality of fNIR relies on the light transmission properties of oxy-compared to deoxy-hemoglobin in the near-infrared (NIR) part of the spectrum. The sensor emits multiple wavelengths of NIR light and then detects how much light of each wavelength passes through the skull and brain and returns to the surface of the head (Figure 1). The relative levels of the wavelengths provide a means of calculating, in real-time, the cortical blood volume and oxygenation changes due to neuronal activation [9]. This measure is essentially the same physiologic signal that fMRI detects. Additional benefits of fNIR include higher real-time accuracy, more robust operation in real-world environments, and vastly shorter (or nonexistent) training times [3,5] than competing EEG or fMRI technologies. Finally, in addition to measuring cognitive activity, the fNIR signal also includes other physiologic parameters, such as heart rate and respiration rate, which have a potentially useful role in the PSI.

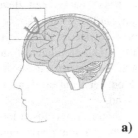
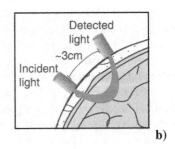

a)   b)

Fig. 1. Incident NIR light passes through scalp and skull to the cortex. Using scatter models, light reaching the cortex can be detected approximately 3 cm away. The amount of light detect is a function of extinction coefficient (attenuation) which in turn is a function of the tissue content. Using different wavelengths of NIR light, it is possible to solve for concentrations of hemoglobin and oxy-hemoglobin.

1.2 Tactile Communications

Visual and auditory modalities are commonly used for effectively presenting information to users; however, once these channels are overloaded, task performance may be reduced due to bottlenecks in the perceptual system. An alternative to these approaches is tactile stimulation, which would act as the output effector for this PSI system. Tactile mechanisms are capable of producing a distinguishable low resolution "image" or tactile icon (tacton) on the skin of the user [1] in a manner that can be discreet or even covert. Past studies have already shown that reaction times were improved with kinesthetic or vibrotactile cues, as opposed to auditory or visual cues [6,7], indicating the ability of users to recognize and distinguish tactile stimuli is greater than that of auditory or visual stimuli.

In addition to the proven ability of subjects to recognize and react to tactile stimuli, using tactile mechanism for communications rather than visual or auditory cues does not interfere with concurrent visual or auditory tasks [10]. Tactile mechanisms as a form of communications can convey messages or even situational awareness information without overloading the visual and auditory senses that are often already in use by the current tasks.

2 Objective

This paper introduces a PSI using functional brain imaging and a tactile feedback system to facilitate communication with an operator. Those most benefited by this particular system would be operators who rely heavily on visual and auditory stimuli for their primary tasks. This validation of a tactile system as a channel for communications presents an effective means to potentially increase task performance of a human user and thereby improve the effectiveness of the computing system. Such a system can optimize performance in an environment where individuals are taxed with high requirements. This is accomplished through informed, intelligent distribution of information presentation across multiple modalities.

Fig. 2 below demonstrates the concept of new information (such as feedback) being presented to the operator (shown as the secondary task). These new tasks require both perceptual systems and working memory systems (the spatial working memory tasks require visual cues and the verbal working memory tasks require auditory cues). The operator is capable of performing the primary task with a secondary task of the other modality (as the green check indicates), but not of the same modality (as the red X indicates). This is further emphasized by the renderings of the brain's cortical activity based on fMRI data, which shows different patterns of activity for each type, indicating the area is already very busy processing information.

Therefore, the addition of tactile feedback to this system presented in Fig. 2 would add another modality for communication to the already overloaded operator. Additionally, because some stimuli can be presented in multiple modalities, the system would be able to present the stimuli appropriately by only using modalities that are not in use for the primary task. This information would sometimes be known just by the nature of the actual task, but may often require functional brain imaging to know how the person is actually processing the information while performing the

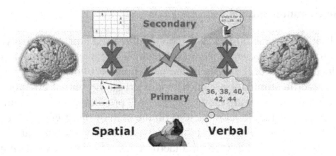

Fig. 2. Diagram of experimental setup for the PSI

task. For example, remembering a telephone number can be done either through a verbal strategy (by silently repeating the numbers) or by a spatial strategy (by visualizing the phone keypad and the path your finger would travel to dial the number). Therefore, it cannot be assumed that a user will always be taxed in the perceptual or memory system that is typically associated with a particular task.

In this study, task performance is monitored with an fNIR PSI interface and compares the use of tactile feedback (tactons) to the use of visual feedback (computer monitors). Performance is measured through time required for cognitive activation as determined by the fNIR oxygenation signal. The study essentially validates the use of tactons as an effective communications modality when compared to the traditionally and commonly used visual modality. By adding tactons to a system as a communications channel, this system increases the number of complementary modalities available for communications to the operator; providing additional channels that do not impinge on existing channels will lead to more effective communications as suggested by the media richness theory [2,4]. The goal of this research is focused on providing the dismounted warfighter with the information necessary to operate and survive in the most effective modality for the situation at hand.

2.1 Methods

The fNIR system to be used in this research, called OTIS, was developed by Archinoetics, LLC (Figure 3). OTIS is a completely non-invasive, continuous-wave fNIR system that is portable and supports up to two sensors that allow for sensing over areas of the scalp with hair, a distinct feature of this fNIR sensing system. Each sensor has two channels with a central emitter and two detectors. The system uses three wavelengths of NIR light and has a sampling frequency of 34.8Hz. [8]. OTIS communicates over Ethernet to a PC where custom software applications process and log the data.

The OTIS sensor will be placed on the subject's head over Broca's area to measure cognitive activity associated with language processing. Accordingly, the subject will be given a task that activates this area such that the tactile feedback indicates to them their success in performing the task. The performance of the subjects will be quantified as time to activation. In preliminary testing, subjects reported finding it

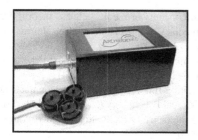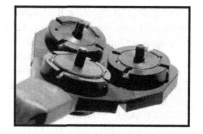

Fig. 3. Current generation of Archinoetics fNIR system and close up of sensor

useful to have feedback in the form of a visual graph indicating their level of success in trying to produce an activation on demand. Retrospective analysis of these trials has confirmed the benefit of this feedback, quantified in terms of an increased number of successful attempts to activate over a given number of trials.

Activation will be determined using custom, real-time cognitive activation detection algorithms. These detection algorithms have adjustable variables and settings that will remain constant between subjects and runs for consistent time-to-activation calculations. Each subject undergoes a calibration process for the fNIR system based on the decided settings for the detection algorithm.

3 Discussion

In addition to improving operator performance and system effectiveness, a PSI system with tactile feedback has multiple applications to improving information processing. The improvement of information processing applies to multiple categories of information content, whether surveillance, readiness status, situational, training, medical, or otherwise.

Validation of tacton discrimination capabilities and the effectiveness of tactons as an alternative means of communication has broad ranging potential in the public sector for any situation in which the audio-visual systems are already occupied. Tactile alerts are already present in many everyday devices, such as cell phones and PDAs, so its use as a communications system would be transparent to the user that already possesses these items. Such a form of tactile alerts can be used to discriminate between critical and non-critical information to be presented to the user via these devices.

References

1. Brewster, S., King, A.: An investigation into the use of tactons to present progress information. In: Costabile, M.F., Paternó, F. (eds.) INTERACT 2005. LNCS, vol. 3585, pp. 6–17. Springer, Heidelberg (2005)
2. Carlson, J.R., Zmud, R.W.: Channel expansion theory and the experiential nature of media richness perceptions. Academy of Management Journal 42(2), 153–170 (1999)
3. Chance, B., et al.: A novel method of fast imaging of brain function, non-invasively, with light. Optics Express, 2(10) (1998)

4. Cooper, R.B., Cooper, R.B.: Exploring the core concepts of media richness theory: The impact of cue multiplicity and feedback immediacy on decision quality. Journal of Management Information Systems 20(1), 263–299 (2003)
5. Coyle, S., et al.: On the suitability of near-infrared (NIR) systems for next-generation brain-computer interfaces. Physiological Measurement 25(4), 815–822 (2004)
6. Diederich, A.: Intersensory facilitation of reaction-time: Evaluation of counter and diffusion coactivation models. Journal of Mathematical Psychology (39), 381–394 (1995)
7. Gielen, C.A.M., Schmidt, R.A.: On the nature of intersensory facilitation of reaction time. Perception and Psychophysics (34), 161–168 (1983)
8. Nishimura, E.M., Stautzenberger, J., Robinson, W., Downs, T.H., Downs III, J.H.: A New Approach to fNIR: OTIS. IEEE Engineering in Medicine and Biology Magazine (2007) (in press)
9. Okada, E., et al.: Theoretical and experimental investigation of near-infrared light propagation in a model of the adult head. Applied Optics 36(1), 21–31 (1997)
10. Sklar, A.E., Sarter, N.B.: Good vibrations: Tactile feedback in support of attention allocation and human-automation coordination in event-driven domains. Human Factors (41), 543–552 (1999)

A Model for Visio-Haptic Attention for Efficient Resource Allocation in Multimodal Environments

Priyamvada Tripathi, Kanav Kahol, Anusha Sridaran,
and Sethuraman Panchanathan

Center for Cognitive Ubiquitous Computing,
Arizona State University, Tempe, AZ, USA
{priyamvada.tripathi, Kanav.Kahol,
Anusha.Sridaran, panch}@asu.edu

Abstract. Sequences of visual and haptic exploration were obtained on surfaces of different curvature from human subjects. We then extracted regions of interest (ROI) from the data as a function of number of times a subject fixated on a certain location on object and amount of time spent on such each location. Simple models like a plane, cone, cylinder, paraboloid, hyperboloid, ellipsoid, simple-saddle and a monkey-saddle were generated. Gaussian curvature representation of each point on all the surfaces was pre-computed. The surfaces have been previously tested for haptic and visual realism and distinctness by human subjects in a separate experiment. Both visual and haptic rendering were subsequently used for exploration by human subjects to study whether there is a similarity between the visual ROI and haptic ROIs. Additionally, we wanted to see if there is a correlation between curvature values and the ROIs thus obtained. A multiple regression model was further developed to see if this data can be used to predict the visual exploration path using haptic curvature saliency measures.

Keywords: Vision, Haptics, Eye movements, Attention, Saliency, Regions of Interest.

1 Introduction

Humans interact with their environment through several modalities: vision, touch, audition, gustatory, olfactory. Among these modalities, vision and touch play an important role in gathering information from the surrounding environment and store representation of the environmental objects. This is so because most of the everyday objects such as cups, glasses, bowls, etc., have two essential modal components: a visual component and a tactile component. These two components overlap extensively and interact synergistically in order to produce coherent representations of these object and to enable humans to make consistent responses to them (Spence & Driver, 2004). For example, a purely visual component such as color may not interact with tactile information at all but a 'composite' feature such as texture will need

D.D. Schmorrow, L.M. Reeves (Eds.): Augmented Cognition, HCII 2007, LNAI 4565, pp. 329–336, 2007.
© Springer-Verlag Berlin Heidelberg 2007

contribution of both tactile and visual system to arrive at a coherent judgment. This distribution can be visualized as a Venn diagram as shown in Fig. 1.

Since it is computationally infeasible to enumerate all the objects with all their pertaining characteristics, attention serves as a prerequisite to any computations that may be performed on such multimodal (in this paper multimodality will only mean visuo-tactile) objects (Ballard, 1986; Tsotsos, 1990, 1991). An image or an object can thus be described in terms of its saliency or regions of interest (ROI). Some attributes in an object are assumed to be more salient than others and tend to attract more attention (tactile or visual) of the observer. Similarly, there are some regions of the object that are more focused upon than others in order to gain the representation of the object. Thus, selective attention processes serve an important role in exploration of novel everyday objects. Figure 2 shows how attention can act as 'moderator' in multimodal explorations by humans.

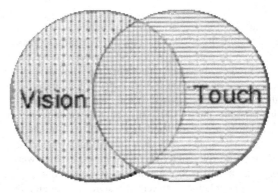

Fig. 1. Venn diagram showing distribution of features in a visuo-tactile object. Vision and Touch can be visualized as overlapping modalities wherein they convey information about purely visual (e.g. color) or tactual features (e.g. hardness) and also of those that combine vision and touch for coherent representation (e.g. texture).

In this paper, we asked the question whether purely spatio-temporal bottom-up exploration of a 3D geometrical feature such as Gaussian curvature will yield any correlation in vision and touch. If a correlation exists, then it paves way for optimal allocation of computational resources in visual and haptic interfaces due to the similarity in ROIs and overlap of perceptual load requirements. Furthermore, a predictive sequence can be developed that uses information from one modality to maximize the performance in other modality.

2 Background and Related Work

Human perceptual system comprises of several modality sub-systems that dictate our interactions with our environment. This distribution in order to extract information from the environment employs mainly two attentional mechanisms to handle the 'bottleneck' of the perceptual system: (a) bottom-up saliency of the attributes or features and (b) top-down or goal driven template search. Bottom-up saliency measures for images and objects have been studied extensively (Wolfe, 1998). In 2001, Itti et al. (Itti, Koch, & Neibur, 1998) constructed a biologically plausible model of visual selection attention that uses 'saliency maps'. Saliency maps, also called conspicuity maps, are explicit representation of saliency values for particular features such as color, luminous intensity, orientation. These features are traditionally assumed to constitute the set of 'basic features' for visual selective attention models. These models scan the locations in the images in order of decreasing saliency. Other features that have been explored for search mechanisms in vision are size, spatial frequency, scale, motion, shape, and depth cues (Pashler, 1998). Curvature has been explored as a possible candidate by several researchers in visual search task where curved object is to be identified from a from several distracters without any curvature (Brown, Weisstein, & May, 1992; Cheal & Lyon, 1992; Sun & Perona, 1993). These studies, unfortunately, are very limited in their exploration. In our point of view, curvature is a 3D concept and needs to be rendered in a 3D environment for results with reasonable perceptual accuracy. Curvature has occasionally been confused with

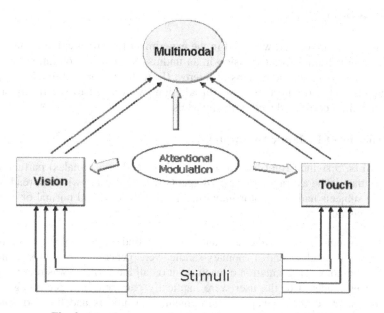

Fig. 2. Attention as a moderator in human perceptual system

change in orientation or illumination changes (Riggs, 1973). Additionally, no studies have actually explored the effect of curvature of haptic attention. Most contemporary studies point out that attention is most likely a post-sensory phenomenon (Mesulam, 1998; Posner & Dehaene, 1994),hence, it is needed that exploration be done of these 3D parameters on both haptics as well as vision.

Ouerhani and Hugli (Ouerhani & Hugli, 2000) explored the usefulness of depth (defined as distance from camera to the object) as a feature in saliency maps in a neurally plausible model of attention and pointed out that the depth contributed immensely in the focus of visual attention since the "depth enhanced model detects depth locations which stand out from their surrounding". Unfortunately, they did not include curvature in the model. Some studies (Jenmalm, Birznieks, Goodwin, & Johansson) have indicated that human subjects automatically adjusted the grasping force to correspond to the amount of curvature present on the object. This seems to signify that there is a very likely correlation between visual and haptic assessment of curvature and also, attentional exploration is sometimes dictated by curvature values of the object.

Thus, it is possible that curvature is an important signifier of the object exploration. In order to study its bottom-up saliency pattern in human subject, we conducted experiments and related the measures so conducted with a multiple regression model. Stimuli were carefully rendered using varying Gaussian curvature values and tested for distinctness and realism (Sridaran, Hansford, Kahol, & Panchanathan, 2007). In order to remove all other features from consideration, we opted for stimuli that will have only curvature as its parameter for exploration.

3 Methodology

A repeated measure design was used in the experiment to extract exploration strategy of humans in (1) touch and (2) vision in an undirected or free exploration condition. The goal was to extract the regions of interest (ROI) for vision and touch in separate explorations and correlate these two. In addition, we wanted to see if any specific curvature values correlated well with any ROIs.

3.1 Experiment 1: Haptic Exploration

Participants. 5 sighted right handed individuals (2 males, 3 females) participated in the experiment. The average age of participants was 27.8 years with a spread of 10.2 years. No subjects had any motor impairment. All subjected had normal or corrected to normal vision.

Material. Simple models like a plane, cone, cylinder, paraboloid, hyperboloid, ellipsoid, simple-saddle and a monkey-saddle were generated for the system. The Gaussian curvature representation of each point on all the surfaces was pre-computed. The surfaces rendered to the user were haptically parameterized according to their Gaussian curvatures in the haptic environment. The models and the corresponding Gaussian curvature signs are listed below:

- Planar Surface : plane, $K = 0$
- Parabolic Surface: Cylinder and Cone: $K = 0$.
- Elliptic Surface: Paraboloid, Ellipsoid , Sphere: $K > 0$
- Hyperbolic Surface: Elliptic Hyperboloid, Simple-saddle, Monkey–saddle: $K < 0$.

Each of these models has a homogenous Gaussian curvature sign. The haptic interface from Sensable® (Phantom Joystick) was used for the surface exploration during the haptic rendering process.

Methodology. The subjects were blindfolded and guided to the center of the surface before the start of exploration and a haptic snap effect was provided for the surfaces to guide the user to stay in the vicinity of the surface throughout. Surfaces were presented in a randomized fashion.

Data was obtained on the number of fixations (defined as a location where subjects stayed for more than 3 ms) and amount of time spent on each fixation point. The data was normalized and relative fixation data was thus obtained.

3.2 Experiment 2: Visual Exploration

Participants. Same participants from the haptic experiment were included.

Material. The images from the haptic objects as rendered were used as a slideshow in Clearview® software in Tobii® tracker. The screen resolution was the same as the haptic rendering screen resolution (1280x800).

Methodology. Subjects were seated in a hands free stool in front of the screen so that their center of fixation is the center of the image. They were required not to move during the experiment. When done, they could press any key to go to the next image. Image order was randomized to avoid any order effect. Relative fixation data was calculated from the gaze data thus obtained.

4 Results

4.1 Calculation of ROIs

Visual ROIs were calculated as a multiplicative function of normalized values of total time spent on a region and number of times the location is visited. Thus, locations were ordered according to the number of times it was visited and then multiplied with their corresponding dwell time i.e. amount of time spent on each location.

Haptic ROIs were calculated in similar to visual ROIs as a function of total time spent on a location and the number of times the location is visited

4.2 Correlation Analysis and Multiple Regression Model

ANOVA(Analysis of Variance) was performed on the visual ROIs and haptic ROIs. The F value obtained was equal to 0.82 and hence, null hypothesis that the means were equal could not be rejected. Typically, ANOVA is used to signify interaction effects between treatments but in this case our objective was to show that distribution of the two data groups (visual ROIs and hapticROIs) is overlapping. A high correlation of the points of ROIs was also observed (r= 0.849). Fig. 3. shows the correlation between Gaussian curvature and haptic ROIs.

Multiple regression model was employed to determine the visual ROIs for the given values of Gaussian curvature and haptic ROIs and used to predict the values of visual ROIs. The visual ROIs and the haptic ROIs values were divided into a training set and testing set. The values were normalized with respect to the total time spent.

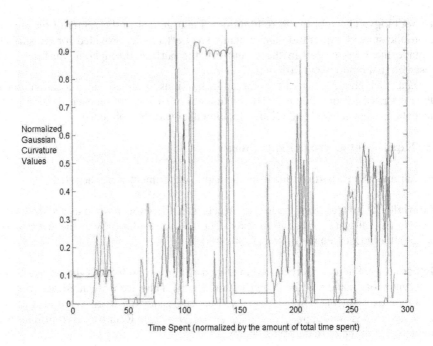

Fig. 3. Gaussian curvature plotted against time spent on each value. Red shows Time spent; blue shows the values for normalized Gaussian curvature.

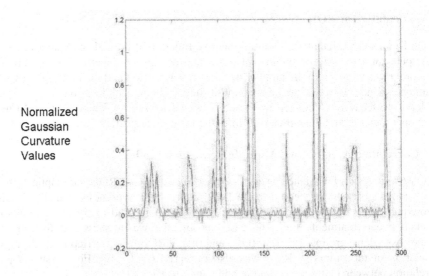

Fig. 4. The predicted values (shown in red) and actual values (shown in blue) for a visual ROI list

The training set employed 70% of all the data capture sessions and the remaining 30% of the data capture sessions were testing set. The test data values were fed to the linear model determined by the regression analysis to determine the predicted values of visual ROIs. Correlation coefficient between predicted values and actual values was determined. In all the ROIs, the correlation between predicted and actual measurement was above 0.89 for each subject and across subjects average correlation value was 0.85. Figure 4 shows an example curve of actual visual ROI (shown in blue) for a subject and the predicted visual ROI from the regression model. The correlation between predicted and actual values in this case was 0.97.

The experiment showed that the concept of saliency maps might be valid for curvature values. Furthermore, this allows allocation of attentional resources across vision and haptics based on the perceptual saliency as a function of curvature in each modality. This can prove very crucial to multimodal environments with high computation and response demands such as tele-surgery and tele-perception which require real-time realistic rendering.

5   Discussion

In this paper, we conduct experiments to compare the regions of interest (ROI) for visual and haptic exploration of surfaces with varying Gaussian curvature. Although, the analysis is somewhat preliminary, it is strongly indicative of the overlap between geometrical features in haptics to its visual exploration. This shows that there is a 'behind the scene' mechanism that attracts our eye gaze in 3D objects. More importantly, such a correlation also supports that interaction between haptics and visual modalities exist beyond the surface characteristics that are confined to visual or haptics modality alone.

Further exploration is needed that can quantitatively evaluate the perceptual load characteristics for such a system. For example, if a feature were to be presented that both modalities *add*, then it can be deduced that variance of such a feature is actually lesser (Ernst & Banks, 2002). Decision noise theory is a possible paradigm to explore the quantitative thresholds for such a distribution.

6   Conclusion

New augmented cognition applications such that flight simulations, remote perception and operation, and surgical simulations have created high demand for interfaces that tackle the information bottleneck for both computer and the user in most efficient manner. This brings in two concepts critical for human perception and human-computer interaction design: attention and multimodality. In spite of the plethora of information that overwhelms our surroundings, we perceive only a small amount that is relevant to us. A fascinating opportunity exists in development of attentive interfaces that employ computational models capable of predicting behavior using multimodal attention. Such systems will be highly beneficial for multimodal human computer interfaces.

References

1. Ballard, D.H.: Cortical connections and parallel processing: Structure and function. In: Arbib, M.A., Hanson, A.R. (eds.) Vision, brain, and cooperative computation, pp. 563–621. MIT Press, Cambridge (1986)
2. Brown, J.M., Weisstein, N., May, J.G.: Visual search for simple volumetric shapes. Perception and Psychophysics 51(4), 42–48 (1992)
3. Cheal, M., Lyon, D.: Attention in visual search: Multiple search classes. Perception and Psychophysics 52(2), 113–138 (1992)
4. Ernst, M.O., Banks, M.S.: Humans integrate visual and haptic information in a statistically optimal fashion. Nature 415(6870), 429–433 (2002)
5. Itti, L., Koch, C., Neibur, E.: A model of saliency-based visual attention for rapid scene analysis. IEEE Transactions on Pattern Analysis and Machine Intelligence 20(11), 1254–1259 (1998)
6. Jenmalm, P., Birznieks, I.I., Goodwin, A., Johansson, R.: Differential responses in populations of fingertip tactile afferents to objects' surface curvatures. Acta. Physiologica Scandinavica A24, 181
7. Mesulam, M.-M.: From sensation to cognition. Brain 121, 1013–1052 (1998)
8. Ouerhani, N., Hugli, H.: Computing visual attention from scene depth. In: Paper presented at the 15th International Conference on Pattern Recognition (2000)
9. Pashler, H. (ed.): Attention. University College London Press, London (1998)
10. Posner, M.I., Dehaene, S.: Attentional networks. Trends in Neuroscience (17), 75–79 (1994)
11. Riggs, L.A.: Curvature as a feature of pattern vision. Science 181, 1070–1072 (1973)
12. Spence, C., Driver, J. (eds.): Crossmodal space and crossmodal attention. Oxford University Press Inc, USA (2004)
13. Sridaran, A., Hansford, D., Kahol, K., Panchanathan, S.: Surface interrogation methods for haptic rendering of virtual objects. Paper presented at the World Haptics 2007, Tsukuba, Japan (March 22-24, 2007)
14. Sun, J., Perona, P.: Preattentive perception of elementary three dimensional shapes. Invest. Ophtalmol. Vis. Sci. 41(Supplement), 1083 (1993)
15. Tsotsos, J.K.: Analyzing vision at the complexity level. Brain and Behavioral Sciences 13, 423 (1990)
16. Tsotsos, J.K.: Computaional resources do constrain behavior. Brain and Behavioral Sciences 13, 506 (1991)
17. Wolfe, J.: Visual search. In: Pashler, H. (ed.) Attention, University College London Press, London, UK (1998)

Towards Attention-Guided Human-Computer Collaborative Reasoning for Spatial Configuration and Design

Sven Bertel

Cognitive Systems Research Group & SFB/TR 8 Spatial Cognition, Universität Bremen,
28359 Bremen, Germany
bertel@informatik.uni-bremen.de

Abstract. In this contribution, we investigate the interrelation between visual focus and higher-level cognitive processing during diagrammatic problem solving. It is argued that eye movement data can be employed for the detection and prediction of model selection in mental model-based reasoning contexts. The argument is substantiated by results from an explorative eye tracking study. Implications for the role of cognitive models in human-computer collaborative reasoning and potential application domains are discussed.

Keywords: Visual focus; focus of attention; eye tracking; problem solving; human-computer collaborative reasoning; computational cognitive modeling.

1 Background

Mental shifts of attentional focus have frequently been related to 'a moving of the mind's eye'. There exists broad psychological, functional anatomical, and neural evidence linking attentional processes to processes in eye movement control. Consequently, it has been argued that both sets of processes should be regarded as interdependent and that attentional shifts may even be fundamentally oculomotor in nature (e.g. [5]; [17]).

Attentional and eye movement patterns may form part of the memory of a spatial scene or configuration (e.g. [13]) and they may influence subsequent memory access and mental reasoning [11]. To some degree, eye movements are also indicative of higher-level cognitive control processes such as in diagrammatic problem solving and of changes of related mental foci. Eye movement data may help assess which spatial or logical problem parts are attended to at which moment during diagram-based problem solving and which mental reasoning strategies are employed ([2]; [10]). Conversely, actively directing a person's visual attention through visual cues can affect his performance in mental problem solving [6].

D.D. Schmorrow, L.M. Reeves (Eds.): Augmented Cognition, HCII 2007, LNAI 4565, pp. 337–345, 2007.
© Springer-Verlag Berlin Heidelberg 2007

2 General Approach

This paper reports on the development of a methodological approach that aims at creating a more appropriate coupling of human and computer-generated reasoning during joint diagram-based problem solving. Example domains include spatial configuration or design tasks. The goal is to enable the computational partner to better adapt to current mental processes and states of the human partner, and thus to allow for more efficient and effective collaboration to emerge.

2.1 Collaborative Human-Computer Problem Solving

Collaborative human-computer reasoning involves a human and a computer-based system that share and manipulate a common representation (e.g. a diagram) while jointly solving a reasoning problem. The setting is asymmetrical in that the parties' reasoning strategies and processing capacities differ [1]. Consequently, good collaboration quality and satisfactory productivity do not come for free. One way to achieve complementarity is to anticipate the other partner's actions; for the computational reasoner this could mean to (a) monitor the human reasoner's actions (e.g. his eye movements or actions on external diagrammatic media), (b) include a cognitive reasoning model with the computer-based system and feed it with the action data, (c) generate hypotheses from the model about the human's current and imminent mental states and likely next actions, and (d) adjust the actions of the computational reasoner accordingly. Among others, hypotheses may address cognitive parameters (e.g. working memory loads or targets of attentional foci), problem parameters (e.g. complexity with respect to mental reasoning), and mental problem solving properties (e.g. current, individual, or general preferences in mental model construction).

2.2 Multi-solution Configuration Problems

Specifically, we address diagrammatic spatial configuration problems that each allow for multiple solution models to be constructed (see Fig. 1 for an example problem). In other words, these problems are underdetermined in that some of the spatial relations involved can be instantiated in more than one way. Research on diagrammatic reasoning as well as psychological research on mental problem solving suggests that with such class of problems the problem solving will be model-based and that a human reasoner will likely not construct all possible solution models. Instead, the construction of a concrete instance (e.g. a variant of one of the possible solution models) will be preferred (e.g. [8]; [9]).

We argue that for well-coupled human-computer reasoning it is a central issue to robustly discriminate which model currently is in the focus of the human's mental reasoning, and to also establish this mental model's main structural and functional properties. If information on the human's currently most probable mental model were readily available at any time, the computational reasoner could generate predictions on further courses of reasoning and on the solution model to be most likely constructed in the end. The more accurate these predictions, the better could computational actions and reactions be then adjusted to the human's reasoning.

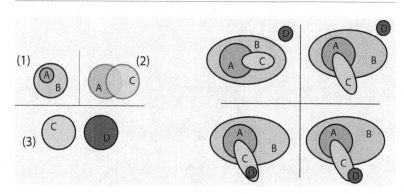

Fig. 1. A topological configuration problem of the kind addressed in this contribution. *Left:* Given are four regions A – D and three topological relations (1) – (3): non-tangential proper part (A, B), partial overlap (A, C), and disconnected (C, D) (given in the RCC-8 calculus; [15]). *Right:* Four different solution models which implement the three relations.

2.3 General Preferences for Specific Solution Models

It is not only on an individual basis that humans prefer the mental construction of certain models over that of other models when solving underdetermined problems: It has been shown that preferences in mental model construction also exist on a general basis across individuals (e.g. [9]). Causes for these preferences have among others been linked to issues of problem complexity, such as to the number of relations that need to be mentally instantiated in a specific model [7]. While such general considerations can certainly help understand mental problem solving mechanisms as such, they are not sufficiently informative for any concrete setting·in which an individual tries to solve a specific problem. Would he construct a model that is preferred by most people, or wouldn't he? The answer can only be provided by looking at the individual and at his reasoning situation.

2.4 Visual Focus and Mental Focus in Diagram-Based Problem Solving

Looking into a reasoner's mind, however, is not easily done, even for restricted domains and tasks. In Section 1, we have discussed a few interrelations between visual focus (as made explicit by fixations of the eye) and mental focus of attention. While attentional and visual foci generally coincide during normal visual perception (*overt* attention) the two can be separated to some extent during a fixation (*covert* attention; [14]).

There exist comparatively few investigations into the interrelations between attentional and visual foci during complex, higher-level, and cognitively demanding tasks, such as with spatial or insight problem solving. It seems safe to assume a somewhat looser connection than exists with strongly data-driven activities (e.g. scene perception or even during object recognition). During problem solving with diagram-based spatial configuration tasks one can expect phases of more data-driven activities (e.g. inspection of a diagram's content) to occur next to phases in which eye

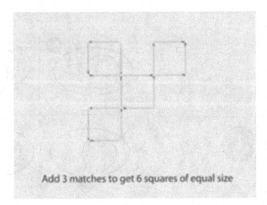

Add 3 matches to get 6 squares of equal size

Fig. 2. A configuration problem that requires mentally modifying a geometric arrangement of matchsticks

movements reflect aspects of higher-level cognitive activities (such as of application of problem solving strategies or shifts of attentional control).

3   Eye Movements During Mental Problem-Solving – An Explorative Study

In a recent eye tracking study, 18 participants were presented with a series of geometric arrangements of matchsticks (see Fig. 2 and 3 for an example). They were asked to mentally reconfigure the arrangements, one at a time, to fit given verbal descriptions. All problems had multiple solutions, and the participants' eye movements were recorded during mental problem solving. Each participant was asked to indicate the point in time when he thought that he had found a solution to a problem. The discovered solution model was subsequently recorded.

3.1   Findings

The study was primarily aimed at detecting general problem solving mechanisms and eye movement patterns that the subjects employed. The measures that were used in the analysis included relative proportions of time and fixations over problem parts (over the entire duration as well as partial) and relative frequencies of 2- and 3-fixation sequences across parts. The analysis was performed after the experiments.

Frequently, the constructed model was found to be a function of the distribution of relative fixation frequencies over parts as well as of relative frequencies of part-part transitions (both for 2- and 3-fixation sequences). Subjects differed qualitatively in their problem solving styles, as well as in their overall performance levels. There is ample evidence for segmented problem solving processes.

Fixation Frequencies for Problem Parts. Simply taking measure of the differences in relative fixation frequencies over different parts of the diagram often seems to be a good indicator for the solution that was mentally constructed. For example, with problems in which matchsticks had to be simply added (such as in case of the problem

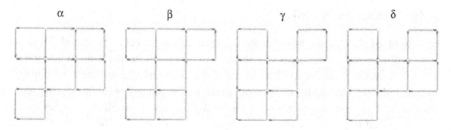

Fig. 3. Four different solution models α – δ for the matchstick problem of Fig. 2

in Fig. 2), fixation frequencies were often higher at places at which matches were eventually added. This effect was found to increase toward the end of a problem solving episode (for an individual problem), thus being in-line with other research results which suggest that while problem inspection may occur mostly early in the process, solution construction activities are reflected more in eye movements towards its end [10].

Fixation Frequencies for Part-Part Transitions. Measures which compare relative frequencies of series of two or three consecutive fixations over different parts seem be able to give stronger predictions of the constructed solution model than measures which simply look at individual problem parts. One hypothesis is that these patterns reflect phases in which a mentally constructed solution is checked against the external configuration, and in which diagram parts (matches or squares) are counted. Also, repetitive region spanning saccades could be used to bind together commonly manipulated diagram parts during mental imagery (e.g. in order to prevent image decay in the perceptual presence of the external diagram).

Differences in Problem Solving Styles. Individuals sometimes differed in problem solving styles. For example, with problems that required to subtract a certain number of items, some subjects were found to focus mostly on those parts that they were to subtract (two to three times more fixations than on parts that stayed) while other subjects focused significantly more on parts that stayed than on parts that they were to subtract. Interestingly, this preference seems to be somewhat consistent for an individual across different tasks, potentially reflecting more general differences in strategy or ability across different problem solvers.

Segmented Problem Solving. The study provided evidence for distinct problem solving phases. Most notably, fixations to parts of the verbal instruction (e.g. to "3 matches" or "6 squares" in the case of "Add 3 matches to get 6 squares of equal size") were often followed by specific patterns across the diagrammatic parts. A possible interpretation for such patterns could reflect functional episodes in which the configuration is checked against the specified description. Data on part-part transitions provides further evidence for problem solving phases that can be functionally distinguished.

3.2 Implications for Modeling

In the light of this exploratory study into the relations between visual focus and mental problem solving it seems that there is in fact good justification to assume that eye movement data can be used as an input for a robust and dynamic modeling of attentional shifts – including shifts that occur during mental problem solving and in particular with regard to spatial or diagrammatic reasoning problems. Further studies will be required to gradually shed more light on details of how the processing levels interact.

Computational models of how humans reason about diagram-based configuration problems can exploit eye movement data on different levels of abstraction. The easiest level apparently just requires simple statistics over fixations in different diagram parts, more sophisticated levels would include a modeling of functional phases and of subgoals during inspection, exploration, and mental construction phases, as well as of an interaction between more perceptual- and more reasoning-driven aspect (for a collection of some ideas on modeling the latter, see [3]).

Grant and Spivey have recently shown [6] that perception can also influence problem solving in that animating the parts of a diagrammatic problem that are crucial to finding a solution can in fact lead problem solvers towards finding one. One can expect in the same spirit that adding animations or other perceptually noticeable changes to a matchstick problem can not only increase or decrease the problem solver's performance level but also influence the model that he will eventually construct. Even more if these changes occur at crucial moments during the problem solving process (e.g. when visual attention is directed anyway to the location or problem part where the changes will occur as compared to attention being dragged there by a perceptual stimulus).

4 Relevance of Problem and of Domain

Applications that may benefit from a computational modeling of interrelations between visual and attentional foci in reasoning include many spatial configuration and layout tasks, also in assistive or tutoring settings. Architectural and product design as well as land-use planning are domains that will likely increasingly require this sort of cognitive adequacy because neither human nor computer can be taken out of the related work processes [4]. These domains have in common that their problems are partly in diagrammatic form and relate to spatial configurations, that they are complex and cognitively demanding and that the typical, professional human involved would welcome dedicated computer-based assistance [12]. Yet, for reasons of esthetics, implicitness of knowledge, style or preferences neither domain nor tasks can be adequately fully formally specified and be handled computationally (cf. *partially unformalized constraint problems*, [16]). Accordingly for much of reasoning in design and spatial configuration, good human-computer cooperation and collaboration are preconditions for effective work.

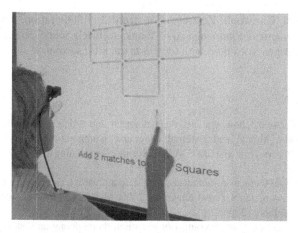

Fig. 4. The next step: Analysis of eye movements during interactive problem solving with matchstick configuration problems

5   Future Work and Discussion

There seems to be a connection between the distribution of visual focus over time during problem solving and the solution model that subjects ultimately construct. More studies are required to investigate further details of this connection, especially towards markers (i.e. characteristic eye movement patterns) that help identify distinct problem solving phases and measures of the current significance of eye movements over problem parts (e.g. does a prolonged fixation signify that a detailed inspection of a specific diagram part occurs, or does the subject simply not attend to diagrammatic content at the moment, does he 'blank', for example during imagery?). Also, further investigation is required on how eye movement patterns change when subjects are allowed to interact with diagrammatic content (e.g. draw on the board). Last, studies of related but more complex tasks are needed to gather information on how the found effects scale with problem size (e.g. Can similar effects be found for spatial layout tasks that involve areal and heterogeneous objects? In which respect do more complex tasks change the modeling requirements and the predictive power?)

Strategies and other findings from the exploratory study are currently being computationally described and are fed back into an interactive spatial reasoning set-up that uses spatial configuration tasks similar to the ones used in the study (based on electronic whiteboards and mobile eye tracking; see Fig. 4). The aim is to establish sets of reasoning and interaction schemes that relate short-term data points to their medium-term reasoning contexts. For example, eye fixations can lead to entirely different interpretations (and ultimately to different actions of the computational reasoning partner) depending on which preferences in mental model construction are predicted.

Acknowledgments. The author gratefully acknowledges support by the *German Research Foundation* (DFG) through the project *R1-[ImageSpace]*, SFB/TR 8 *Spatial Cognition*. Many thanks to Muhammad Ahmed, Sandra Budde, Mary Hegarty, Jan

Hövelmann, and Christoph Zetzsche for fruitful collaboration, and to Thomas Barkowsky for practical comments. Also, thanks to Erich Schneider and colleagues of LMU Munich for generous help with the *Qlotz* tracking system.

References

1. Bertel, S.: Show me how you act on a diagram and I'll tell you what you think. In: Reasoning with Mental and External Diagrams: Computational Modeling and Spatial Assistance. Papers from the 2005 AAAI Spring Symposium (SS-05-06), AAAI, Menlo Park, CA (2005)

2. Bertel, S.: Visual focus in computer-assisted diagrammatic reasoning. In: Barker-Plummer, D., Cox, R., Swoboda, N. (eds.) Diagrams 2006. LNCS (LNAI), vol. 4045, pp. 241–244. Springer, Heidelberg (2006)

3. Bertel, S.: Some notes on the control of attention, its modeling and anticipatory cognitive computing. In: Proc. 2007 AAAI Spring Symposium on Control Mechanisms for Spatial Knowledge Processing in Cognitive / Intelligent Systems, AAAI, Menlo Park, CA (2007)

4. Bertel, S., Vrachliotis, G., Freksa, C: Aspect-oriented building design: Towards computer-aided approaches to solving spatial constraints in architecture. In: Allen, G. (ed.) Applied Spatial Cognition: From Research to Cognitive Technology pp. 75–102. Lawrence Erlbaum Associates, Mahwah (In press)

5. Corbetta, M.: Frontoparietal cortical networks for directing attention and the eye to visual locations: identical, independent, or overlapping neural systems? In: Proc. Natl. Acad. Sci. U.S.A. vol. 95, pp. 831–838 (1998)

6. Grant, R.E., Spivey, J.M.: Eye movements and problem solving: guiding attention guides thought. Psychological Science 14(5), 462–466 (2003)

7. Halford, G.S., Wilson, W.H., Phillips, S.: Processing capacity defined by relational complexity: Implications for comparative, developmental, and cognitive psychology. Behavioral and Brain Sciences 21, 803–865 (1998)

8. Johnson-Laird, P., Byrne, R.: Deduction. Lawrence Erlbaum, Hillsdale (1991)

9. Knauff, M., Rauh, R., Schlieder, C.: Preferred mental models in qualitative spatial reasoning: A cognitive assessment of Allen's calculus. In: Proceedings of the Seventeenth Annual Conference of the Cognitive Science Society, pp. 200–205. Lawrence Erlbaum Associates, Mahwah (1995)

10. Knoblich, G., Ohlsson, S., Raney, E.G.: An eye movement study of insight problem solving. Memory & Cognition 29(7), 1000–1009 (2001)

11. Laeng, B., Teodorescu, D.: Eye scanpaths during visual imagery reenact those of perception of the same visual scene. Cognitive Science 26, 207–231 (2002)

12. Meniru, K., Rivard, H., Bédard, C.: Specifications for computer-aided conceptual building design. Design Studies 24, 51–71 (2003)

13. Noton, D., Stark, L.: Eye movements and visual perception. Scientific American 224, 34–43 (1971)

14. Posner, M.I.: Orienting of attention. Quarterly Journal of Experimental Psychology 32, 3–25 (1980)

15. Randell, D.A., Cui, Z., Cohn, A.G.: A spatial logic based on regions and connection. In: Nebel, B., Swartout, W., Rich, C. (eds.) Principles of Knowledge Representation and Reasoning: Proc. of the 3rd International Conference (KR-92), pp. 165–176. Morgan Kaufmann, San Francisco (1992)

16. Schlieder, C., Hagen, C.: Interactive layout generation with a diagrammatic constraint language. In: Habel, C., Brauer, W., Freksa, C., Wender, K.F. (eds.) Spatial Cognition II. LNCS (LNAI), vol. 1849, pp. 198–211. Springer, Heidelberg (2000)
17. Shepherd, M., Findlay, J.M., Hockey, R.J.: The relationship between eye movements and spatial attention. Quarterly J. of Experimental Psychology 38A, 475–491 (1986)

Automated SAF Adaptation Tool (ASAT)

Roy Stripling[1], Joseph T. Coyne[1], Anna Cole[2], Daniel Afergan[2], Raymond L. Barnes[2], Kelly A. Rossi[2], Leah M. Reeves[3], and Dylan D. Schmorrow[4]

[1] US Naval Research Laboratory, 4555 Overlook Ave, SW, Washington, DC 20375
[2] Strategic Analysis, Inc., 3601 Wilson Blvd, Suite 500, Arlington, VA 22201
[3] Potomac Institute for Policy Studies, 901 N. Stuart St, Suite 200, Arlington, VA 22203
[4] Office of Naval Research, 875 North Randolph St, Arlington, VA 22203
{roy.stripling, joseph.coyne}@nrl.navy.mil,
{acole, dafergan, lbarnes,krossi}@sainc.com,
lreeves@potomacinstitute.org, schmord@onr.navy.mil

Abstract. The purpose of this paper is to describe a new, user-friendly tool that will enable researchers and instructors to setup and run virtual environment scenarios that adapt to the VE user's real-time performance and cognitive status. This tool, the Automated SAF Adaptation Tool (ASAT), will work with existing performance and cognitive state assessment software, and with existing semi-automated forces (SAF) behavior engines. ASAT will collect processed performance and cognitive state data from the assessment software and trigger SAF behavior setting manipulations that were pre-selected by the SAF operator. A key feature of ASAT is the ability to setup and execute these real-time manipulations without the need to alter code in either the assessment software or the SAF engines.

Keywords: semi-automated forces, SAF, real-time, adaptation, virtual environment, training, cognitive state.

1 Introduction

At present, Virtual Environment (VE) training packages do not support adaptive training – the ability of the system to modify the ongoing tactical scenario based on real-time assessments of the trainee's performance and/or cognitive state. It has been hypothesized that the ability to execute such "on-the-fly" modifications, if properly implemented, would enhance training experiences by optimizing the trainee's cognitive state for training and by tailoring the training experience to individual's or team's evolving skill level [1, 2, 3]. However, currently there is no adequate or practical adaptive training system in which to test this hypothesis.

To date, our work with adaptive VEs has focused on military infantry training systems. These systems leverage complex behavior-model architectures to provide "semi-automated" behaviors for the computer generated forces (CGF). The most commonly used behavior engine for military simulation and VE training is Joint Semi-Automated Forces (JSAF). Newer SAF architectures are also in development. We have worked with both JSAF and OTBSAF (the testbed for the system that will

D.D. Schmorrow, L.M. Reeves (Eds.): Augmented Cognition, HCII 2007, LNAI 4565, pp. 346–353, 2007.
© Springer-Verlag Berlin Heidelberg 2007

be released as OneSAF). A detailed description of these SAF architectures is beyond the scope of this manuscript. However, it is useful to point out that they allow the SAF operator to set up scenarios by placing CGF individuals, squads, and vehicles throughout the virtual environment.   The SAF engines also provide complex Graphical User Interface (GUI) controls and menus, which allow the operator to adjust a variety of behavior-relevant settings including CGF competency, range of engagement, underlying cognitive model, and response to particular events such as gunshots. Manipulating these and other attributes during a scenario and in response to the level of performance or to the cognitive state of individual or teams of trainees would constitute adaptive training.   An operator using the SAF's GUI could manipulate these settings, but the complexity of the GUI and the limited rate of human processing and motor abilities limit the ability of the operator to implement these changes in real-time. Additionally, the SAF operator cannot collect, process, and interpret the many streams of behaviorally and physiologically based performance data that reflect trainees' cognitive status and skill level.   Automated systems that do assess these aspects of trainee performance have been developed and are the continued focus of additional research. Detailed description of such measures and systems are also beyond the scope of this paper. However, such measures include measures of trainee arousal [4], and engagement [5, 6] among others. The key tool that is missing before robust user-friendly closed-loop training environments can be produced is an automated method for triggering adaptive manipulations within complex SAF applications.

We recently demonstrated that it is possible for an automated system to collect, process, and trigger adaptive manipulations in a SAF application (OTBSAF) in real-time. For this demonstration, we collected ECG (electrocardiographic data) from two-man teams immersed in a virtual infantry trainer. The ECG data was processed in real-time to derive a measure of physiological arousal using the methods described by [4]. Persistent high or low arousal levels from individuals or from the two man team triggered a variety of automated behavior setting changes in OTBSAF, including, at its most extreme, activating and sending in an increasing number of enemy CGFs. These manipulations in the SAF settings were transmitted via UDP messages to a Linux computer running OTBSAF. This approach, however, left much to be desired and was found to be impractical for several reasons. First, it did not produce stable behavior in JSAF, the SAF engine more commonly in use today. Second, it required source-code access and modifications to the SAF environments. Third, it required several weeks of iterative coding to produce a small set of potential manipulations that could be triggered. Fourth, hard-coding the manipulations limited the range of scenarios that could be generated for use in the closed-loop training demonstration. The last of these problems is particularly worrisome because it restricts the flexibility of the training system, rendering it obsolete as soon as new enemy tactics or scenarios for training are desired. Collectively, these problems combine to produce a very cumbersome and user-unfriendly environment in which to conduct research and training.

We are now pursuing a new approach that will enable the rapid development of a large set of operator-defined manipulations without requiring code changes to the SAF applications. This approach will also work with independently-developed software products that produce real-time behaviorally- and/or physiologically-derived measures of performance, and will work with any military training or mission rehearsal scenario that can be developed in the SAF applications. The end product of this effort will be a sufficiently user-friendly executable that can be used for a broad variety of research and training operations. Of particular importance, with further development this application will also be able to incorporate methods for auto-selecting unique combinations of automated manipulations based on educationally-sound logic rules. These logic rules would specify the type and timings of manipulations that are appropriate in the current training context AND in the context of the trainees' performance and cognitive status. The development of educational logic rules is beyond the scope of the current effort.

In the near term, this approach is expanding on available open-source code to develop the Automated SAF Adaptation Tool (ASAT). ASAT, functioning as a stand-alone executable, will reach across platforms to receive behaviorally- and/or physiologically-derived measures of performance and activate, at the appropriate time, user-defined, pre-recorded SAF manipulations based on either user- or vendor-specified performance thresholds. ASAT currently collects performance data by reading such data from ASCII formatted files or by reading the data from user-specified fields displayed on the performance assessment application's own GUI. In the future, ASAT will also collect performance data via networked transmission from these applications that conform to ASAT API specifications,

2 Performance Assessment Input Module

One of the key features of the ASAT tool is the ability to interact and use data from a range of real-time performance and physiological sources. The current ASAT design allows for data to be collected from a user-specified source through one of two methods. These methods include reading data from an ASCII (American Standard Code for Information Interchange) file or reading data from a program developed in the LabVIEW programming environment (National Instruments). Both methods allow for the data to be read by ASAT as it is being recorded to a file or updated on the LabVIEW GUI.

The majority of systems that collect continuous physiological data append the information to a file for later analysis as the information is collected. This data may be collected in application specific files or in files with standardized file formats. ASCII data is a common format for this type of data, and ASAT seeks to exploit this feature by allowing data to be read in from an ASCII file source. ASAT will perform this function by copying the data file and reading the last lines of the file. The ASAT system will not read from the original data file to reduce the chances of errors and file corruption associated with multiple programs reading and writing to the same file at the same time. ASAT allows users to specify how often they would like to read the performance data into the system (which should be dependent on how frequently the source application generates the data and saves it to file).

The ASCII file input component of the ASAT tool will help users preview files, select the appropriate data column to be used and also store the preferences for later use. The system also allows more advanced users to use the stored settings to

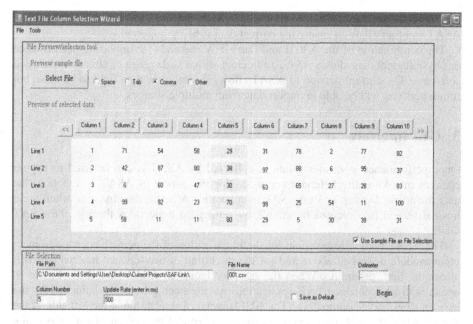

Fig. 1. Graphical interface for inputting an ASCII file into ASAT

minimize the set up time. An advanced user may only need to enter the new file name associated with the data to setup the data input. Figure 1 below presents a screen capture depicting the file preview tool used to select and input ASCII data into the ASAT package.

The second source of performance or physiological data that ASAT is currently being configured to use as an input source is data from a LabVIEW program. The LabVIEW interface requires minimal system resources compared to the ASCII tool and is a common programming environment for many researchers developing performance assessment tools.

As shown in Figure 2 the user specifies the LabVIEW program name and reference object within LabVIEW. Similar to the ASCII interface, the user can also specify the update rate used to import the data and can pull data in from LabVIEW faster than the

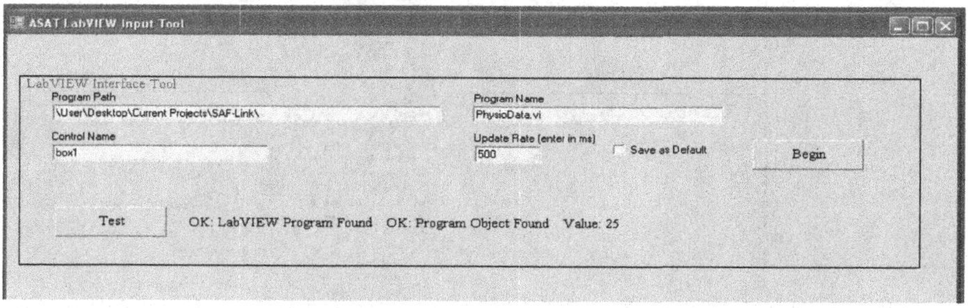

Fig. 2. Graphical interface for importing LabVIEW data into ASAT

ASCII method. The LabVIEW tool also allows the user to test the link between ASAT and LabVIEW to ensure the correct data is being imported.

The combination of the ASCII and LabVIEW methods for importing performance or physiological data allows ASAT to interact with a wide range of already developed software. The current version of ASAT allows for only one data field to be used, but future versions will be able to import data from multiple sources.

3   GUI Interface

Once performance assessment data is collected by ASAT it can be used to trigger changes in SAF entity behavior settings. For this aspect of ASAT to function, the user must first develop and save SAF manipulation Macros, then indicate when these macros should be executed by ASAT by setting up logic rules through the ASAT GUI.

The ASAT GUI is responsible for the initialization of the performance assessment input module described above and for the recording of user-created macros that will affect the SAF program. When the operator launches ASAT, the GUI (Figure 3) opens with an embedded SAF application (having been previously launched by the user on a networked computer). The GUI launches a sidebar along the left side of the screen, while the SAF program will take up the rest of the screen. Besides opening the performance assessment input module, or "logger", the GUI allows the user to create, store, and load behaviors that can be implemented when the scenario reaches certain conditions.

A macro is a mechanism that records a series of user inputs events (mouse moves, mouse clicks, and keyboard presses) as a single executable series of events that can later be played back by the computer. This allows the automated adjustment of SAF entity behavior settings through the SAF GUI at a faster rate and with greater repeatability than an actual user could achieve.

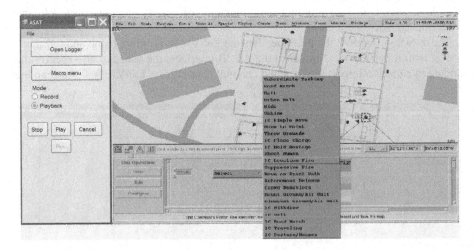

Fig. 3. ASAT GUI with JSAF running

ASAT also offers a macro manipulation window (Figure 4) that allows the ASAT operator to establish logical rules that determine when to execute previously created macros. Users create conditional logic statements by selecting either a physiological or performance variable and an operator, and then entering a threshold value into the text field. After they have created a conditional logic statement, they specify which macro should be run when the conditions are met. The window gives the option to add more rules to the equation (using statements such as AND, and OR) or to finish the equation. Previously created rules are displayed in a panel at the top center of the window. By combining the two menus, the operator is able to record actions and then play them back on command or automatically during certain circumstances. This allows the actions to be identical each time and eliminates many outside variables involved in virtual environment training.

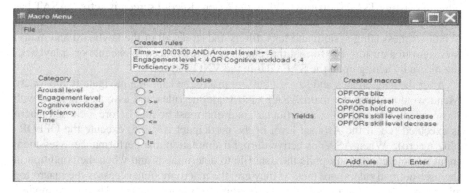

Fig. 4. ASAT Macro manipulation window

4 Macro Recording and Execution

To enable ASAT to carryout its task in a user-friendly manner we are leveraging an open-source network remote control application called Virtual Network Computing (VNC). VNC was first developed by AT&T Laboratories in Cambridge, and is now maintained and further developed by RealVNC in the UK (http://www.realvnc.com/). VNC is open-source software that can simultaneously run on multiple operating systems and enable any computer on a network to view and remotely control the GUI of another computer connected to the same network. VNC uses the remote framebuffer (RFB) protocol to transmit keystrokes and mouse events, along with screen updates between a VNC server and a VNC viewer (Richardson 2006). In the context of the ASAT application, the VNC server is the Linux-based machine that has the ability to generate and change VE scenarios using a SAF application. The ASAT GUI, running on Microsoft Windows, has a VNC Viewer control that allows the user to create a sequence of actions (macros) in JSAF that will automatically execute once cues are received from the performance assessment logger module (as described above).

VncSharp, an open-source client library and custom control, is being utilized to embed a VNC Viewer and add VNC functionality to the ASAT application.

VncSharp was written by David Humphrey, Matt Cyr and Chuck Borgh at Seneca College as a project under the Centre for Development of Open Technology initiative (http://cdot.senecac.on.ca/projects/vncsharp/index.html). It is an implementation of VNC's RFB protocol written in Microsoft's C# language for the .NET framework. VncSharp provides a conduit for ASAT to programmatically take advantage of the methods and properties provided by VNC while writing software in the Visual Studio .NET development environment.

When ASAT is launched, the panel on the right of the ASAT GUI shows the remote machine's GUI (JSAF, for example). This panel is the VncSharp Windows control, which serves as the VNC Viewer for ASAT. The VncSharp Windows control screen is continually updated, and all keystrokes and mouse events in this ASAT panel are transmitted back to the JSAF machine. This allows the user to create a scenario in JSAF (running on a remote machine) from ASAT, in addition to making edits to existing JSAF scenarios. When the Macro Record screen is active, ASAT has a procedure independent of VNC that programmatically taps into the Microsoft Windows messaging system and logs, filters and stores all of the keyboard and mouse messages in a custom file format that can later be referenced to execute or "playback" the macro by acting upon the SAF GUI in the VNC Viewer.

After the user creates and saves a custom macro, he can then navigate to the Macro Menu window from the main ASAT GUI to define rules and associate macros with those rules. For each rule, a particular condition must be met before a chosen macro is executed (i.e. if the Arousal level of the participant is < 0.5, execute the OPFORs blitz macro). When ASAT is active during a simulation, the performance assessment input module continually polls the data file to determine if and when the condition in the user-defined rule(s) are met. If they are, the macro module accesses the macro log file created during the macro record procedure for the given rule. The macro module then directs the focus of the program to the VNC Viewer and automates keyboard and mouse events using Microsoft Win32 API's and a Microsoft .NET Framework Class Library, SendKeys. When the mouse and keyboard events are automated and sent to the VNC Viewer within ASAT, they are directly transmitted to the JSAF machine to alter the training scenario based on performance and neuro/physiological measures acquired during the simulation.

5 Conclusions

ASAT will provide a means of rapidly developing robust closed-loop integrated training systems that can continue to leverage the well-developed SAF architectures that currently drive many military training simulations. In doing so, it will provide a robust tool for testing many worthwhile hypotheses regarding the use of Augmented Cognition approaches in training and educational environments. For example, ASAT can support the development and testing of training systems which sense an individuals attention levels and then adjust the VE to maintain those attention levels within a specified range. Of broader significance, ASAT is not conceptually restricted to use with SAF architectures, but should work with any GUI based application that enables human operators to modify the application's settings during operation. Thus the ultimate impact of ASAT may reach far beyond the military training and education communities.

References

1. Schmorrow, D., Cohn, J.V., Stripling, R., Kruse, A.A.: Enhancing Virtual Environments Using Sensory-Multiplexing. At: Interservice/Industry Training, Simulation and Education Conference (I/ITSEC) Annual Meeting, Orlando FL (2004)
2. Raley, C., Stripling, R., Kruse, A., Schmorrow, D., Patrey, J.: Augmented Cognition Overview: Improving Information Intake Under Stress. In: Proceedings of the Human Factors and Ergonomics Society Annual Meeting (HFES 2004), New Orleans LA (2004)
3. Cohn, J.V., Stripling, R., Kruse, A.A.: Investigating the Transition from Novice to Expert in a Virtual Training Environment using Neuro-Cognitive Measures. At: 1st Annual Meeting on Augmented Cognition, Las Vegas NV (2005)
4. Hoover, A., Muth, E.: A Real-Time Index of Vagal Activity. Int. J. Human-Computer Interaction 17, 197–209 (2004)
5. Freeman, F.G., Mikulka, P.J., Scerbo, M.W., Scott, L.: An Evaluation of an Adaptive Automation System Using a Cognitive Vigilance Task. Bio. Psych. 67(3), 283–297 (2004)
6. Pope, A.T., Bogart, E.H., Bartolome, D.S.: Biocybernetic System Evaluates Indexes of Operator Engagement in Automated Task. Bio. Psych. 40(1-2), 187–195 (1995)
7. Richardson, T.: The RFB Protocol version. 3.8. In: RealVNC Ltd (October 2006) http://www.realvnc.com/docs/rfbproto.pdf

Unobtrusive Multimodal Emotion Detection in Adaptive Interfaces: Speech and Facial Expressions

Khiet P. Truong, David A. van Leeuwen, and Mark A. Neerincx

TNO Human Factors, Dept. of Human Interfaces, P.O. Box 23, 3769 ZG Soesterberg,
The Netherlands
{khiet.truong, david.vanleeuwen, mark.neerincx}@tno.nl

Abstract. Two unobtrusive modalities for automatic emotion recognition are discussed: speech and facial expressions. First, an overview is given of emotion recognition studies based on a combination of speech and facial expressions. We will identify difficulties concerning data collection, data fusion, system evaluation and emotion annotation that one is most likely to encounter in emotion recognition research. Further, we identify some of the possible applications for emotion recognition such as health monitoring or e-learning systems. Finally, we will discuss the growing need for developing agreed standards in automatic emotion recognition research.

Keywords: emotion detection, emotion recognition, classification, speech, facial expression, emotion database.

1 Introduction

In human-human communication, we give emotional signals to each other all the time: when we talk and when we write (e.g., through emoticons), we want to create a feeling of mutual understanding and share our feelings and intentions with each other. Emotions are part of human nature. Machine's inability to feel is one of the main reasons why communications and interactions between humans and machines fail. Therefore, researchers have been trying to automatically detect emotions in order to improve human-machine interaction. In this way, interfaces can be designed to adapt to the user's emotions: for example, a computer assisted language learning system may sense the frustration in the student's tone of voice and facial expressions, and may decide to lower the level of difficultness or to switch to another exercise in order to keep the student motivated. When we talk to each other face to face, we can see emotions expressed in face, body gestures etc. and we can hear emotions expressed in vocal sounds. Facial expressions and speech are considered to be very accessible, visible and non-obtrusive modalities and therefore, we will focus on these two channels.

The term 'emotion' is a term that can have many senses and interpretations. Other terms that can be used to refer to 'emotion' are 'affective', 'expressive', 'emotional state' or 'mood'. We will use 'affective', 'expressive' and 'emotional state' interchangeably with 'emotion'. 'Mood' on the other hand is usually described as an emotion that can last

D.D. Schmorrow, L.M. Reeves (Eds.): Augmented Cognition, HCII 2007, LNAI 4565, pp. 354–363, 2007.
© Springer-Verlag Berlin Heidelberg 2007

for a longer period of time. In short, we will continue to use the term 'emotion' in its broad sense, meaning that we will use 'emotion' to describe a broad range of feelings that humans can have and express and which can influence humans in their behavior [1].

This paper is structured as follows: Section 2 gives an overview of emotion recognition studies that have been carried out on speech and facial expressions. In Section 3, we will elaborate on some general difficulties in emotion research. Section 4 describes possible real-life emotion recognition applications. And finally, we conclude this paper with a discussion and general conclusions in Section 5.

2 Short Overview: State of the Art

Emotions can be measured through different modalities. Usually, physiological measures such as heart rate or skin conductivity (e.g., [2, 3, 4]) are considered obtrusive, while speech and facial expressions are relatively non-obtrusive measures. Therefore, the focus will be on emotional analyses of speech and facial expressions.

2.1 Automatic Emotion Recognition from Speech

By making variations in the melody of an utterance, by changing the speaking rate or by changing the loudness etc., humans can produce emotional speech which seems to be a prerequisite for effective human-human communication. In voice-based automatic emotion recognition, we are more interested in *how* words are spoken rather than *what* words are spoken (although knowing *what* words are spoken may also help emotion recognition, e.g., swear words). In the course of time, many studies have investigated voice-based emotion recognition (see Table 1). The acoustic-phonetic correlates of emotional speech have been exhaustively investigated (e.g., [5-9]). Based on previous studies we can observe that often prosody-related features are used such as statistics of F0 (fundamental frequency of speech), statistics of intensity, speech rate, F0/intensity contour and duration. Further, quality-related speech features such as Mel-Frequency Cepstrum Coefficients (MFCC), Hammarberg Index, centre of spectral gravity, the energy distribution in the spectrum, jitter and shimmer are also frequently used. The emotions are modeled through these features and a modeling technique; frequently used modeling techniques include Linear Discriminant Analysis (LDA), Support Vector Machines (SVM), Hidden Markov Models (HMM), Gaussian Mixture Models (GMM), Neural Networks (NN) and K-Nearest Neighbors (KNN). Further, note the small number of subjects used in most of these studies. In order to perform subject-independent classification experiments and to make reliable statements about the results, more subjects should be used.

The acquisition and the use of realistic emotional speech data in emotion recognition remain challenges. Most of the studies in Table 1 have used acted or semi-spontaneous speech data that is elicited through a Wizard-of-Oz experiment (subjects interacting with a system, not knowing that the system is actually being operated by a human being). For speech analysis, a clean speech signal is preferred, i.e., background noise, overlap or crosstalk in speech, clipping etc. should be avoided. However, the more realistic the setting is in which the data is acquired, the harder it is to avoid noisy data (see Fig. 1).

Table 1. Short overview of automatic emotion recognition studies based on speech (where data can be acted real or obtained via woz=Wizard Of Oz, SI=SubjectIndependent, SD=SubjectDependent)

Study	Data	SI/ SD	Speech features	Method+Accuracy
Banse 1996 [5]	14 emotions, 12 subjects (acted)	?	F0, energy, speech rate, long-term spectrum	LDA: 25-53%
Ang 2002 [6]	2 emotions (woz)	?	F0, energy, speech rate, duration, pauses, spectral tilt	Decision tree: 75%
Nwe 2003 [7]	6 emotions, 12 subjects (acted)	SD	LFPC (Log Frequency Power Coefficients)	HMM: 77%-89%
Vidrascu 2005 [8]	2 emotions, 404 subjects (real)	?	F0, energy, duration, spectral features, disfluency	SVM: 83%
Batliner 2005 [9]	4 emotions, 51 subjects (woz)	SI	F0, energy, duration	LDA: 78%

In addition to finding acoustic profiles for basic emotions, researchers have been investigating acoustic correlates of emotion dimensions. The two most frequently used dimensions in the emotional space are that of activation (or arousal, active-passive) and evaluation (valence, positive-negative). Acoustic correlates found on the activation scale are much stronger than the correlates found on the evaluation scale. It seems to be much more difficult to describe negativity or positivity in terms of acoustic features.

In summary, although the classification results in Table 1 show accuracies that are well above chance, they are based on artificial conditions and therefore, we must conclude that automatic emotion recognition in speech is still in its development phase.

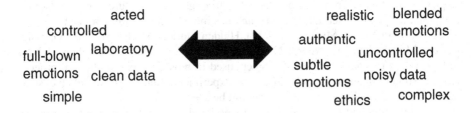

Fig. 1. Emotion research: from laboratory to real-life

2.2 Automatic Emotion Recognition from Facial Expressions

The movements of certain (combinations of) landmarks in the face can reveal much about the expressed emotions in the face: e.g., raised eyebrows typically indicate surprise, frowned eyebrows are usually used to express anger or dislike and smiles are usually characterized by an upward lip movement. The process of automatically recognizing a facial expression can be divided into three sub-processes: 1) detection of the face, 2) feature detection and extraction and 3) classification of emotions. The best known method for facial data extraction is the facial action coding system (FACS, see [11]). The FACS system describes facial movements in terms of Action Units (AU). This system consists of a taxonomy of 44 AUs with which facial expressions can be described, and has attracted many researchers from the field of computer vision to develop automatic facial expression analyzers based on AUs.

In Table 2, we show a short summary of more recent facial expression recognition studies; for a more exhaustive overview, readers are referred to [12]. In many aspects, the approach and challenges in facial emotion recognition studies resemble voice-based emotion recognition studies, e.g., small number of emotions, acted data etc. Difficulties with noisy data include e.g., bad illumination or background issues, different head poses and movements, facial hair and glasses.

Table 2. Short overview of emotion recognition studies based on facial expressions (SI=SubjectIndependent, SD=SubjectDependent)

Study	# Classes of Emotions/Database	SI/SD	Facial features/modeling	Method+Accuracy
Pantic 2000 [13]	7 emotions (posed)	?	Action Units	Hybrid: Fuzzy+NN: 91%
Cohen 2003 [14]	7 emotions, 210 subjects (posed)	SI	Motion Units	Tree-Augmented-Naïve Bayes: 73%
Sebe 2004 [15]	4 emotions, 28 subjects (realistic)	SI	Motion Units	KNN: 95%
Den Uyl 2005 [16]	7 emotions (posed)	?	Active Appearance Model	NN: 85%

2.3 Multimodal Automatic Emotion Recognition

An increasing number of researchers believe that multi-modality is a key factor in automatic emotion recognition. In one of the first bimodal emotion recognition studies, De Silva et al. [17] found that some emotions were better recognized by humans through the auditory modality than the visual modality, and vice versa: anger, happiness, surprise and dislike were more visual dominant, and sadness and fear were more audio dominant. Since some modalities may carry complementary information and since humans also make use of multimodal information, it seems natural to fuse different modalities, which may lead to higher classification accuracies.

In Table 3, we can observe that indeed classification accuracies increase when audiovisual information (AV) is used instead of individual audio (A) or video channels (V). Usually, we make a distinction between fusion on feature-level and decision-level. On feature-level, features from different modalities can be concatenated to each other to form one large N-dimensional feature vector. Feature selection techniques may then be used to remove redundant features. Fusion on decision-level means that the features of the different modalities are processed separately, and are fused when the separate classifiers give outputs/scores which are usually in terms of posterior probabilities or likelihoods. These scores are then subsequently fused by summing, or taking the product of the scores etc. Fusing classifiers and data streams is not straightforward; we will discuss in Section 3.3 the difficulties that may arise in the fusion process.

Other studies have not only used speech and facial expressions, but also other physiological measures such as skin response, heart rate etc. [2-4]. However, physiological measures are usually measured with specialized hardware and sensors that are attached to the body which can be perceived as obtrusive. In general, the use of certain multimodal features depends on the application that one has in mind and the allowed degree of obtrusiveness.

Table 3. Short overview of bimodal emotion recognition studies based on speech and facial expressions (A=audio, V=video, AV=audiovisual, SI=SubjectIndependent, SD=Subject Dependent)

Study	Data	SI/ SD	Fusion method	Accuracy
Chen 1998 [18]	6 emotions, 2 subjects (acted)	??	Feature-level (concatenation)	75% (A), 69% (V), 97% (AV)
De Silva 2000 [19]	6 emotions, 2 subjects (acted)	SD	Dominant rule-based fusion	72% (AV)
Sebe 2006 [20]	11 emotions, 38 subjects (acted)	SD	Feature-level, Bayesian topology	45% (A), 56% (V), 89% (AV)

3   General Difficulties in Automatic Emotion Recognition

Apart from specific speech related and facial expressions related difficulties which were discussed in Section 2.1 and 2.2 respectively, there are also some more general difficulties to tackle in automatic emotion recognition research.

3.1   How Should We Annotate Emotion?

As the summaries of emotion recognition studies show (Table 1, 2 and 3), most of these studies still use categorical emotion labels. However, these labels are not always useful for real, genuine spontaneous emotion data since these labels tend to represent the extremes of each emotion category that are rarely encountered in spontaneous speech data. Further, humans can also express degrees of happiness or sadness. Taking this into account, a dimensional approach to emotion representation can offer an elegant solution. An advantage of this approach is that labels and categories of emotions have become redundant; we can express emotions now in terms of degrees of activation and evaluation. However, few studies have performed detection of degrees or shades of emotions in terms of emotional dimensions.

There remains discussion about how to obtain ground truth emotion annotations. On the one hand, we can define a ground truth emotion as an emotion that is perceived by people and that is agreed upon by most of the receivers. On the other hand, we can define a ground truth emotion as the experienced, true emotion as felt by the person her/himself. However, there can be a discrepancy between the perceived and experienced emotion: people may not always express their (true) emotions, especially when they are in conversation and obey the unwritten conversational rules. An option would be to let the subjects annotate their own emotional expressions (self-annotations) and compare these with the annotated emotions as perceived by other subjects.

3.2 Lack of Spontaneous Multimodal Data

One of the major obstacles in emotion research is the lack of annotated, spontaneous emotion data. Consequences are that most emotion recognition systems are trained on relatively small datasets containing a small number of subjects and that the classification results do not transfer very well to other data sets or real-life situations. However, we have seen that it is difficult to acquire analyzable signals in real-life situations (see Section 2.1, 2.2 and Fig. 1). Also note that for speech analysis, it is important that the content is independent of the expressed emotion to avoid confounding, e.g., [21].

One of the largest spontaneous audiovisual emotion databases (to date) is the Belfast Naturalistic database [22] which consists of TV clips. Other ways of collecting or eliciting (semi-) spontaneous emotions include showing movies or still pictures [23], listening to music [24], playing games [3] or interacting with virtual characters [25]. Playing (video) games seems to be particularly suitable for collecting emotion data: game developers are increasingly instructed to develop video games that in some way can trigger a range of emotions [26]. Also, manipulated games offer better control over the elicited emotion.

Finally, we should enable easier comparison and interpretation between studies by collecting a representative emotion database that can serve as a basis for benchmarking.

3.3 Fusion of Multimodal Measures

Table 3 showed that fusion of multimodal features could improve the performance of an emotion recognition system substantially. But, in most cases, fusion of multimodal features is not straightforward due to the different properties and behaviors of the features. For instance, the segmental units over which the features are measured are most likely to differ for many features which make it difficult to synchronize the features, e.g., different frame rates or lag times. Further, how should we deal with feature streams that have missing data while other streams have continuous output: e.g., speech features are usually measured over non-silent segments while heart rate can be measured continuously. And how should the system cope with conflicting outcomes of the classifiers as this can occur frequently in real-life data where blended emotions are not rare [27].

It seems that some researchers prefer a more human-like approach to fusion in emotion recognition [10, 20]: they prefer to fuse features on feature-level, which simulates humans who process multimodal information simultaneously and not separately. However, decision-level fusions are more informative and more explaining, e.g., the behavior of each modality during the recognition process can be more controlled and can be made more visible for feedback purposes. Further, decision-level fusions are somewhat easier to perform and have proven to be powerful in e.g., speaker recognition.

3.4 Evaluation of Emotion Recognition Systems in a Detection Framework

In emotion classification, the classifier's task is usually defined as "classify a given sound/image in one of these N emotion categories". An average accuracy percentage, based on calculations on the confusion matrix, is usually given as a single perform-ance measure. However, this average accuracy measure depends on the number of emotion categories and the proportions of the used trials of each emotion category which is not very useful for making comparisons between studies. Instead of *classifi-cation*, we prefer to speak in terms of *detection* in which the classifier's task is de-fined as "does this given sound/image sound/look like emotion X, yes or no?". In this case, we can adopt the detection framework and evaluate the discrimination perform-ance with a single measure Equal Error Rate (EER, which is defined as the point where the false alarm rate is equal to the miss rate). Further, it should also be clear whether the detection/classification experiment was performed subject-independently so we can interpret the results better. At this moment, comparing performances be-tween emotion recognition systems is difficult which is partly due to the lack of shared datasets and shared evaluation standards.

4   Emotion Recognition in Adaptive Interfaces

It is clear that many efforts are taken to investigate automatic emotion recognition, but what exactly drives researchers in pursuing an automatic emotion recognition sys-tem? From a scientific point of view, we would like to put our knowledge about hu-man emotion to the test and build a machine with human-like traits that enables an improved human-machine interaction: typically, this involves adapting interfaces to the user via emotion recognition. We are also interested in improving automatic speech recognition (ASR) systems by employing emotion-sensitive acoustic models (since it is generally known that ASR performances decrease when affective speech is uttered). Emotion recognition can also be used in computer-mediated communication (i.e., video conferencing, audio chat) in e.g., the e-health domain: monitoring a pa-tient's emotional state from a distance during a medical consult or therapy can be very useful for a doctor. Other environments that may benefit from automatic emotion rec-ognition include call centers, meetings (meeting browsers [28]), crisis management and surveillance.

Finally, adaptive interfaces employing emotion recognition can adjust their inter-faces in games or e-learning systems to the player's or student's emotional state in or-der to increase his/her motivation. Grootjen et al. [29] have been investigating auto-matic assessment of stress and task load in order to develop an emotion-sensitive adaptive interface that can adapt to the operator's stress level so that tasks of a stressed operator can be allocated to another operator. They have been collecting mul-timodal measures of operators performing tasks on a navy ship. Working on that data, they have experienced many of the similar issues discussed above: speech analysis is difficult due to background noises consisting of loud beeps, facial expression analysis is difficult due to the pose of the head and background issues (see Fig. 2), fusion of multimodal measures is difficult because of their different time scales etc. With the development of advancing emotion recognition technology that can cope with these problems, opportunities for future interesting and useful applications increase.

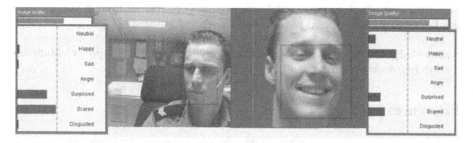

Fig. 2. The FaceReader trying to classify data from Grootjen et al. [29]. Left: ambiguous output. Right: the FaceReader is sensitive to background which was manually removed to improve classification output.

5 Discussion and Conclusions

We have discussed some of the problems that one can encounter in automatic emotion recognition research with the focus on speech and facial expressions analysis. Some of the difficulties can be partly solved by agreeing upon standards for the emotion community, and some of the difficulties can be solved by developing advanced technologies that can deal with noisy data. By describing these difficulties and problems for the development of an emotion recognition system, we do not want to discourage researchers. Rather, our intention is to encourage researchers in the emotion community to elaborate on the problems and to agree upon standards. A lot of work is being carried out by a European project HUMAINE [30] that aims at laying foundations for the development of 'emotion-oriented' systems. Consequently, if we agree upon standards such as the definition of "emotion", evaluation measures and annotation issues, we can further develop data sets that can be used for benchmarking emotion recognition systems. One of the reasons why it is difficult to agree upon emotion standards may be related to the subjectivity and dependency of emotion phenomena. Further research should indicate to what extent emotion recognition and production is subject, culture or context dependent so we can take this into account in our research.

It is clear that building an automatic emotion recognition system can be very complex, especially if we want to incorporate an accurate and complete model or theory of emotion. However, is it always necessary or realistic to pursue such an ideal system that is based on a complete and complex model of emotion? Researchers must keep in mind that detection of 'simple' striking emotions in context (e.g., 'panic') can also be of high practical value for adaptive interfaces.

One of the conclusions that we can draw from the short overviews of uni and multimodal emotion recognition studies is that we have arrived at a point where we should bridge the gap between working and training emotion models with simulated emotion data and applying these models to real-life emotion data. Furthermore, we should enable easier comparisons between emotion recognition studies by developing some standards for an automatic emotion recognition framework. Researchers are now increasingly working with authentic emotion data and the results of these emotion recognition systems are promising but still a lot of improvements can be made. It is rather incredible that humans are able to make judgments about someone's emotions based on a bulk of multimodal information. For now, we think it is fair to say that humans still 'have the best feel for emotions'.

Acknowledgements. This study is supported by the Dutch BSIK project MultimediaN (http://www.multimedian.nl).

References

1. Cowie, R., Schröder, M.: Piecing together the emotion jigsaw. In: Machine Learning for Multimodal Interaction, pp. 305–317 (2005)
2. Kapoor, A., Picard, R.W.: Multimodal affect recognition in learning environments. In: Proceedings of the ACM International Conference on Multimedia, pp. 677–682 (2005)
3. Kim, J., André, E., Rehm, M., Vogt, T., Wagner, J.: Integrating information from speech and physiological signals to achieve emotional sensitivity. In: Proceedings of Interspeech, pp. 809–812 (2005)
4. Zhai, J., Barreto, A.: Stress Recognition Using Non-invasive Technology. In: Proceedings of the 19th International Florida Artificial Intelligence Research Society Conference FLAIRS, pp. 395–400 (2006)
5. Banse, R., Scherer, K.R.: Acoustic profiles in vocal emotion expression. Journal of Personality and Social Psychology 70, 614–636 (1996)
6. Ang, J., Dhillon, R., Krupski, A., Shriberg, E., Stolcke, A.: Prosody-based automatic detection of annoyance and frustration in Human-Computer Dialog. In: Proceedings of the ICSLP International Conference on Spoken Language Processing, pp. 2037–2040 (2002)
7. Nwe, T.L., Foo, S.W, De Silva, L.C.: Speech emotion recognition using hidden Markov models. Speech Communication 41, 603–623 (2003)
8. Vidrascu, L., Devillers, L.: Detection of real-life emotions in call centers. In: Proceedings of Interspeech, pp. 1841–1844 (2005)
9. Batliner, A., Steidl, S., Hacker, C., Nöth, E., Niemann, H.: Tales of tuning - prototyping for automatic classification of emotional user states. In: Proceedings of Interspeech, pp. 489–492 (2005)
10. Pantic, M., Rothkrantz, L.J.M.: Towards an Affect-Sensitive Multimodal Human-Computer Interaction. Proceedings of the IEEE 91, 1370–1390 (2003)
11. Ekman, P., Friesen, W.V.: Facial action coding system: A technique for the measurement of facial movement. Consulting Psychologists Press, Palo Alto (1978)
12. Pantic, M., Rothkrantz, L.J.M.: Automatic Analysis of Facial Expressions: The State of the Art. IEEE Transaction on Pattern Analysis and Machine Intelligence 22, 1424–1445 (2000)
13. Pantic, M., Rothkrantz, L.J.M.: Expert system for automatic analysis of facial expression. Image and Vision Computing Journal 18, 881–905 (2000)
14. Cohen, I., Sebe, N., Chen, L., Garg, A., Huang, T.S.: Facial Expression Recognition from Video Sequences: Temporal and Static Modeling. Computer Vision and Image Understanding 91, 160–187 (2003)

15. Sebe, N., Sun, Y., Bakker, E., Lew, M.S., Cohen, I., Huang, T.S.: Towards Authentic Emotion Recognition. In: IEEE SMC International Conference on Systems, Man, and Cybernetics, pp. 623–628 (2004)
16. Den Uyl, M., Van Kuilenburg, H.: FaceReader: an online facial expression recognition system. In: Proceedings of 5th International Conference on Methods and Techniques in Behavorial Research, pp. 589–590 (2005)
17. De Silva, L.C., Miyasato, T., Nakatsu, R.: Facial emotion recognition using multi-modal information. In: Proceedings of the ICICS International Conference on Information, Communications and Signal Processing, pp. 397–401 (1997)
18. Chen, L.S., Tao, H., Huang, T.S., Miyasato, T., Nakatsu, R.: Emotion recognition from audiovisual information. In: Proceedings of the IEEE Workshop on Multimedia Signal Processing, pp. 83–88 (1998)
19. De Silva, L.C., Ng, P.C.: Bimodal Emotion Recognition. In: Proceedings of the IEEE International Conference on Automatic Face and Gesture Recognition, pp. 332–335 (2000)
20. Sebe, N., Cohen, I., Gevers, T., Huang, T.: Emotion Recognition Based on Joint Visual and Audio Cues. In: Proceedings of the ICPR International Conference on Pattern Recognition, pp. 1136–1139 (2006)
21. Chen, L.S.: Joint processing of audio-visual information for the recognition of emotional expressions in human-computer interaction. Phd thesis (2000)
22. Douglas-Cowie, E., Cowie, R., Schröder, M.: A new emotion database: Considerations, sources and scope. In: Proceedings of ISCA ITRW Workshop on Speech and Emotion, pp. 39–44 (2000)
23. Lang, P.J.: The emotion probe - studies of motivation and attention. American Psychologist 50, 371–385 (1995)
24. Wagner, J., Kim, J., André, E.: From physiological signals to emotions: implementing and comparing selected methods for feature extraction and classification. In: Proceedings of the IEEE ICME International Conference on Multimedia & Expo, pp. 940–943 (2005)
25. Cox, C.: SALAS Sensitive Artificial Listener induction techniques. Paper presented to HUMAINE Network of Excellence Summer School (2004), Retrieved 5 Februay 2007 from http://emotion-research.net/ws/summerschool1/SALAS.ppt#259
26. Lazarro, N.: Why we play games: 4 keys to more emotion. Paper retrieved February 5, 2007 from http://www.xeodesign.com/xeodesign_whyweplaygames.pdf
27. Douglas-Cowie, E., Devillers, L., Martin, J., Cowie, R., Savvidou, S., Abrilian, S., Cox, C.: Multimodal databases of everyday emotion: facing up to complexity. In: Proceedings of Interspeech, pp. 813–816 (2005)
28. AMI project, http://www.amiproject.org
29. Grootjen, M., Neerincx, M.A., Weert, J.C.M., Truong, K.P.: Measuring Cognitive Task Load on a Naval Ship: Implications of a Real World Environment. In: Proceedings of ACI (this volume) (2007)
30. HUMAINE project, http://emotion-research.net/

Embedding Hercule Poirot in Networks: Addressing Inefficiencies in Digital Forensic Investigations

Barbara Endicott-Popovsky[1] and Deborah A. Frincke[2]

[1] University of Washington
[2] Pacific Northwest National Labs
endicott@u.washington.edu, deborah.frincke@pnl.gov

Abstract. Forensic investigations on networks are not scalable in terms of time and money [1]. Those investigations that do occur consume months of attention from the very experts who should be investing in more productive activities, like designing and improving network performance [1]. Given these circumstances, organizations often must select which cases to pursue, ignoring many that could be prosecuted, if time allowed. Recognizing the exponential growth in the number of crimes that employ computers and networks that become subject to digital evidence procedures, researchers and practitioners, alike, have called for embedding forensics—essentially integrating the cognitive skills of a detective into the network [2, 3, 4]. The premise is that the level of effort required to document incidents can thus be reduced, significantly. This paper introduces what technical factors might reflect those detecting skills, leading to solutions that could offset the inefficiencies of current practice.

Keywords: Network forensics, digital forensics, computer crime, augmented cognition.

1 Introduction to the Problem

Unlike most crime scenes where crime tape isolates the scene allowing experienced forensic investigators the luxury of time to gather admissible evidence, a digital crime scene is an active network with the network administrators functioning as first responders. Often they are unaware of courtroom evidence gathering requirements [1, 3]. Practitioners who do consider collecting network forensic data face a choice between expending extraordinary effort (time and money) collecting forensically sound data, or simply restoring the network as quickly as possible. They most often make the expedient choice—responding to distraught users by restoring network function immediately, ignoring the rigors of collecting and preserving forensically sound data [3]. This translates to key evidentiary files most likely altered in the process, limiting their value in the courtroom and opening them to legal challenge [5].

This paper explores this problem and the forces for change that will require rethinking network design to include embedded forensics that substitute for the crime

D.D. Schmorrow, L.M. Reeves (Eds.): Augmented Cognition, HCII 2007, LNAI 4565, pp. 364–372, 2007.

scene detective. We believe the methods of augmented cognition can offer insight into this transformation and initiate exploration of this idea in the context of our existing research.

1.1 Motivation for Change

In today's world, digital evidence gathered hastily, without regard to its admissibility, may be admitted anyway, with law enforcement and legal professionals often unaware of the potential legal problems that could arise [5]. A review of several hundred pages of computer forensic testimony in cases from 2000 to present, confirmed this concern [6]. Technical competence ranged from minimal to highly professional, reflecting the state of the legal system with regard to digital forensics. Not only are those responding to a crime scene unprepared, the fact that there are no agreed-upon professional standards for network forensic procedures means the court system and legal professionals are likewise unprepared.

While legal arguments on both sides of the bar—defense and prosecution—have been technically unsophisticated to date, it is not expected that the *status quo* will remain. Several trends are motivating change.

To identify a few:

1) The threat spectrum is growing and indicates a movement toward organized crime as the predominant beneficiary of online criminal activities [7]. This means more online crime and bigger losses. As an example, estimates of the impacts to the world economy indicate that the dollar amount of online theft exceeds the profits of e-commerce by almost two to one [8].

2) In light of recent legislation, legal counsel, in the interest of establishing evidence of due care, have begun urging organizations to invest in procedures and technology that will allow collection of forensically sound data defensible in a court of law [9]. This is precipitating efforts by organizations such as NIST and IFIP to converge on digital forensics standards that can be relied upon in the courtroom. [10]

3) As a result, organizations face an urgent need to 're-think' incident response and the role of digital forensics among their network strategies if they wish to deter the growing threat by pursuing, and assisting in the capture of, online criminals. [11]

1.2 Examining Two Criminal Cases

In [1] the authors explored two successfully prosecuted computer crimes that demonstrate the need for a preventive and proactive response to malicious intrusion. The comparison indicates the growing costs and consequences of professional criminals beginning to dominate online crime, as well as the challenge of finding experts to execute forensic investigations. The findings are summarized in Table 1.

Table 1. Criminal Case Comparison

Characteristics	Script Kiddy[1] Case	Professional Criminal Case
Type of attack	Exploitation of a network vulnerability to perform a denial of service attack	Online automated auction scam
Damages	$400,000	$25 million
Investigator time	417 hours	9 months
Investigation costs	$27,800	$100,000 (partial)
Consequences	Community service	3 & 4 years in prison
Investigator	Sys admins learning forensics	Expert recruited by the FBI
Forensic readiness	Reactive	Reactive.

Analysis of the results suggests that the investigations required to successfully prosecute these cases, are not scalable. The costs per incident are too high, take too much organizational time and result in comparatively little consequence to the offender. The study further concluded that there is a need to "operationalize" the concept of organizational network forensic readiness, defined as 'maximizing the ability of an environment to collect credible digital evidence while minimizing the cost of an incident response' [2]. This is essentially the act of 'embedding a detective' in networks--capturing the expertise of the crime scene investigator, including the procedures needed to collect admissible evidence, in lieu of *ad hoc* investigations by non-law enforcement.

Without relying on training network administrators to become law enforcement professionals, this means rethinking strategies for protecting networked systems and ultimately redesigning them to include the characteristics of good detection.

1.3 Changing Strategies

In [11], the authors proposed a strategic framework (Table 2), derived from Carnegie Mellon's 3R model for survivable systems, as a vehicle for rethinking network protection strategies [12]. By the addition of a 4th R–*Redress*—defined as the ability to hold intruders accountable—the focus of network protection changes from purely defensive to include offensive strategies. A 4R approach changes the desired outcome of an attack from "patch and recover" to include identification of the attacker. As a consequence, it also expands the duties of those responsible for securing networks to include employing the skills of a detective at a crime scene [11].

Implementing a 4R strategy in an organization will necessitate re-examination of current security policies, procedures, methods, mechanisms, and tools in order to ensure compliance with courtroom admissibility standards and to include the requirements of a skilled detective. This implies a need for a comprehensive approach for incorporating digital forensic investigation into networked systems.

---

[1] A script kiddy is a recreational hacker with little skill who uses readily available, already-developed hacking tools for online mischief.

Table 2. 4R Strategies for defendingforensically ready networks

Strategy	Tools
Resistance Ability to repel attacks	• Firewalls • User authentication • Diversification
Recognition 1) Ability to detect an attack or a probe 2) Ability to react / adapt during an attack	• Intrusion detection systems • Internal integrity checks
Recovery 1) Provide essential services during attack 2) Restore services following an attack	• Incident response • ("forensics" - *the what*) • Replication • Backup systems • Fault tolerant designs
Redress 1) Ability to hold intruders accountable 2) Ability to retaliate	• Forensics - *the who* • Legal remedies • Active defense

1.4 The Research Gap

As early as 2001, researchers participating in the annual *Digital Forensics Research Workshops* (*http://www.dfrws.org/*) identified the lack of a conceptual framework for proactive approaches to digital forensics from the 'organization-as-first-responder' viewpoint. Instead the primary research focus has been on forensic methods, tools and techniques, largely from a law enforcement perspective [13]. Table 3 summarizes the distribution of DFRWS research from 2002 to 2006:

Table 3. Distribution of presentations DFRWS 2002-2006

Research Category	Number of Presentations
Education	2
Evidence analysis and management	16
File system forensics	3
Investigation	6
Network forensics	13
Standards and methods	12
Comprehensive framework	1
Tools	7

As one of the premiere venues for digital forensics research, the DFRWS is indicative of the research emphasis in the field of digital forensics to date. The gap identified in 2001—the lack of a conceptual framework for digital forensics—has not yet been resolved, particularly from a user's perspective [14].

2 Life Cycle Methodology

To begin to address this gap, in [1] we proposed an implementation framework—the life cycle methodology shown in Fig. 1. The NFDLC (Network Forensics Development Life Cycle) describes, from an organization view, how the skills of a detective can be embedded in systems. The methodology is based on the NIST Information Systems Development Life Cycle (ISDLC) that incorporates security across the life cycle [15] and is integrated with detection skill requirements, including compliance with legal considerations, such as evidence admissibility rules.

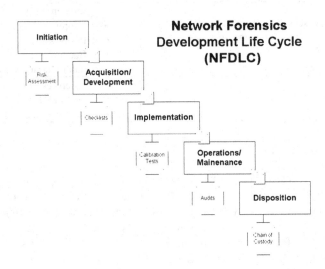

Fig. 1. Modifications to the ISDLC to embed digital forensics

As a result, the following changes to the ISDLC were recommended [14]:

Initiation phase: The risk assessment task would expand to include a determination of what aspects of a network would warrant digital forensic protection. Discussions with practitioners led to the conclusion that not all elements of a network would warrant the investment in embedded forensics [16]. Determination of where forensic investments should be made would involve an analysis of legal risk and liability.

Acquisition/Development phase: Checklists, like those developed by other researchers [4, 17-19], would be appropriate to determine what forensic procedures/tools/technologies should be embedded in the network. In many instances, these will require modification to include the skills of a detective. An example from our current research will be discussed subsequently.

Implementation phase: Calibration testing would be added. Today's manufacturers of network devices may provide general specifications, but few guarantee actual device behavior. The consequences of failing to validate behavior could lead to inadmissible evidence through legal challenge and failed legal action. Calibration can provide the needed validation of device reliability and predictability [5].

Operation/Maintenance phase: Calibration audits would be added to confirm results of previous calibration tests because as the network grows and changes, re-testing will be necessary.

Disposition phase: Chain of custody procedures would be incorporated to ensure preservation of potential evidence residing in retired systems.

3   Progress to Date

Detailed content of the NFDLC methodology is under development. We began with calibration testing in the Implementation phase because we saw an immediate need. Existing network devices, such as switches and taps with span port capability, are used already to collect network traffic data for the courtroom. If they are not calibrated, expert testimony can be compromised as described in [5].

A generalized framework for developing calibration tests, the OCTDF (Fig. 2), evolved from tests devised for a specific forensic tap [5]. This has spawned an avenue of inquiry that we continue to pursue as we scale the OCTDF to more complex network devices and in different application contexts [20].

Observability Calibration Test Development Framework (OCTDF)

1)   *Step 1*: Identify Potential Challenge Areas and Environment
   Identification is accomplished by briefly modeling interactions of interest given a particular scenario; then using that information to identify whether, or not, lost network data could damage evidence value. The result will be a set of pairs of behavior to be observed, and the circumstances under which that observation is expected to take place.

2)   *Step 2*: Identify Calibration Testing Goals
   Given each pairing of behaviors to be observed, and the likely circumstance for observation, testing goals are identified that are supportive of demonstrating evidence value.

3)   *Step 3*: Devise a Test Protocol.
   From the testing goals identified in Step 2, a testing protocol is devised that will provide appropriate calibration for the device in question.

Fig. 2. Framework for calibration test protocols

Our attention has turned to development of the remainder of the methodology, which we've anthropomorphized through the metaphor of 'embedding a detective in the network.' The network becomes the detective. While network data is being collected today at various nodes, its use as evidence is incidental to its prime function—network management. We contend existing network tools will require modification to include detection considerations. An example would be intrusion detection systems (IDS) that today alert network administrators to possible incursions.

Intrusion detection systems (IDS) were designed to augment cognition of network administrators managing security on networks. They provide alerts that a possible intrusion has occurred. They are tuned to either signatures of known intrusion scenarios or anomalous behavior and are designed primarily to provide data for human decision-making. The data comes from a variety of sources—i.e., audit log, systems logs, host OS—originally designed to assist with administering systems, but never intended to be employed as evidence-gathering devices for the courtroom.

If IDS systems were to assume the role of embedded detective, complete with an understanding of admissibility requirements, they would need to be modified to reflect new requirements. Table 4 describes five basic characteristics of IDS systems and the corresponding changes that would have to occur.

Table 4. Modifications to IDS ssytems

IDS Characteristics	Current Requirement	Augmented to Embed Detective
System philosophy	Alert decision makers to a potential intrusion	Identify intrusion and begin forensic data collection
Detection methodology *Anomalous behavior*	Alerts when anomalous behavior occurs	Will require additional data to determine if anomaly is an intrusion
Signature detection	Alerts when known misuse/intrusion signatures detected	Collects forensic data when malevolent signature identified
Data storage	Random archiving and retention periods	Uniform archiving and retention periods
Sensor location	Near valuable data assets and strategic network nodes	Near assets determined by risk analysis to warrant a 4R strategy approach

Additional considerations might include:

1) Degree of autonomy in response—this will affect forensics in many ways, in that (a) the response itself may render forensic data inadmissible, (b) the response may require integration with a human to make decisions even in simple matters like handling the forensic data—not everyone may be legally authorized to see/handle all data, and (c) the response will more than likely cross domains, adding complexity to the task of the integrated detective.
2) Source of authority for data collection—the way data is gathered, who can see it, what data can be combined, etc, depends heavily on the source of authority for gathering that data as well as "who" gathered it. Does the detective make inferences based on all data? Does the detective decide not to pick up some data, or have an ability to request additional authority?

From our preliminary analysis, as users begin to automate more and more IDS/forensics systems, we have identified the issue of how IDS systems handle the legal and technological issues arising from cross/overlapping domains as an important research challenge to pursue.

4 Conclusions and Future Work

As courtroom admissibility requirements become important considerations for networked systems, 'embedding a detective in the network' is a useful metaphor for the changes that will be required. For systems to become forensically ready, substituting the 'embedded detective' for costly and non-scalable *ad hoc* investigations will necessitate a change in network protection strategies to include discovering the culprit, as opposed to simply restoring network function as quickly as possible when an intrusion occurs. The new strategy implies modification of existing security policies, tools, technologies and procedures to accommodate these additional requirements. A good example is IDS technology, which today provides some augmented cognition capabilities to network administrators, but will necessitate enhancement if the role of the detective is included.

We anticipate that organizations will find that selective implementation of forensic readiness is good security policy. Possible benefiting scenarios include pursuit of an insider/intruder for the purpose of legal action and documentation of due care in the event of civil litigation claiming networked systems are not adequately secured and defended.

Future work will involve:

1) Continued development of all phases of the NFDLC methodology.
2) Conceptualization and design of a forensically ready IDS system that embeds the skills of a detective.
3) Implementation of the NFDLC in a newly designed client network to assess the feasibility of limited forensic readiness.

References

1. Endicott-Popovsky, B.E., Ryan, D., Frincke, D.: The New Zealand Hacker Case: A Post Mortem. In: Proceedings Safety and Security in a Networked World: Balancing Cyber-Rights & Responsibilities, Oxford Internet Institute, Oxford, England (September 2005), Retrieved from the World Wide Web: http://www.oii.ox.ac.uk/research/cybersafety/?view=papers
2. Tan, J.: Forensic Readiness, @Stake, Cambridge, MA (2001)
3. Dittrich, D., Endicott-Popovsky, B.E.: INFO498 Introduction to Computer Security Incident Response, University of Washington, Seattle, WA (Fall, 2003)
4. Rowlinson, R.: Ten Steps to Forensic Readiness. International Journal of Digital Evidence 23(3) (Winter 2004)
5. Endicott-Popovsky, B.E., Chee, B., Frincke, D.: Role of Calibration as Part of Establishing Foundation for Expert Testimony. In: Proceedings 3rd Annual IFIP WG 11. Orlando, FL (January 2007)
6. Lawson, M, Lawson R.: Expert Witness Testimony. Global CompuSearch, LLC, Spokane, WA (2000-2003)
7. CSI/FBI: CSI/FBI Computer Crime and Security Survey, Computer Security Institute, San Francisco, CA (2005)

8. Bailey, K.: Trouble in Cyberspace: Why this Conference is Important, NWSec, Seattle, WA (February 2007), Retrieved from the World Wide Web http://students. washington.edu/greyhat/mainsec.html
9. Gates, P.: Seminar in Data Security, Seattle, WA (March 2005)
10. NIST: Computer Forensics Tool Testing (CFTT) Project, Retrieved from the World Wide Web: http://www.cftt.nist.gov/
11. Endicott-Popovsky, B.E., Frincke, D.: Adding the Fourth 'R': A Systems Approach to Solving the Hacker's Arms Race. In: Hawaii International Conference on System Sciences (HICSS) 39 Symposium: Skilled Human-intelligent Agent Performance: Measurement, Application and Symbiosis, Kauai, HI, (January 2006). Retrieved from the World Wide Web: http://www.itl.nist.gov/iaui/vvrg/hicss39/4_r_s_rev_3_HICSS_2006.doc
12. Ellison, R.J., Fisher, D.A., Linger, R.C., Lipson, H.F., Longstaff, T.A., Mead, N.R.: Survivable Network Systems: An Emerging Discipline. CMU/SEI 97-TR-013, Software Engineering Institute, Carnegie-Mellon University, Pittsburgh, PA (May 1999)
13. Mocas, S.: Building Theoretical Underpinnings for Digital Forensics Research. Compsec Online: Digital Investigations 1(1) (2003)
14. Endicott-Popovsky, B., Frincke, D.: Embedding Forensic Capabilities into Networks: Addressing Inefficiencies in Digital Forensics Investigations. In: Proceedings Seventh IEEE Systems, Man and Cybernetics Information Assurance Workshop, pp.133–139. United States Military Academy, West Point, NY (June 2006)
15. Grance, T., Hash, J., Stevens, M.: Security Considerations in the Information System Development Life Cycle. U.S. Department of Commerce, NIST Special Publication, pp. 800–864 (2004)
16. Bailey, K., Winn, J.: Personal Interviews (March 2006)
17. Yasinsac, A., Manzano, Y.: Policies to Enhance Computer and Network Forensics. In: Proceedings 2001 IEEE Workshop on Information Assurance and Security, United States Military Academy, West Point, NY (June 2001)
18. Wolfe-Wilson, J., Wolfe, H.B.: Management Strategies for Implementing Forensic Security Measures (electronic version). Information Security Technical Report 8(2), 55–64 (2003)
19. Carrier, B., Spafford, E.: Getting Physical with the Digital Investigation Process [electronic version], International Journal of Digital Evidence, vol. 2(2) (Fall 2003)
20. Endicott-Popovsky, B.E., Fluckiger, J.D., Frincke, D.A.: Establishing Tap Reliability in Expert Witness Testimony: Using Scenarios to Identify Calibration Need. In: Proceedings 2nd International Workshop on Systematic Approaches to Digital Forensic Engineering, Seattle, WA, (April 2007)

The Future of Augmented Cognition Systems in Education and Training

Erica D. Palmer and David A. Kobus

Pacific Science & Engineering Group
9180 Brown Deer Road
San Diego, CA 92121
{ericapalmer, dakobus}@pacific-science.com

Abstract. As adaptive interfaces increase in sophistication and application, augmented cognition systems are becoming accessible to a wider variety of users in real-world settings. The potential for using closed-loop augmented cognition systems in education and training is immense, and will be instrumental in meeting growing demands for distance learning and remote training. Augmented cognition technologies can be applied in numerous ways to dynamically tailor instruction to the user's cognitive style and skill level. Examples of such applications are discussed, along with their implications for enhanced educational and training programs of the future.

Keywords: Augmented cognition, education, training.

1 Introduction

At any given moment, humans are faced with a potentially overwhelming amount of sensory information arriving from multiple modalities. Perceptual and cognitive systems are critical for filtering and selecting information relevant to the individual's current goal state, performing the necessary operations, and formulating appropriate responses. In many situations, components of these systems can become overburdened, resulting in decreased efficiency and performance decrements. Augmented cognition seeks to identify where potential limitations exist in components of the perceptual and cognitive systems, and to detect them when they occur during task performance using sensitive physiological measures.

Closed-loop augmented cognition systems go a step further by using physiological measures in an ongoing fashion to control the delivery of mitigations when needed to maintain an acceptable level of task performance. St. John & Kobus [1] outline two common paradigms, *adaptive* and *integral*, used in augmented cognition research for enhancing user performance. In the adaptive paradigm, the application of the mitigation is contingent upon the user's physiological or cognitive state, rather than implemented continuously. In this paradigm the mitigation is only useful during specific states and therefore is only applied during these periods. A continuous application of the mitigation would result in periods of less than optimal performance; otherwise the need to monitor physiological or cognitive state would not be necessary. In contrast, the integral paradigm proposes that monitoring and utilizing the user's

D.D. Schmorrow, L.M. Reeves (Eds.): Augmented Cognition, HCII 2007, LNAI 4565, pp. 373–379, 2007.
© Springer-Verlag Berlin Heidelberg 2007

psychophysiology is a continuous and integral part of the augmented task. Unlike the adaptive paradigm, mitigations are not used to return the user to optimal performance level or limit the impact of task demands when problematic conditions arise. Rather, they are key components of the task process that continuously modify which or when information is presented to users.

A key aspect of augmented cognition therefore is the monitoring of the user's physiological state in real-time. A number of non-invasive physiological measures are currently being used or investigated for augmented cognition purposes. Among those are heart rate and variability, skin conductance, eye movements, eye blinks, pupil dilation, head movement, electroencephalographic (EEG) measures, evoked or event-related brain potentials (EPs or ERPs), and functional near infrared (fNIR) measures. Used in augmented cognition systems, these tools have already begun to contribute to more effective task performance. For example, Tremoulet et al [2] demonstrated significantly reduced error rates and decreased time in decision making during a Tactical Tomahawk Weapons Control System simulation as a result of a closed-loop system in which presentation of alerting tasks was dictated by ongoing EEG, electrocardiogram, and galvanic skin response measures. Another example of a successful closed-loop system comes from work by Snow and colleagues [3] in the context of improving performance of a single operator controlling multiple Uninhabited Combat Air Vehicles. Participants showed significant performance benefits when they received mitigations driven by changes in real-time fNIR signals as compared to a baseline condition with no mitigation.

While augmented cognition systems offer very exciting possibilities both for research and for real-world applications, moving such systems out of the lab and into operational environments is not without its challenges. For example, the sensors and accompanying equipment that are used to obtain physiological measures are often expensive, uncomfortable, cumbersome, limit mobility, and cannot be used without extensive training. In addition, the ability to process physiological data in real-time is critical for closed-loop applications. This includes developing techniques for online identification and removal of noise and artifacts in the data that can obscure the signals of interest. Such artifacts can result from user movement or from various kinds of electrical signals in the environment.

Fortunately, technological advances are helping to bring real life application of augmented cognition systems closer to fruition. For example, EEG systems are now available that record electrical signals from the brain and transmit them wirelessly to a light-weight, portable receiver [4]. This leaves the user free to move around and perform tasks in a natural manner. Recently, significant advances have been made in real-time artifact removal for EEG [5], which will contribute to the feasibility of obtaining useable EEG data in operational environments. In addition, newer EEG systems have specially designed electrodes that do not require the extensive scalp abrading and prep work necessitated by traditional EEG electrodes. Eye tracking systems are also continuously improving. Whereas older systems required the user's head to remain stationary, recent developments make it possible to obtain eye and head movement data while the user is moving. Along with increases in mobility, physiological monitoring systems are also beginning to see improvements in comfort, ease of application, and real-time processing of data, all critical for their use in real-world applications. In addition, affordable personal computers are now becoming powerful enough to compute and store the massive amounts of data obtained from physiological sensors.

This increased accessibility means that augmented cognition technologies can soon be applied to a number of different settings, including the home, classrooms, job sites, and military training facilities. Thus, one exciting and important use of these technologies is the development of a closed-looped system to facilitate and enhance educational and training applications.

2   Application to Education and Training

With advances in web-based technology, distance learning has become increasingly common. Course material is presented and student progress is assessed entirely over the web. In an effort to take advantage of available technology and to improve the learning experience, interactive demonstrations and learning practices are becoming routine features of online courses. As a result, the learning experience becomes more individualized, and the curriculum has been developed to address the "average" student. Augmented cognition systems, particularly closed-loop systems, have the potential to take interactive web-based courses to a new level, adjusting the information flow rate and difficultly to best match the needs and ability of each student. Augmented cognition systems may also be used to identify how best to supplement or complement traditional classroom learning with individualized instruction in the form of educational applications that could be used at home.

The military too has taken advantage of the distance learning paradigm. Web-based learning helps fulfill the frequent need to train individuals at remote locations and in the absence of live trainers or role-players for team-based training. Military personnel are expected to master an increasingly vast array of skills and become proficient at numerous tasks, often with insufficient time or resources available for training. Thus, improvements in training programs will be very valuable. Similar issues arise in the area of healthcare. Training resources, whether for medical professionals or for caretakers, are often insufficient, and consequences of ineffective training can be serious. Augmented cognition systems could be an important part of reducing mistakes through improved training programs and practices. Such systems may also provide a new method of evaluating training levels that participants achieve.

2.1   Skill Level Assessment

An important part of education and training programs is tailoring the material to the needs of the student or trainee. Therefore, a means of altering presentation of material by assessing an individual's proficiency, strengths, and weaknesses "on the fly" would be highly desirable. Different levels of expertise have been conceptually defined, ranging from "novice" to "master" [6]. It should be possible to identify patterns of physiological responses that reflect an individual's level of expertise along this continuum. Indeed, differences in patterns of brain activity have been observed among individuals with different skill levels [7], and within individuals before and after extensive practice with a task [8]. Similarly, ongoing physiological measures of alertness, effort, and workload can help to assess an individual's progress in learning.

These patterns of physiological responses can be used to dictate, in an ongoing fashion, how the material to be learned is presented. Greater support would be provided when a student's physiological measures reflected lower levels of expertise, while presentation of material would proceed with less support when a higher level of expertise was indicated. Support might take the form of slower rate of presentation, more redundancy in the material, or fewer assumptions about pre-existing knowledge, just to name a few possibilities. This kind of adaptive learning could improve efficacy and efficiency in a variety of educational and training settings.

2.2 Detection of Error Types

In educational and training applications that use behavioral measures such as response accuracy to assess performance, it can be valuable to have more information about the types of errors that are made. For example, it would be useful to distinguish "slips", or accidental/unintended responses, from mistakes that reflect difficulty with the material or task. Consider a training program in which individuals learn to rapidly classify types of aircraft that are presented briefly on a radar screen, and indicate the class by button press. Errors in classification could occur if the trainee, in an attempt to respond quickly, simply slips and presses the wrong button for his/her intended response. Alternatively, the trainee could be having difficulty distinguishing the different aircraft types.

Luu and Campbell [9] report the use of a neurophysiological measure, the Error-Related Negativity (ERN), in conjunction with behavioral data to help distinguish slips from other types of mistakes. Real-time application of such measures during a training exercise could help to guide the training; a large proportion of slips might trigger additional training on the mappings between aircraft types and buttons, while a large proportion of mistakes could prompt additional training on distinguishing the different types of aircraft. Similar closed-loop systems could be applied to educational programs, for example in teaching children to match letters and sounds or to perform multiplication problems. Such a system would not only provide material to the student at an optimal pace, but it would assess how and why errors occurred so the instruction would be modified to best address problem areas.

2.3 Presentation of Written Material

Even as learning media progress from text books to online applications, a great deal of emphasis is placed on written material. An important part of developing effective and efficient education and training programs will therefore depend on optimizing presentation of text. Again, this is an area where physiological measures and closed-loop augmented cognition systems could be of great value. For example, eye tracking could be used during presentation of text to determine an individual's reading speed, and to modulate the rate of text presentation accordingly. Similarly, workload, attention, and alertness could be monitored with EEG, and presentation of text could be adjusted accordingly. A study by Buswell [10] (as cited in [11]) has shown that the number of regressive eye movements and duration of fixations are highly correlated with reading difficulty. These measures hold great promise as potential metrics for monitoring reading difficulty in augmented systems.

Taken together, such measures would not only modulate rate of presentation of material, but also trigger actions to restore alertness, change the modality of presentation (e.g., intersperse spoken material into written text), determine the level of difficulty of the text being presented, or provide support materials when difficulties are detected. Such mitigations would be applicable to education and training settings alike, and provide another means of using augmented cognition systems to individualize instruction.

2.4 Modulation of Material Type

There is evidence for individual differences in preference for and facility with visual vs. spatial material [12]. Further, within an individual, there are working memory systems for verbal and spatial material that are at least partly dissociable [13]. Transient evoked-potential responses have been identified that differ between verbal and spatial versions of the same task [14]. Instructional applications that use augmented cognition can capitalize on these facts through ongoing modulation of the type of material presented based on an individual's changing capacity to use each material type.

An example of such an application is in the development of instructional materials to teach medical professionals and caretakers how to use certain medical devices. Traditionally, instructional materials have relied heavily on verbal presentation, often in the form of text. With the advent of multimedia capabilities, these materials can now more readily incorporate visuospatial components, such as visual "tours" of buttonology, animations, or videos of users carrying out specific functions or tasks. Adding augmented cognition technology could allow flexible emphasis on, or switching between, verbal and visuospatial modes of presentation, based on real-time neurophysiological measures of the user's cognitive capacity for each type of material.

2.5 Team Training

While there are numerous possibilities for using augmented cognition to improve individual training and education programs, there are also important applications for team-based training [15]. For example, in team training exercises, task responsibilities are often distributed among team members. Using physiological measures such as EEG, it would be possible to measure workload simultaneously in all team members. An augmented cognition system could be developed to intervene when a specific team member's workload exceeds some pre-determined threshold, temporarily reassigning one or more of that team member's tasks to another team member(s) with a lower measured workload.

In training for some team-based activities or tasks, it may be the case that a live instructor or full set of team members or other role player is not available. This occurs frequently in military applications, in which individuals may be relatively isolated in remote locations. Well executed team-based operations are critical to the military, however, so it is important for individuals to train for and practice their roles in such operations even when live instructors or role players are not present. Simulated role players can serve this purpose, and an augmented cognition system can both ensure that the simulated role players fit the needs of the live team member, and act as trainer. This can be accomplished by using physiologically determined measures of the individual's skill level and workload to provide adaptively challenging and supported training and practice.

2.6 Possible Commercial Applications

With success in school becoming an increasingly important predictor of success in later life, the demand for products that improve a student's academic performance is enormous. Thus, there is great potential for commercial applications that can provide optimally tailored instruction that is not available in large classes with a single teacher, or through many current distance learning courses. The individualized learning experience made possible with augmented cognition systems is unique, and holds promise for the development of educational software that can enhance classroom or online learning of specific subject matter, or improve basic skills such as reading, spelling, and math. As the technology behind physiological sensor systems continues to advance and become more accessible, educational programs that incorporate augmented cognition systems will become marketable to schools, learning centers, and individuals alike.

Similarly, commercially available training programs that utilize augmented cognition technology will hold great appeal for organizations looking for effective, lower-cost alternatives to traditional training practices. A company that manufactures medical devices, for example, could put themselves at considerable advantage over their competition by offering along with a new device a sophisticated training program that incorporates augmented cognition principles and technologies to optimize and validate user training. Such a training program could reduce errors by incorporating into the training program a means to assess a user's mastery of the material and ensure that adequate proficiency is achieved.

3 Summary

The ultimate goal of the science of augmented cognition is to develop technologies capable of extending the information management capacity or information throughput to the user in applied environments. The fields of education and training are the next likely targets for augmented cognition technology after it reaches commercial viability. Education and training are moving toward an increasingly computational medium. With distance learning and remote training in high demand, instructional systems will need to adapt to this new nonhuman teaching interaction while ensuring the quality of instruction. Augmented cognition technologies could be applied to educational and training settings and guarantee students an optimal teaching strategy adapted to their individual cognitive styles. This application of augmented cognition promises to have great impact on society at large.

References

1. St. John, M.F., Kobus, D.A.: Practical considerations for applied research in augmented cognition. In: Schmorrow, D., Stanny, K. (eds.) Augmented Cognition: A Practitioners Guide (in press)
2. Tremoulet, P., Barton, J., Crave, P., Gifford, A., Morizio, N., Belov, N., Stibler, K., Regli, S.H., Thomas, M.: Augmented cognition for Tactical Tomahawk Weapons Control System operators. In: Schmorrow, D., Stanney, K., Reeves, L. (eds.) Foundations of Augmented Cognition, 2nd edn. pp. 313–318. Arlington, VA: Strategic Analysis, Inc. & the Augmented Cognition International Society (2006)
3. Snow, M.P., Barker, R.A., O'Neill, K.R., Offer, B.W., Edwards, R.E.: Augmented cognition in a prototype uninhabited combat air vehicle operator console. In: Schmorrow, D., Stanney, K., Reeves, L. (eds.) Foundations of Augmented Cognition, 2nd edn. pp. 279–288. Arlington, VA: Strategic Analysis, Inc. & the Augmented Cognition International Society (2006)
4. Honeywell Laboratories. DARPA Improving Warfighter Information Intake under Stress - Augmented Cognition Phase III Final Report (September 16, 2005)
5. Poolman, P., Frank, R.M., Bell, R.M.A.: Advanced integrated real-time artifact removal framework. In: Schmorrow, D., Stanney, K., Reeves, L.(eds.) Foundations of Augmented Cognition, 2nd edn. pp. 102–110. Arlington, VA: Strategic Analysis, Inc. & the Augmented Cognition International Society (2006)
6. Hoffman, R.R.: How can expertise be defined?: Implications of research from cognitive psychology. In: Williams, R., Faulkner, W., Fleck, J. (eds.) Exploring Expertise, pp. 81–100. Macmillan, New York (1998)
7. Gevins, A., Smith, M.E.: Neurophysiological measures of working memory and individual differences in cognitive ability and cognitive style. Cerebral Cortex (10), 829–839 (2000)
8. Petersen, S.E., van Mier, H., Fiez, J.A., Raichle, M.E.: The effects of practice on the functional anatomy of task performance. In: Proceedings of the National Academy of Sciences (95), pp. 853–860 (1998)
9. Luu, P., Campbell, G.: Oops, I did it again: Using neurophysiological indicators to distinguish slips from mistakes in simulation-based training systems. In: Proceedings of the 11th International Conference of Human-Computer Interaction, Las Vegas, NV (July 22-27, 2005)
10. Buswell, G.T.: Fundamental reading habits: A study of their development. Education Monographs (21) (1922)
11. Schiff, W.: Perception: An Applied Approach. New Jersey: Houghton Mifflin Company (1980)
12. Riding, R.J.: The nature and effects of cognitive style. In: Sternberg, R.J., Zhang, L. (eds.) Perspectives on Thinking, Learning, and Cognitive Styles, pp. 47–72. Erlbaum, Mahwah (2001)
13. Baddeley, A., Hitch, G.: Working memory. In: Bower, G. (ed.) Recent Advances in Learning and Motivation, pp. 47–90. Academic Press, New York (1974)
14. McEvoy, L.K., Smith, M.E., Gevins, A.: Dynamic cortical networks of verbal and spatial working memory: Effects of memory load and task practice. Cerebral Cortex (8), 563–574 (1998)
15. Nicholson, D.M., Lackey, S.J., Arnold, R., Scott, K.: Augmented cognition technologies applied to training: A roadmap for the future. In: Schmorrow, D.D. (ed.) Foundations of Augmented Cognition, pp. 931–940. Lawrence Erlbaum Associates, Mahwah (2005)

An Adaptive Instructional Architecture for Training and Education

Denise M. Nicholson[1], Cali M. Fidopiastis[1], Larry D. Davis[1],
Dylan D. Schmorrow[2], and Kay M. Stanney[3]

[1] Institute for Simulation and Training, University of Central Florida,
[2] Office of Naval Research,
[3] College of Engineering and Computer Science, University of Central Florida
{dnichols, cfidopia, ldavis}@ist.ucf.edu, SCHMORD@ONR.NAVY.MIL,
Stanney@mail.ucf.edu

Abstract. Office of Naval Research (ONR) initiatives such as Human Performance Training and Education (HPT&E) as well as Virtual Technologies and Environments (VIRTE) have primarily focused on developing the strategies and technologies for creating multimodal reality or simulation based content. Resulting state-of-the-art training and education prototype simulators still rely heavily on instructors to interpret performance data, and adapt instruction via scenario generation, mitigations, feedback and after action review tools. Further research is required to fully close the loop and provide automated, adaptive instruction in these learning environments. To meet this goal, an ONR funded initiative focusing on the Training and Education arm of the HPT&E program will address the processes and components required to deliver these capabilities in the form of an Adaptive Instructional Architecture (AIA). An overview of the AIA as it applies to Marine Corps Warfighter training protocols is given as well as the theoretical foundations supporting it.

Keywords: adaptive training systems, augmented cognition, simulation.

1 Introduction

The role of the warfighter has changed significantly over the past decade, yet many current training strategies rely upon inflexible, dedicated training systems that necessitate extensive instructor involvement throughout the learning process [9]. More deployable and flexible multiuse workstations that are cost effective and reduce manning requirements under increased mission demands have been proposed for the Marine Corps warfighter [6]. The core of such workstations is an Adaptive Instructional Architecture (AIA). More specifically, the AIA structure is based upon the central hypothesis that learning methods and technologies which are 1) based on an understanding of task and domain specific knowledge, skill, and attitude needs, 2) driven by continual assessment and diagnosis of individual and team capabilities and potentials, and 3) implemented as adaptive/individualized selection and training solutions produce more efficient and effective combat behavior across the spectrum of Marine Corps missions. Thus, under the current ONR funded initiative of HPT&E,

D.D. Schmorrow, L.M. Reeves (Eds.): Augmented Cognition, HCII 2007, LNAI 4565, pp. 380–384, 2007.
© Springer-Verlag Berlin Heidelberg 2007

the AIA research effort seeks to support flexible adaptive training of Marines engaged in more expected forms of combat as well as irregular or nontraditional warfare.

More recently, empirical results from ONR funded initiatives (e.g., VIRTE) have included viable methodologies for measuring the cognitive state of the user. The use of neuropsychological sensing devices such as EEG and fNIR within an Augmented Cognition framework has further advanced the capabilities of learning systems to monitor brain changes as learners progress from novice to expert states [4]. The closed-loop system whereby the users' cognitive state drives the adaptation of the training is a key component to the development and the effectiveness of such multiuse workstations [14]. Further theoretical support for the augmented cognition framework comes from extensive research in the domains of experiential learning and cognitive load theory, which have also been applied to warfighter training paradigms [7].

2 Experiential Learning

Learning by definition is the process by which memories are constructed, while memory is the outcome of learning [13]. Thus, within learning theory, the process of successful learning requires an interaction between the training tools expressing the to-be-learned subject matter and the neural constraints of the learner. Further, contextualized learning environments are pivotal in retraining persons with cognitive deficits caused by traumatic brain injury [17, 5]. Providing a realistic and interactive training protocol may optimize the knowledge acquisition capabilities of the learner, which may in turn decrease training time [3].

The potential advantages of an experiential learning paradigm are that the user is mentally engaged while gaining familiarity with tools of the trade. As shown in figure 1, simulated real-world conditions allows for skill set engagement while delivering naturalistic outcomes caused by the learners' behavior. In turn the learners can reflect

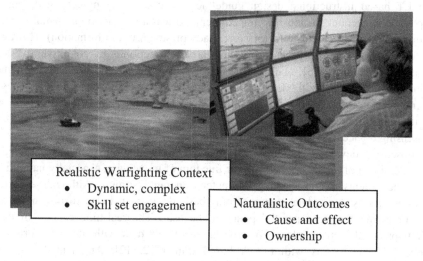

Fig. 1. Advantages of an experiential learning environment

on the outcomes of their problem solving strategies, which allows them to build their knowledge base of military relevant occupational requirements. In addition, the adaptive nature of the training environment will allow for increasing complexity that allows for further expansion of the learners skill set and working knowledge [7]. In the view of positive regard, the person may also build respect for his or her own capability and responsibility as a team member, which may also motivate learning.

3   Cognitive Load Theory

Underlying the concept of experiential learning is the interaction of a biologically mediated learning system with external training delivery protocols. The nature of this interaction has been speculated from either side of the interface through theories of memory to best practices in pedagogy. For example, the construct of a "schema" or knowledge structures that can guide attention and direct behavior through the acquisition and retrieval of context relevant information have been postulated as a structural ideation for long-term memory [1, 11]. More recently, the concept has been extended to instructional design methodologies [15] in the form of Cognitive Load Theory (CLT).

The concern between instructional design and human brain architecture is one of facilitating comprehension and problem solving through appropriately structured instructions and optimized multimodal data presentations [10]. CLT maintains that any instructional delivery system must account for the limitations in the brain processing capabilities (e.g., attention and working memory) of the user. Increases in cognitive load imposed by complex learning environments may not leave enough processing capacity for appropriate levels of learning to occur [8].

CLT based instructional design guidelines for creating computer-aided training applications account for intrinsic impediments to learning (e.g., poor spatial rotation ability), as well as extrinsic factors (e.g., lack of supportive information). However, direct measurement of brain processing areas susceptible to cognitive overload remains problematic [16]. The measurement issues are similar to those of augmented cognition and operationally defining cognitive state along with subsequent changes in cognitive state associated with learning. Both CLT and augmented cognition are brain architecture based paradigms that can be more explicitly researched utilizing biosensing devices.

Biosensing devices commonly used in augmented cognition studies are pictured in Figure 2. Each of the devices allows for freedom of movement, especially naturalistic head movements, when viewing computer generated stimuli. Although computer monitors are shown, data capture from these devices includes displaying visual stimuli within the frontoparallel plane of the user. The real-time capture of these psychophysical metrics allows for correlation of this data with human information processing capabilities within AIA based trainer [2, 12]. Augmented cognition

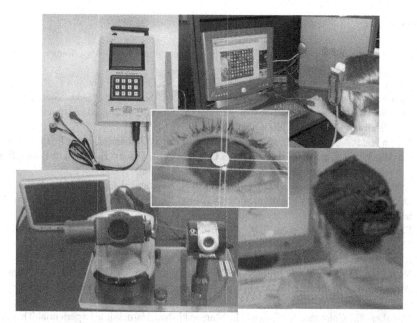

Fig. 2. Biosensing devices commonly used in Augmented Cognition research. Clockwise. Wearable Arousal Meter (Clemson University), Near Infrared Imaging (Archinoetics), Mobile EEG (B-Alert System), and Head and Eye tracking (Applied Science Laboratories).

methodologies coupled with CL theory allows the basis for testable hypotheses that can further direct the design cycle of the AIA.

4 Conclusions

The workstation of the 21st Century Marine Corps warfighter must not only deliver effective training to a single learner, it must adapt to each learner and present a multiplicity of potential occupational situations to many learners with reliability and fidelity. The AIA infrastructure potentially delivers a cost efficient solution; however, more research into the design requirements of such a system are pending. Experiential learning and cognitive load theories will assist in driving this research. Together with an augmented cognition framework, the bridge between instructional design and neural based learning theories will allow us to more clearly define constructs such as cognitive state and its relationship to learning.

Acknowledgements. This work was supported by the Office of Naval Research as part of the Human Performance Training and Education (HPT&E) program and through a Presidential Equipment Grant from the University of Central Florida. The authors would like to thank the members of the Applied Cognition and Training in Immersive Virtual Environments (ACTIVE) lab for assisting with this work in progress.

References

1. Bartlett, F.C.: Remembering: A Study in Experimental and Social Psychology. Cambridge University Press, Cambridge (1932)
2. Berka, C., Levendowski, D., Hale, K., Fuchs, S.: Objective Measures of Situational Awareness Using Neurophysiology Technology. In: Schmorrow, D.D., Stanney, K.M., Reeves, L.M. (eds.) Foundations of Augmented Cognition, 2nd edn. Strategic Analysis Inc, Virginia, pp. 145–154 (2006)
3. Kirschner, P.A., Sweller, J., Clark, R.E.: Why Minimal Guidance During Instruction Does Not Work: An Anlaysis of the Failure of Constructivist, Discovery, Problem-Based, Experiential and Inquiry based Teaching. Edu. Psych. 41, 75–86 (2006)
4. Kruse, A.A., Schmorrow, D.D.: Foundations of Augmented Cognition. In: Schmorrow, D.D. (ed.) Foundations of Augmented Cognition, pp. 441–445. Lawrence Erlbaum, Mahawah (2005)
5. Fidopiastis, C.M., Stapleton, C.B., Whiteside, J.D., Hughes, C.E., Fiore, S.M., Martin, G.A, Rolland, J.P., Smith, E.M.: Human Experience Modeler: Context-Driven Cognitive Retraining to Facilitate Transfer of Learning. Cyberpsychol. Behav. 9, 183–187 (2006)
6. Nicholson, D., Stanney, K., Fiore, S., Davis, L., Fidopiastis, C., Finkelstein, N., Arnold.: An Adaptive System for Improving and Augmenting Human Performance. In: Proc Aug Cog 2 (2006)
7. Menaker, E., Coleman, S., Collins, J., Murawski, M.: Harnessing Experiential Theory to Achieve Warfighter Excellence. In: Proceedings of the Interservice/Industry Training, Simulation, and Education Conference (I/ITSEC), Orlando (2006)
8. van van Merrënboer, J.J, Kirschner, P.A., Kester, L.: Taking the Load Off a Learner's Mind: Instructional Design for Complex Learning. Edu. Psych 38, 5–13 (2003)
9. Osga, G.A.: 21st Century Workstations – Active Partners in Accomplishing Task Goals. In: Proceedings of the Human Factors and Ergonomics Society 44th Annual Meeting. Human Factors and Ergonomics Society, Santa Monica (2000)
10. Pollock, E., Chandler, P., Sweller, J.: Assimilating Complex Information. Learn Inst. 12, 61–68 (2002)
11. Schank, R.C.: Conceptual Information Processing. Elsevier, New York (1975)
12. Schmorrow, D.D.: Foundations of Augmented Cognition, vol. II. Lawrence Erlbaum, Mahawah (2005)
13. Squire, L.R.: Memory and Brain. Oxford University Press, New York (1987)
14. St. John, M., Kobus, D.A., Morrison, J.G., Schmorrow, D.D.: Overview of DARPA Augmented Cognition Technical Integration Experiment. In: Schmorrow, D.D. (ed.) Foundations of Augmented Cognition, pp. 446–452. Lawrence Erlbaum, Mahawah (2005)
15. Sweller, J.: Instructional Design in Technical Areas. Australian Council for Educational Research, Australia (1999)
16. Whelan, R.R.: Neuroimaging of Cognitive Load in Instructional Multimedia. Ed Res Rev (2006) (in press)
17. Ylvisaker, M.: Traumatic Brain injury Rehabilitation, Children and Adolescents. 2nd edn. Butterworth-Heinemann, Boston (1998)

AFFectIX – An Affective Component as Part of an E-Learning-System

Karina Oertel, Robin Kaiser, Jörg Voskamp, and Bodo Urban

Fraunhofer Institute for Computer Graphics, Division Rostock,
Joachim-Jungius-Straße 11, 18059 Rostock, Germany
{karina.oertel, robin.kaiser, jörg.voskamp,
bodo.urban}@igd-r.fraunhofer.de

Abstract. This paper presents a system component, so called AFFectIX, as an affix to an e-learning system which was that way enhanced with affective abilities. AFFectIX is based on an emotion recognition sensor system and aims to reply negative emotions during human-computer interaction and to provoke an optimum emotional level for the learning process. It was implemented as a first prototype and evaluated by an ad-hoc sample of ten participants. First findings indicate a slight tendency for more satisfaction and learning success.

Keywords: Affective Computing, Usability, Emotion Recognition, E-Learning.

1 Introduction

Despite the ongoing development in technology over the past decades, computers widely still do not consider emotions of their users, even though many studies showed how important they are for communication, cognition and more satisfied and effective human-computer interaction [8] [11]. In particular e-learning systems concentrate mainly on the learning target up to now, whereas human expert tutors also focus on the emotional component of learning [5] and current research [2] [4] [1] demonstrate that negative emotions like boredom or angriness reduce cognitive effort, cause performance problems and in consequence hinder the achievement of learning goals whereas positive emotions increase the learning success and improve abilities for problem solving significantly.

In this paper we are focusing on the interplay between emotions and computers in the learning domain and present an affective component, so called AFFectIX, as an affix to an e-learning system. AFFectIX recognizes emotions by the integration of a sensor system and the application of a classifier to model affective states, both were developed at Fraunhofer IGD Rostock [6]. Based on these results it is selecting and executing predefined actions during interaction with users to reply negative emotions and provoke an optimum emotional level for the learning process.

In an empirical study three questions should be clarified: (1) Are users more pleased when using the affixed system? (2) Will a greater learning success achieved? (3) Do users of the affixed system have more positive and less negative emotions? The first two questions were proofed by using questionnaires regarding satisfaction

D.D. Schmorrow, L.M. Reeves (Eds.): Augmented Cognition, HCII 2007, LNAI 4565, pp. 385–393, 2007.
© Springer-Verlag Berlin Heidelberg 2007

and factual knowledge respectively. Question three was checked by the Affective Monitor, which was implemented to log affective states, their residence time, and the status of AFFectIX as well.

2 Emotion Recognition

2.1 Model of Emotions

Valence-Arousal-Performance. AFFectIX and the used sensor system as well are based on the most common circumplex model of emotions [13], a dimensional approach for classifying emotions. It assumes the existence of the dimensions valence (positive or negative) and arousal (the intensity of feeling) utilized to describe different emotions in a continuous manner (see fig. 1). The Yerkes-Dodson law demonstrates an **empirical** relationship between **arousal** and performance with a bell-shaped curve. It dictates that performance increases with cognitive arousal but only to a certain point: when levels of arousal become too high, performance will decrease. A **corollary** is that there is an optimal level of arousal for a given task. In contrast, a slight positive valence seems to be the optimum for performing a task [2].

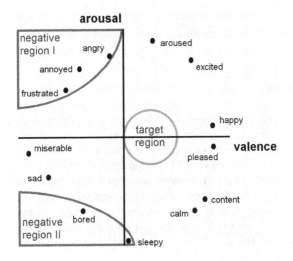

Fig. 1. Regions of Emotion

Negative Emotions. For the learning process, two negative regions in the valence-arousal-space can be defined that should be avoided (see fig. 1). By negative valence and positive arousal region 1 is described, which stands for emotions like frustration and angriness. Emotions like boredom and sleepiness are represented by region 2, located in an emotion-space characterized by negative valence and negative arousal.

Target Emotions. The target region for emotion (see fig. 1), specified by a slight positive valence and neutral arousal, provides a maximum of efficiency and productivity in learning. Besides, the user will probably feel more comfortable during the learning process [2].

2.2 Sensor System

Emotion recognition represents the first step in building affective applications. To detect emotions and deduce emotional states we decided to analyze physiological data since emotions are coupled with changes of physiological parameters and needed bio-sensors are convenient, requiring minimal effort on the user's part. The used emotion recognition sensor system EREC [6] belongs to so-called affective wearables, which can be intuitively operated with a battery pack and consists of a sensor glove, a chest belt and a data collection unit. Integrated in the glove are sensors for heart rate, galvanic skin response and skin temperature for real-time measurements. Evaluated sensor data are wirelessly sent to the data collection unit where they are subject to error checks and further analyses. The enhanced data are then available to a PC or stored on an exchangeable memory card.

2.3 Classification

To deduce affective states from physiological data a procedure is needed, which map sensor signals to valence- and arousal-values according to our emotional model. In the first processing step, measured data are delivered from sensors and made available for following processing steps while utilizing the OmniRoute framework developed at Fraunhofer IGD Rostock. In the next step, the same filters are applied, that were used in the data mining process before, in order to support same value ranges. Finally, trained classifiers are applied. It has shown, that output for the most probable emotion should not be given as a basic emotion (i.e. anger, joy), but rather as a continuous value lying between 0 to 1 respectively for valence and arousal. This helps to assess the results in relation to specific tasks. With data mining techniques we are able to fuse the acquired multi-modal data and derive the desired information on the user in real-time. Tests confirm a prediction performance for basic emotions up to 70% (random classifiers reaches about 20%).

3   AFFectIX

3.1   Architecture

Elements and Relations. AFFectIX consists of the following components: (1) a emotion recognition module which integrates the above mentioned sensor system and the classification scheme; (2) a catalogue of actions to reply negative emotions; (3) a module for selection of appropriate actions; (4) a module for execution of theses actions; and (5) a user model, from which (1) – (4) are implemented so far (see fig.2). Main source for the execution module is the selection module which gets input from the catalogue of actions. The learning environment and the affective component are connected via a special communication channel and represented by one user interface the learners are interacting with.

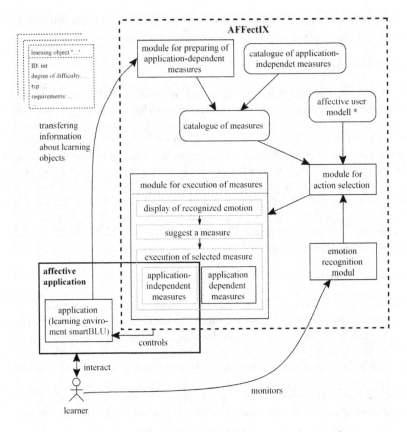

Fig. 2. Architecture of AFFectIX, (*) was not implemented

Procedure. Before the interaction between learners and the affixed e-learning system can started, the preparation of the catalogue of actions has to be finished. After the system start[1] AFFectIX is active and the permanent tracking of physiological data begins. Based on the physiological data the emotional states are recognized by the recognition module. Depending on these results the action selection module selects appropriate actions. Finally, the selected actions were executed. This process consists of three steps according to [4]: (1) the display of recognized emotion; (2) the offer of selected action; and (3) the performance of action.

3.2 Basic System

The learning environment SmartBLU [14] provides an e-learning system for the Internet. SmartBLU has been developed since 1996 at Fraunhofer IGD Rostock. It offers a wide range of functionality for learners, authors, tutors and administrators to create and provide online-courses.

---

[1] The active mode of AFFectIX is recognizable as an icon in system tray and could be controlled by a special menu.

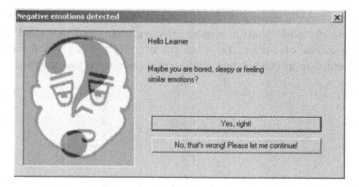

Fig. 3. Example for displaying a recognized emotion

3.3 Catalogue of Actions

A catalogue of affective actions describes actions to support the user in managing negative emotions. Besides a distinction of measures for both region 1 and 2, actions are separated into application-independent or application-dependent actions. Examples for application-independent actions used by AFFectIX are motivational statements, the possibility to express displeasure, the suggestion of a short break or even a way to treat the computer with hammer, flamethrower and chain saw to reduce stress. These actions could according to [3] further differentiated into passive supports that are used to manipulate moods without necessarily addressing or discussing the emotions themselves including media, activities etc. and active support that occurs when people's emotions were addressed directly. Application-dependent actions, bound to the given e-learning system or at least to the application domain, are mainly changes of lessons or of manner to present the subject (e.g. an animation instead of pure text) or the start of a questionnaire to check the learners learn progress.

3.4 Selection of Actions

With a technology for detecting different emotions, well-defined regions of negative and target emotions and a catalogue of actions as well, it is still open what the affective procedure looks like. We suppose to select replying actions depending on predominant emotions which are characterized by residence time mainly. Moreover the selection depends on the availability of actions: while application-independent actions could be continuously offered application-dependent actions have to consider constraints of application and relations between actions as well.

3.5 Execution of Actions

Step 1: Display of recognized emotion. To initialize the process for executing actions we decided to display the recognized emotion for 3 reasons: (1) to convey emotions as an essential ability of affective computing which could already motivate a change of mood; (2) to let the user verify the recognized emotion; and (3) to consider that in learning environments the use of avatars who do not have to be necessarily virtual characters are obviously leads to a more effective, funny and motivated interaction. The display consist of a comic face (one per negative region), which illustrates the recognized emotion in combination with a color code for it and a verbal paraphrase (see fig. 3).

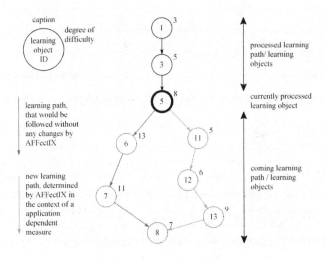

Fig. 4. Changes of learning path

Step 2: Offer of selected action. According to the display of recognized emotion (see fig.3) a selected action was offered whereas the comic face illustrates the target emotion. The proposed action could be confirmed or rejected by the user.

Step 3: Execution of action. If the user confirms a selected action it will be executed whereas the observation of affective states is continued in case of rejection. Figure 4 illustrates the change of learning path as main instrument for execution of application-dependent actions.

4   Experimental Study

4.1   Setup

To track and record the process of emotion recognition and the residence time in different emotional states or regions the Affective Monitor as a further module of AFFectIX was developed. The Affective Monitor displays the values of valence and arousal and the resulted mapping to one of the three emotional regions (see figure 1) for every classification. Furthermore the past time since last action and the dominance (percent) of one emotional region were shown. Additionally it presents the mean of residence time in each region, the average of valence and arousal, and the number of measures in the regions. Corresponding precise values were documented one in a second and reset after an execution of an action.

4.2 Method

Participants and Tasks. Ten participants (3 female, 7 male), who were randomly separated into two groups, took part. Group 1 was supported by AFFectIX whereas group 2 was not. Both of them had to wear the sensor glove and execute representative tasks. The e-learning content (selected lessons for beginners about financial accounting) was able to explore within 30 minutes and do not require any further knowledge. It contains a set of different lessons, a test module and multimedia learning objects.

Procedure. The test started by a short introduction and the activation of the sensor system and the Affective Monitor. Then a short slideshow of pictures using the International Affective Picture System (IAPS) was shown to determine the individual classification space. After that the tasks were executed and questionnaires have to be fulfilled finally.

Measures and Questionnaires. The *state of emotion* was acquired by the emotion recognition module and represented by the Affective Monitor. For *user satisfaction* a questionnaire was used containing 8 questions to be rated on a 5point scale. Moreover there were additionally questions for group 1 (affective group) to get assessments especially for the use of AFFectIX. The *learning success* was evaluated by using multiple choice questions within the test module.

5 Preliminary Results

5.1 Results

State of Emotion. Measures for the affective group were more often in negative region 1 as for group 2, but for region 2 it was contrary (see table 1). Moreover emotional states of participants of control group were more often measured in the target region than it is for group 1. So we could not see that learners supported by AFFectIX are less of negative emotions or more often in positive or neutral mood.

Table 1. Results for state of emotion

	participants (ID)											
	group 1 (affective group)						group 2 (control group)					
	0	2	4	6	9	Ø	1	3	5	7	9	Ø
valence	-0.65	-0.98	-0.83	-0.67	-0.30	-0.42	0.67	0.51	0.31	0.01	0.37	0.17
arousal	-0.48	0.30	0.17	0.03	0.07	0.09	-0.49	0.14	0.51	0.79	0.70	0.33
region 1	0	23	24	0	21	14	7	31	5	34	15	18
region 2	41	0	5	0	7	11	0	0	1	1	1	1
target region	0	0	0	0	0	0	0	0	1	0	1	0

User Satisfaction. The questionnaire data show that the fun factor of the course was rated higher by the affective group whereas the participants of the control group were more satisfied with the course and rated it's worth higher (see table 2).

Table 2. Results for user satisfaction (abstract)

questions	participants (ID)											
	group 1 (affective group)						group 2 (control group)					
	0	2	4	6	9	Ø	1	3	5	7	9	Ø
relevance of course	-1	0	1	1	1	0.4	1	-2	1	2	1	0.6
fun	0	1	1	1	0	0.6	0	0	0	1	-1	0.0
satisfaction	0	-1	0	1	1	0.2	1	-1	1	1	1	0.6
accuracy of recognition	1	0	-2	-	2	0.2	-	-	-	-	-	-
helpfulness of actions	-1	-	-	-	-1	-1.0	-	-	-	-	-	-

Learning Success. Table 3 shows that a greater learning success was achieved by group 1 and that the actions of AFFectIX apparently do not hinder the learning or exploring process.

Table 3. Results for learning success

	participants (ID)											
	group 1 (affective group)						group 2 (control group)					
	0	2	4	6	9	Ø	1	3	5	7	9	Ø
test results	72%	97%	94%	74%	97%	87%	97%	51%	90%	92%	62%	78%

5.2 Discussion

The obtained data indicate a slight tendency for more satisfaction and learning success as well by participants using AFFectIX, even though neither less negative emotions nor more positive ones could be measured. Taken together, the provided results can be considered as first assumptions regarding interaction with an affective e-learning system which have to be examined more closely. They also point at the difficulties of designing an interactive system what is not only affective but also adaptive regarding the users and tasks. Moreover, the current research reveal some important issues to be dealt with if constructive work for an affective system has be done: (1) What does emotions recognition rates below 100 percent mean for strategies of emotion response?; (2) What strategy should be applied if emotion response failed or was rejected by user?; (3) What and wherefrom information about application and user should be obtained to generate adequate system response?; (4) Are possibly domain-specific models of emotion relevant?

6 Conclusions

The presented paper demonstrates AFFectIX as our first prototype of a system component that seems capable of providing active emotional support to learners interacting with an affective e-learning system. AFFectIX couples emotion recognition technology with a new approach for emotional response that potentially leads to an engaging and productive interaction. Still even from our small explorative study some lessons for how to design an affective system can be extracted. First, convey of recognized emotion to the user seems to be good strategies for emotional dialogue in HCI and help to overcome the problem of emotion recognition rates of about 70 percent as well. Second, selection and control of application-depended actions for emotional response are possibly main challenges of building affective systems that require a deep understanding of respective application domain and application-specific criteria (e.g. dialogue elements, alternative or redundant navigation paths, hierarchy and priority of content). Third, the affective system will probably work best when it learns the individual preferences of its user, including possibly characteristics of the user's personality.

References

1. Jaques, P.A., et al.: Applying Affective Tactics for a Better Learning. In: European Conference on Artificial Intelligence. Valencia, pp. 109–113 (2004)
2. Kaiser, R.: Prototypical development of an affective component for an e-learning system. Master thesis, University of Rostock, Germany, Department of Computer Science (2006)
3. Klein, J., Moon, Y., Picard, R.W.: This Computer Responds to User Frustration: Theory, Design, and Results. Interacting with Computers 14(2), 119–140 (2002)
4. Kort, B., Reilly, R., Picard, R.W.: An Affective Model of Interplay Between Emotions and Learning: Reengineering Educational Pedagogy – Building a Learning Companion. In: Advanced Learning Technologies (2001)
5. Lepper, M.R., Chabay, R.W.: Socializing the Intelligent Tutor: Bringing Empathy to Computer Tutors. In: Learning issues for intelligent tutoring systems, pp. 242–257. Springer, Heidelberg (1988)
6. Peter, C., et al.: A Wearable Multi-Sensor System for Mobile Acquisition of Emotion-Related Physiological Data. In: Tao, J., Tan, T., Picard, R.W. (eds.) ACII 2005. LNCS, vol. 3784, pp. 691–698. Springer, Heidelberg (2005)
7. Oertel, K., et al.: EmoTetris for Recognition of Affective States. In: HCI International [Proceedings on CD-Rom] (2005)
8. Picard, R.W.: Affective Computing. MIT Press, Cambridge, Massachusetts (1997)
9. Picard, R.W.: Affective Computing for HCI. In: Proceedings of 8th International Conference on Human-Computer Interaction. pp. 829–833 (1999)
10. Picard, R.W.: Toward Computers that Recognize and Respond to user Emotion. IBM Systems Journal 39, 705–719 (2000)
11. Reeves, B., Nass, C.: The media equation: How people treat computers, television, and new media like real people and places. Cambridge University Press, New York (1996)
12. Reynolds, C., Picard, R.W.: Designing for Affective Interactions. In: Proceedings of the 9th International Conference on Human-Computer Interaction. New Orleans (2001)
13. Russell, J.A.: A circumplex model of affect. Journal of Personality and Social Psychology 39, 1161–1178 (1980)
14. SmartBLU: Learning Management System smartBLU. Accessed (September 30, 2006) http://www.smartblu.de

Performance Compared to Experience Level in a Virtual Reality Surgical Skills Trainer

Christoph Aschwanden[1], Lawrence Burgess[1], and Kevin Montgomery[2]

[1] Telehealth Research Institute, John A. Burns School of Medicine,
651 Ilalo St., Honolulu, Hawaii 96813, USA
{caschwan, lburgess}@hawaii.edu
[2] Stanford-NASA National Biocomputation Center, 701 Welch Road,
Suite 1128, Palo Alto, CA 94304, USA
kevin@biocomp.stanford.edu

Abstract. A virtual reality (VR) manual skills experiment was conducted comparing Human performance measures to experiences indicated on a questionnaire handed out. How much do past experiences influence human performance on a VR surgical skills simulator? Performance measures included; time, accuracy, efficiency of motion and errors. Past experiences are among video games and computer proficiency. Results showed little or no relations between experience level and performance. Significant results could only be established for computer gaming experience versus task completion time, $F(1, 22) = 3.3$, $p = .083$. Participants familiar with computer gaming were able to carry out tasks faster than their counterparts.

Keywords: Skills Training, Experience, Performance, Surgery, Laparoscopy, Endoscopy, Gaming, Joystick, Virtual Reality, Simulation, Time, Accuracy, Efficiency, Motion, Errors, HCI, VRMSS, SPRING.

1 Introduction

Minimally invasive surgery has been shown to have advantages over conventional open methods with decreased postoperative morbidity and more rapid healing. Laparoscopic procedures now represent the 'gold standard' for various abdominal surgical procedures [1], and endoscopic procedures are commonplace in other surgical specialties. Both utilize endoscopes and instruments to access a cavity, but the term laparoscopic is used for abdominal or pelvic endoscopic procedures. Microscopic procedures also require specialized skill training and are utilized to some extent in most surgical specialties. Training is necessary to ensure skills acquisition prior to patient contact to maintain the highest standards of patient care, and to maintain skills for infrequently performed procedures. With the steady validation and assimilation of simulation training into medical education, there is also the ethical imperative to utilize such training whenever possible before laying hands on the patient [2].

Beginning endoscopic surgeons are faced with two nuances to the procedure. Unlike open surgery, laparoscopic and endoscopic surgeons have to work in three

D.D. Schmorrow, L.M. Reeves (Eds.): Augmented Cognition, HCII 2007, LNAI 4565, pp. 394–399, 2007.

dimensions (3-D) while viewing an operation on a 2-D video monitor. This change decreases depth perception which can increase technical errors. Secondly, an instrument must be manipulated through a single entry point into the cavity, which creates a pivot or fulcrum point. This limits instrument maneuverability and also causes the surgeon to have decreased access and visibility, which can lead to an increase in technical errors. Due to these technical issues, training is necessary to reduce the incidence of potential complications during surgery.

Currently employed training environments include inanimate box trainers as well as virtual reality simulators. Advantages to box trainers are the following: low cost which increases access and availability; the use of actual laparoscopic instruments and a video camera and monitor, which helps with pivot point training and transitioning from 3-D to 2-D on a monitor. Its weaknesses in comparison to VR trainers are the following: lacks automated objective scoring which increases the need for instructors; lacks graphics and immersive features which reduces gaming characteristics of user interactivity, competition, and "fun"; lacks intermediate or advanced task training. Detailed performance assessment on inanimate box trainers requires subjectively monitored human evaluation. This process is not only costly but also error-prone [3]. VR simulators collect data automatically and therefore more data can be accurately recorded [1;4;5].

In a first step to validate a virtual reality surgical skill trainer created, a usability study has been conducted to assess satisfaction levels with the skills trainer. During the study, experiences of participants using the system were collected in order to compare the data to performance measures. Experiences were among video games and computer proficiency. Performance measures included time, accuracy, efficiency of motion and errors.

2 Related Work

The impact of hand dominance, gender, and experience with computer games on the performance in virtual reality laparoscopy shows computer gaming experience as well as right hand dominance to have an impact on laparoscopic performance [6-8]. Prior experience with billiards has also been shown to improve performance in VR simulators [8]. In another study, right-handed subjects were found to perform better with either hand in terms of error rate and first time accuracy [9].

In non-VR based studies, improvement was shown after generalized and task specific laparoscopic skills training, with no difference observed between left and right-handed surgeons [10;11].

Based on results from those studies, participants for the surgical skills exercise are expected to exhibit increased performance if they had prior computer gaming experience compared to those with none or little.

3 VR Skills Study

A virtual reality manual skills experiment was conducted comparing Human performance measures to experiences indicated on a questionnaire handed out.

3.1 Participants

The VR skills study took place November 13-15, 2006 in the lobby of the Medical Education Building, John A. Burns School of Medicine, University of Hawaii. Faculty, staff, students and visitors were randomly asked to volunteer and participate in a surgical skills study evaluating a manual surgical skills simulator. Twenty-four subjects were recruited during the three day session. Participants were among various age groups and professions.

3.2 Materials

The study consisted of a consent form, a surgical skills trainer and a questionnaire to assess experiences and satisfaction levels.

The VRMSS [12;13] is a surgical skills training environment created by the Telehealth Research Institute in collaboration with Stanford University using SPRING, a real-time soft-tissue simulation platform for building and running surgical simulators to be used in medical education of surgeons [14]. VRMSS allows for Haptics interaction with a 3D training environment for surgical skills acquisition. Two Phantom Omnis are used to keep costs low. Task configurations include dominant, non-dominant hand as well as bimanual training. Environment layouts are comprised of normal, microscopic and endoscopic views. A foot pedal supports zooming. See Figure 1 for details.

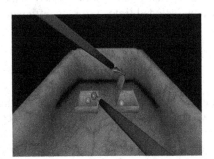 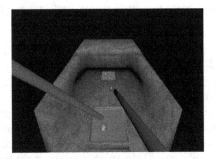

Fig. 1. Virtual Reality Motor-Skills Simulator Scenarios. Left: Transfer skills training with hinged cup in basic environment. Right: Transfer skills training with blood suction in microscopic environment using a foot pedal for zooming.

The questionnaire handed out was based on the Questionnaire for User Interaction Satisfaction (QUIS), a tool developed by a multi-disciplinary team of researchers in the Human-Computer Interaction Lab (HCIL) at the University of Maryland at College Park [15]. QUIS is designed to assess a users' subjective satisfaction with specific aspects of a human-computer interface. QUIS7 was extended to address the utilized virtual reality interface. Questions asked were among (1) past experiences, (2) overall user reactions, (3) screen, (4) learning, (5) multimedia and (6) virtual environment.

3.3 Procedure

At the beginning, each participant received a consent form and information about the study conducted. Participants were then asked to sit down at the VRMSS to execute the surgical skills exercises.

The VRMSS experiment consisted of two parts; participants were first introduced to the virtual reality surgical skills simulator using a tutorial-type scenario explaining the instruments and tasks to perform. A second scenario was designated as the actual experiment for performance data recording. Performance measures for both scenarios were among (a) time, (b) accuracy, (c) efficiency of motion and (d) errors committed.

After the VRMSS session, subjects were given the QUIS questionnaire to assess their experience and satisfaction level with the surgical skills training environment.

3.4 Results

Averaged performance measures have been compared to past experiences indicated on the QUIS questionnaire. The following experiences were selected for analysis. Subjects would check the box to state that they had personally used and were familiar with a system:

- Computer Games
- Trackball
- Joystick
- Pen Based Computing
- Graphics Tablet

Participant's occupation (medical vs. non-medical) was recorded as well. Performance measures chosen:

- Task duration (time: how fast did a participant finish)
- Failed placements in target area (accuracy)
- Instrument-Wall Collisions for dominant & non-dominant hands (errors)
- Instrument path length for dominant & non-dominant hands (efficiency)

Data analysis showed little or no correlations between past experiences and performance measures. One-Way ANOVA displayed significance at the .1 level for "Computer Gaming" experience and "Task Duration" only, $F(1, 22) = 3.3$, $p = .083$. No other relations could be established.

3.5 Discussion

It appears experiences with trackball, joystick, pen and graphics tablet do not transfer to increased performance on the VRMSS. A participant's occupation, medical or non-medical, does not show differences in score.

However, results indicate significance at a marginal level for computer gaming experience versus task completion time. Participants familiar with computer gaming were able to carry out tasks faster than their counterparts.

4 Contributions and Future Directions

Results have confirmed findings with previous publications describing computer gaming experience to be beneficial for surgical skills training [7]. Gaming experience transfers to increase speed in task execution on the VRMSS at a significant level, $F(1, 22) = 3.3$, $p = .083$.

No connection between computer input devices (trackball, joystick, pen, graphics tablet) and VRMSS performance was found. Input devices listed do not appear to enhance surgical training outcomes. No differences were observed between participants with medical and non-medical occupation.

Further studies are planned to explore and compare surgical proficiency with performance measures such as accuracy, efficiency and errors committed. We will address questions on how surgeons compare to novices during surgical skills assessment.

References

1. O'Toole, R.V., Playter, R.R., Krummel, T.M., Blank, W.C., Cornelius, N.H., Roberts, W.R., Bell, W.J., Raibert, M.: Measuring and developing suturing technique with a virtual reality surgical simulator. J. Am. Coll. Surg. 189(1), 114–127 (1999)
2. Ziv, A., Wolpe, P.R., Small, S.D., Glick, S.: Simulation-Based Medical Education: An Ethical Imperative. Academic Medicine 78(8), 783–788 (2003)
3. Woodrum, D.T., Andreatta, P.B., Yellamanchilli, R.K., Feryus, L., Gauger, P.G., Minter, R.M.: Construct validity of the LapSim laparoscopic surgical simulator. Am. J. Surg. 191(1), 28–32 (2006)
4. Gallagher, A.G., Smith, C.D., Bowers, S.P., Seymour, N.E., Pearson, A., McNatt, S., Hananel, D., Satava, R.M.: Psychomotor skills assessment in practicing surgeons experienced in performing advanced laparoscopic procedures. J. Am. Coll. Surg. 197(3), 479–488 (2003)
5. Stylopoulos, N., Cotin, S., Maithel, S.K., Ottensmeye, M., Jackson, P.G., Bardsley, R.S., Neumann, P.F., Rattner, D.W., Dawson, S.L.: Computer-enhanced laparoscopic training system (CELTS): bridging the gap. Surg. Endosc. 18(5), 782–789 (2004)
6. Korndorffer Jr., J.R., Stefanidis, D., Scott, D.J.: Laparoscopic skills laboratories: current assessment and a call for resident training standards. Am. J. Surg. 191(1), 17–22 (2006)
7. Grantcharov, T.P., Bardram, L., Funch-Jensen, P., Rosenberg, J.: Impact of hand dominance, gender, and experience with computer games on performance in virtual reality laparoscopy. Surg. Endosc. 17(7), 1082–1085 (2003)
8. Stefanidis, D., Korndorffer, J., Blank, W.C., Dunne, J.B., Sierra, R., Touchard, B.A., Rice, D.A., Markert, R.J., Kastl, P.R., Scott, D.J.: Psychomotor testing predicts rate of skill acquisition for proficiency-based laparoscopic skills training. Surgery 140(2), 252–262 (2006)
9. Hanna, G.B., Drew, T., Clinch, P., Shimi, S., Dunkley, P., Hau, C., Cuschieri, A.: Psychomotor skills for endoscopic manipulations: differing abilities between right and left-handed individuals. Ann. Surg. 225(3), 333–338 (1997)
10. Powers, T.W., Bentrem, D.J., Nagle, A.P., Toyama, M.T., Murphy, S.A., Murayama, K.M.: Hand dominance and performance in a laparoscopic skills curriculum. Surg. Endosc. 19(5), 673–677 (2005)

11. Powers, T.W., Murayama, K.M., Toyama, M., Murphy, S., Denham III., E.W., Derossis, A.M., Joehl, R.J.: Housestaff performance is improved by participation in a laparoscopic skills curriculum. Am. J. Surg. 184(6), 626–629 (2002)
12. Aschwanden, C., Sherstyuk, A., Burgess, L., Montgomery, K.: A Surgical and Fine-Motor Skills Trainer for Everyone? In: Touch and Force-Feedback in a Virtual Reality Environment for Surgical Training, pp. 19–21. IOS Press, Amsterdam (2006)
13. Aschwanden, C., Hara, K., Burgess, L., Montgomery, K.: Virtual Reality Simulation for Surgical Skills Training in Medical Education, University of Hawaii John A. Burns School of Medicine (2007)
14. Montgomery, K., Bruyns, C., Brown, J., Thonier, G., Tellier, A., Latombe, J.C.: Spring: A General Framework for Collaborative. In: Real-Time Surgical Simulation, pp. 296–303. IOS Press, Amsterdam (2002)
15. Harper, B.D., Slaughter, L., Schneiderman, B.: Questionnaire for User-Interaction Satisfaction (QUIS) (2007) http://lap.umd.edu/quis

Exploring Neural Trajectories of Scientific Problem Solving Skill Acquisition

Ronald H. Stevens[1], Trysha Galloway[1], and Chris Berka[2]

[1] UCLA IMMEX Project, 5601 W. Slauson Ave. #255, Culver City, CA 90230
immex_ron@hotmail.com,
tryshag@gmail.com
[2] Advanced Brain Monitoring, Inc, Carlsbad, CA 92008
chris@b-alert.com

Abstract. We have modeled changes in electroencephalography (EEG) - derived measures of cognitive workload, engagement, and distraction as individuals developed and refined their problem solving skills in science. Subjects performing a series of problem solving simulations showed decreases in the times needed to solve the problems; however, metrics of high cognitive workload and high engagement remained the same. When these indices were measured within the navigation, decision, and display events in the simulations, significant differences in workload and engagement were often observed. In addition, differences in these event categories were also often observed across a series of the tasks, and were variable across individuals. These preliminary studies suggest that the development of EEG-derived models of the dynamic changes in cognitive indices of workload, distraction and engagement may be an important tool for understanding the development of problem solving skills in secondary school students.

Keywords: EEG, Problem solving, Skill Acquisition, Cognitive Workload.

1 Introduction

Skill development occurs in stages that are characterized by changes in the time and mental effort required to exercise the skill (Anderson, 1982, 1995, Schneider and Shiffrin, 1977). Given the complexities of skill acquisition it is not surprising that a variety of approaches have been used to model the process. For instance, some researchers have used machine learning tools to refine models of skill acquisition and learning behaviors in science and mathematics. Such systems rely on learner models that continually provide updated estimates of students' knowledge and misconceptions based on actions such as choosing an incorrect answer or requesting a multimedia hint. Although such learner models are capable of forecasting student difficulties (Stevens, Johnson, & Soller, 2005), or identifying when students may require an educational intervention, they still rely on relatively impoverished input due to the limited range of learner actions that can be detected by the tutoring system (e.g., menu choices, mouse clicks).

D.D. Schmorrow, L.M. Reeves (Eds.): Augmented Cognition, HCII 2007, LNAI 4565, pp. 400–408, 2007.
© Springer-Verlag Berlin Heidelberg 2007

There is a large and growing literature on the EEG correlates of attention, memory, and perception (Fabiani, 2001, Smith, 1999, Berka, 2004, Berka 2006). However, EEG researchers have generally elected to employ study protocols that utilize training-to-criterion to minimize variability across subjects and ensure stable EEG parameters could be characterized. In most studies, the EEG data is not even acquired during the training process, leaving an untapped and potentially rich data source relating to skill acquisition.

While advanced EEG monitoring is becoming more common in high workload / high stress professions (such as tactical command, air traffic controllers), the ideas have not been comprehensively applied to real-world educational settings due to multiple challenges. Some of these challenges are: 1) the acquisition of problem solving skills is a gradual process and not all novices solve problems in the same way, nor do they follow the same path at the same pace as they develop domain understanding; 2) given the diversity of the student population it is difficult to assess what their relative levels of competence are when performing a task making it difficult to accurately relate EEG measures to other measures of skill and 3) the strategic variability makes analyzing the patterns of students' problem solving record too complicated, costly, and time consuming to be performed routinely by instructors; nevertheless, there are many aspects of science education that could benefit from deriving data from advanced monitoring devices and combining them with real-time computational models of the tasks and associated outcomes conditions.

This manuscript describes a beginning synthesis of 1) a probabilistic modeling approach where detailed neural network modeling of problem solving at the population level provides estimates of current and future competence, and, 2) a neurophysiologic approach to skill acquisition where real-time measures of attention, engagement and cognitive work load dynamically contribute estimates of allocation of attention resources and working memory demands as skills are acquired and refined.

2 Methods

The IMMEX™ Problem Solving Environment
The software system used for these studies is termed IMMEX™ which is based on an extensive literature of how students select and use strategies during scientific problem solving (VanLehn, 1996, Haider & Frensch, 1996).

To illustrate the system, a sample biology task called Phyto Physasco provides evidence of a student's ability to identify why the local potato plants are dying. The problem begins with a multimedia presentation explaining the scenario and the student's challenge is to identify the cause. The problem space contains 5 Main Menu items which are used for navigating the problem space, and 38 Sub Menu items describing local weather conditions, soil nutrients, plant appearance, etc. These are decision points, as when the student selects them, s/he confirms that the test was requested and is then presented the data. When students feel they have gathered the information needed to identify the cause they attempt to solve the problem.

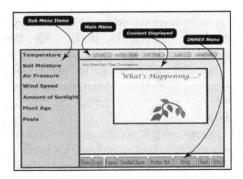

Fig. 1. Sample IMMEX™ simulation. In the Phyto Physasco simulation, potato plants are dying and the student must identify the cause by examining weather conditions, nutrients, etc. Students navigate throughout the problem space using the Main Menu and select data to make decisions using the Sub Menu Items.

The IMMEX database serializes timestamps of how students use these resources. As students solve IMMEX cases, the menu items selected are then used to train competitive, self-organizing ANN (Stevens & Najafi, 1993, Stevens et al, 1996). We use the outputs of this classification to define strategic snapshots of each student's performance. Students often begin by selecting many test items, and consistent with models of skill acquisition (Ericsson, 2004), refine their strategies with time and select fewer tests, eventually stabilizing with an approach that will be used on subsequent problems. As expected, with practice solve rates increase and time on task decreases. The rate of stabilization, and the strategies stabilized with are influenced by gender (Stevens & Soller, 2005), experience (Stevens et al, 2004), and individual or group collaboration.

IMMEX problem solving therefore represents a task where it is possible to construct probabilistic models of many different aspects of problem solving skill acquisition across problem solving domains. The constraints of working memory are likely to be particularly relevant during such skill acquisition where working memory capacity can frequently be exceeded. The possibility of combining these models with EEG workload metrics opens a new window to monitor the cognitive demands and the balances of different working memory capacities needed as students gain experience and begin to stabilize their strategies.

The B-Alert® system

A recently developed wireless EEG sensor headset has combined a battery-powered hardware and sensor placement system to provide a lightweight, easy-to-apply method to acquire and analyze six channels of high-quality EEG. Standardized sensor placements include locations over frontal, central, parietal and occipital regions (sensor sites: F3-F4, C3-C4, Cz-PO, F3-Cz, Fz-C3, Fz-PO). Data are sampled at 256 samples/second with a bandpass from 0.5 Hz and 65Hz (at 3dB attenuation). Quantification of the EEG in real-time, referred to as the B-Alert® system, is achieved using signal analysis techniques to identify and decontaminate fast and slow eye blinks, and identify and reject data points contaminated with excessive muscle activity, amplifier saturation, and/or excursions due to movement artifacts. Wavelet analyses are applied to detect excessive muscle activity (EMG) and to identify and decontaminate eye blinks (Berka 2004, Berka 2007).

Subjects and Study

Subjects (n=12) first performed a single 30-minute baseline EEG test session to adjust the software to accommodate individual differences in the EEG (Berka, 2004). They then performed multiple IMMEX problem sets targeted for 8th-10th grade students. These include Phyto Phyasco, the biology problem described above and a mathematics problem called Paul's Pepperoni Pizza Palace. Subjects generally performed at least 3 cases of each problem set allowing the tracking of strategies and cognitive changes across cases as students gained experience. Then we aligned the EEG output metrics on a second-by-second basis with the problem solving actions to explore the within-task EEG metric changes. For this alignment, we used software (Morea, Techsmith, Inc.) that captures output from the screen, mouse click and keyboard events as well as video and audio output from the users (Figure 2).

The output of the B-Alert software includes EEG metrics (ranging from 0.1-1.0) for distraction (HDT), engagement (HE), and workload (HWL) calculated for each

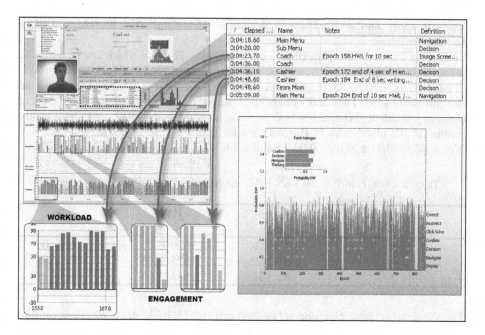

Fig. 2. Relating EEG Workload and Engagement Indexes with Problem Solving Events. The upper left figure is a screen shot of a user (not described in the text) engaged in IMMEX problem solving while keyboard and mouse events are simultaneously recorded; below shows the real-time output of the B-Alert cognitive indexes. Samples of the workload and engagement data streams have been linked with specific events in the log.. In the lower right corner, the timestamps of IMMEX data requests and displays are integrated with the EEG workload indices and then plotted against the one-second epochs of the task. The upper left histograms average the workload indices for each of the IMMEX events including the one second prior to and after the event.

1-second epoch using quadratic and linear discriminant function analyses of model-selected EEG variables derived from power spectral analysis of the 1-Hz bins from 1-40Hz (Berka 2007).

These metrics have proven utility in tracking both phasic and tonic changes in cognitive states, and in predicting errors that result from either fatigue or overload (Berka 2005, Berka 2007). The cognitive indices are expressed as histograms for each 1-second epoch of the problem solving session and show the probability of HWL, HE, or HDT. By integrating the time stamps of data requests with those of the B-Alert system, the navigation, decision, and display-related events can be overlaid onto the cognitive indices.

Increases in Problem Solving Skills Are Not Accompanied by Decreases in Workload or Engagement

We first measured the seconds needed to solve the first, second, and third case of Paul's Pepperoni Pizza (n=7) and calculated the average HWL and HE across the three performances. As shown in Table 1, the time needed to complete the task significantly decreased, however, there were no significant changes in either HWL or HE.

Students Apply Similar Workload to Similar Problems and More Workload to More Difficult Problems

Five of the students also performed 3 cases of Phyto Phyasco which is also a middle school IMMEX problem. There were no significant differences between the HWL ($0.64 \pm .05$ vs. $0.63 \pm .05$, p =.42) and HE ($0.51 \pm .07$, $0.51 \pm .04$, p = .92) across the two problem sets. Two individuals also solved the more difficult high school chemistry problem Hazmat. For both of these individuals the HWL was significantly greater for the three cases of Hazmat than for Paul's Pepperoni Pizza. (Subject 103: $0.76 \pm .02$ vs. $0.71 \pm .03$, p< 0.001; Subject 247: $0.57 \pm .02$ vs. $0.49 \pm .03$, p< 0.005).

Table 1. Changes in Time on Task, HWL and HE With Problem Solving Experience

Performance	Speed (seconds)	HWL	HE
1	422 ± 234	$.629 \pm .07$	$.486 \pm .09$
2	241 ± 126	$.625 \pm .08$	$.469 \pm .08$
3	136 ± 34	$.648 \pm .06$	$.468 \pm .09$

The Navigation and Decision-related Events in IMMEX May Be Behaviorally Relevant

For the initial studies we divided the performance into segments related to problem framing, test selections, confirmation events where the student decides whether or not to pay the fee for the data, and closure where the student decides on the problem solution. The examples for this section were derived from one student who was performing the IMMEX mathematics problem Paul's Pepperoni Pizza. The student missed solving the first case, correctly solved the second case, and then missed the third case indicating that an effective strategy had not yet been formulated.

The problem framing event was defined as the period from when the Prolog first appeared on the screen until the first piece of data information is chosen. For this subject the HWL decreased from the first to the third performance (.72 ± .11 vs. .57 ± .19, t = 28.7, p < .001), and engagement increased .31 ± .30 vs. .49 ±.37 t = 4.3, p <.001). The decreased workload was similar to that observed in other subjects; the increasing HE may relate more to the student missing the problem. During the decision-making process, students often demonstrated a cycling of the B-Alert cognitive indexes characterized by relatively high workload and low engagement which then switched to lower workload and higher engagement (Figure 3). The cycle switches were often, but not always associated with selection of new data.

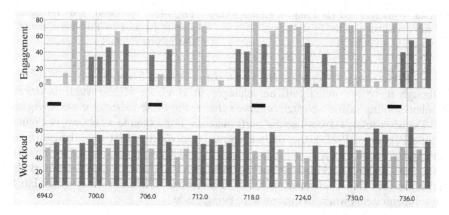

Fig. 3. Fluctuations in HWL and HE during Problem Solving. The bar indicates the epochs where the student made a test selection.

The closing sequences of a problem are a complex process where the student first makes an irrevocable decision to attempt a solution. Then, the he must make a selection choice from an extensive list of possible solutions. Finally, they must confirm their choice. After that they receive feedback on their success / failure; the students have two such solution attempts. The dynamics of HWL and HE for one student's first and second solution attempts of Paul's Pepperoni Pizza are shown in Fig. 4.

In the 10 seconds before deciding to solve the problem (epochs 354 – 364 (I)) there was HWL which decreased as the student made his decision (II, III). Two seconds before the student clicked on and confirmed his choice (epoch 377, IV) there was an increase in engagement which was maintained as the student realized that the answer was incorrect (V).

The workload and engagement dynamics were different on the second solution attempt. Here there was less continuous HWL in the 10 seconds leading up to the decision to solve the problem (Epochs 582- 592, (I, II). At epoch 593 the choice to continue was confirmed, and two seconds before making this decision engagement increased and was maintained during the selection and confirmation process. Between epochs 593 and 596 an incorrect answer was chosen and confirmed (III, IV). At epoch 597 the selection was made and the student learned of the incorrect answer (V).

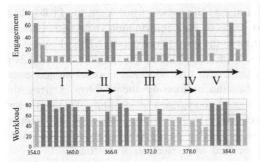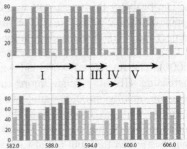

Fig. 4a. Workload and Engagement Events Related to Problem Closure on the First Attempt

Fig. 4b. Workload and Engagement Events Related to Problem Closure on the Second Attempt

Across Performance Changes in HE for Decision-Related Events

Although there are not significant changes in HWL or HE as students develop problem solving skills, we often observed changes in these indices for the Navigation and Decision-related events across performances. For example as shown in Figure 5 (Paul's Pepperoni Pizza), the student correctly solved the first case, had difficulty solving the second case (missing the first try), and then failed to solve the next two cases. The overall workload and engagement levels did not change for this student across the four cases; however, there was a continual increase in the levels of HE for the submenu items where decisions were being made.

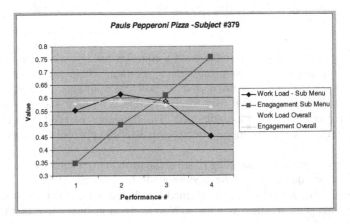

Fig. 5. Changes in Overall HWL and HE and Sub Menu Linked HWL and HE Across Performances

3   Discussion

In this paper we have described a web-based data acquisition architecture and event interleaving process that allows us to map EEG-derived cognitive indices to behaviorally relevant aspects of the students problem solving. An unusual feature of these studies was the application of these technologies to every-day classroom activities that are quite distinct from highly controlled laboratory tasks.

Given the anticipated differences between individual students experience and knowledge, we have focused our initial studies on comparing differences within individuals as skills are developed, rather than compare across individuals. As expected, HWL increased when students were presented with problem sets of greater difficulty. Less expected, however, was the finding that as skills increased, the levels of HWL did not decrease accordingly; suggesting significant mental commitment may be involved during strategic refinement.

By focusing the analyses around relevant problem solving events such as menu navigation and decision making, the changing dynamics of cognitive workload and engagement could be identified. By recording videos of the problem solving process and the user on a second by second basis and interleaving them with EEG cognitive indices through log files generated by IMMEX, the majority of the HWL and HE fluctuations could be linked to observable events such as decision-making and note-taking. Initial studies suggest that decreasing workload and increasing engagement at different events of the problem solving process, such as problem framing and closure, may indicate the student experiencing difficulties and suggest bottlenecks in the learning process. These studies indicate the development of EEG-derived models of the dynamic changes in cognitive indices of workload, distraction, and engagement could be an important tool for understanding the development of problem solving skills in secondary school and university students. Long-term, such models may help target interventions to specific aspects of problem solving where the mental states of an individual reveal barriers to acquiring problem solving skills.

Acknowledgements. Supported in part by grants from the National Science Foundation (NSF-ROLE 0231995, DUE Award 0126050, ESE 9453918) and the U.S. Department of Education (R305H050052).

References

1. Anderson, J.R.: Acquisition of cognitive skill. Psychological Review 89, 369–406 (1982)
2. Berka, C., Levendowski, D.J., Cvetinovic, M.M., Davis, G.F., Lumicao, M.N., Popovic, M.V., Zivkovic, V.T., Olmstead, R.E.: Real-Time Analysis of EEG Indices of Alertness, Cognition and Memory Acquired with a Wireless EEG Headset. International Journal of Human-Computer Interaction 17(2), 151–170 (2004)
3. Berka, C., Levendowski, D.J., Ramsey, C., Davis, K., Lumicao, G., Stanney, M.N., Reeves, K., Harkness, L., Regli, S., Tremoulet, P.D., Stibler, K.: Evaluation of an EEG-Workload Model in an Aegis Simulation, Biomonitoring for Physiological and Cognitive Performance during Military Operations. In: Caldwell, J., Jo Wesentsten, N. Proceddings of SPIE, vol. 5797, pp. 90–99 (2005)
4. Berka, C., Levendowski, D.J., Lumicao, M., Yau, A., Davis, G., Zivkovic, V.: EEG Correlates of Task Engagement and Mental Workload in Vigilance, Learning and Memory Tasks. Aviation Space and Environmental Medicine. 78(5, Section II, Suppl.) (May 2007) (in press)

5. Ericsson, K.A.: Deliberate Practice and the Acquisition and Maintenance of Expert Performance in Medicine and Related Domains. Academic Medicine 79(10), S70–S81 (2004)
6. Fabiani, M., Gratton, G., Coles, M.G.: Event-related Brain Potentials. In: Cacioppo, J.T., Tassinary, L.G., Berntson, G.G. (eds.) Handbook of Psychophysiology, pp. 53–84. Cambridge University Press, Cambridge (2000)
7. Haider, H., Frensch, P.A.: The role of information reduction in skill acquisition. Cognitive Psychology 30, 304–337 (1996)
8. Poythress, M., Russell, C., Siegel, S., Tremoulet, P.D., Craven, P.L., Berka, C., Levendowski, D.J., Chang, D., Baskin, A., Champney, R., Hale, K., Milham, L.: Correlation between Expected Workload and EEG Indices of Cognitive Workload and Task Engagement. In: Proceedings of 2nd Annual Augmented Cognition International Conference, San Francisco, CA (In press)
9. Schneider, W., Shiffrin, R.M.: Controlled and automatic human information processing I: Detection, search, and attention. Psychological Reviews 84, 1–66 (1977)
10. Stevens, R., Casillas, A.: Artificial Neural Networks. In: Mislevy, R.E., Williamson, D.M., Bejar, I. (eds.) Automated Scoring of Complex Tasks in Computer Based Testing: An Introduction, Lawrence Erlbaum, Mahwah (2006)
11. Stevens, R., Johnson, D.F., Soller, A.: Probabilities and Predictions: Modeling the Development of Scientific Competence. Cell Biology Education 4(1), 42–57 (2005)
12. Stevens, R., Soller, A., Cooper, M., Sprang, M.: Modeling the Development of Problem Solving Skills in Chemistry with a Web-Based Tutor. In: Lester, J.C., Vicari, R.M., Paraguaçu, F. (eds.) ITS 2004. LNCS, vol. 3220, pp. 580–591. Springer, Heidelberg (2004)
13. Stevens, R., Wang, P., Lopo, A.: Artificial neural networks can distinguish novice and expert strategies during complex problem solving. JAMIA 3(2), 131–138 (1996)
14. Stevens, R.H., Najafi, K.: Artificial Neural Networks as Adjuncts for Assessing Medical Students' Problem-solving Performances on Computer-based Simulations. Computers and Biomedical Research 26, 172–187 (1993)
15. VanLehn, K.: Cognitive Skill Acquisition. Annual Review. Psychology. 47, 513–539 (1996)

Towards a Closed-Loop Training System: Using a Physiological-Based Diagnosis of the Trainee's State to Drive Feedback Delivery Choices

Amy Bolton[1], Gwendolyn Campbell[2], and Dylan Schmorrow[3]

[1] Strategic Analysis Inc., 3601 Wilson Blvd., Suite 500, Arlington, VA 22201
[2] NAVAIR Orlando Training Systems Division, 12350 Research Pkwy., Orlando, FL 32826
[3] Office of Naval Research, 875 Randolph St., Suite 1425, Arlington, VA 22203
abolton@sainc.com, Gwendolyn.campbell@navy.mil,
Schmord@onr.navy.mil

Abstract. Designers of a closed loop scenario based training systems must have specifications to drive the decisions of whether or not performance feedback is appropriate in response to student behavior, the most effective content of that feedback, and the optimal time and method of delivery. In this paper, we propose that physiological measures, when interpreted in conjunction with information about the learning objective, task environment and student performance, could provide the data necessary to inform effective, automated decision processes. In addition, we present an overview of both the relevant literature in this area and some ongoing work that is explicitly evaluating these hypotheses.

Keywords: Simulation based training, physiological measures, feedback, training interventions.

1 Introduction

Optimal delivery of instruction is both critical and challenging in dynamic, scenario-based training (SBT) computer simulations such as those used by the military. Tasks that human instructors must perform during these sorts of simulated training exercises can impose a heavy burden on them. Partially due to advances in the state-of-the-art in training technology and partially due to the military's desire to reduce the number of personnel required, it may be possible to support functions that overburdened instructors perform by automating much of the SBT process in a closed-loop computer simulation. Unfortunately though, after more than 50 years of literature documenting research conducted in the area of training interventions, few empirically-supported guidelines have emerged to direct the choice and implementation of effective, automated training interventions including the types of measures that should be captured to inform the interventions. Designers of a closed loop SBT system must have specifications to drive the decisions of whether or not feedback is appropriate in response to student behavior, the most effective content of that feedback, and the optimal time and method of delivery. In this paper, we propose that physiological

D.D. Schmorrow, L.M. Reeves (Eds.): Augmented Cognition, HCII 2007, LNAI 4565, pp. 409–414, 2007.

measures, when interpreted in conjunction with information about the learning objective, task environment and student performance, could provide the data necessary to inform effective, automated decision processes. In addition, we will present an overview of both the relevant literature in this area and some ongoing work that is explicitly evaluating these hypotheses.

2 Feedback: Why and What?

One of the biggest challenges in training is making the inferential leap from student behaviors and performances that can be observed to the underlying knowledge, skills and abilities (KSAs) that are presumed to generate those outputs. We want to be able to make valid inferences because the "why" to giving feedback is, typically, to correct deficiencies in those underlying KSAs. Unfortunately, as linguists have been pointing out for decades, performance is an imperfect indicator of underlying capability. A correct action does not necessarily imply that the student has the required KSAs. Similarly, an error does not necessarily imply that the student does not. A set of behaviors, especially behaviors exhibited during a training exercise, is often a conglomeration of guesses, intentional actions and maybe even a few slips (Norman, 1981; Reason, 1990). If there was some way to sort these all out and recognize which actions were guesses, which were intentional, and which were accidental, instructors and training systems would be in a much better position to deliver the most effective feedback.

Recent advances in neurophysiological assessment suggest that EEG data may provide one source of insight into the specific nature of a trainee's individual actions and help distinguish deliberate and learned responses from exploratory "guesses" and unintentional slips. For example, previous fMRI and EEG research suggests that certain incorrect actions are followed by a negative deflection with a mediofrontal distribution that peaks at about 50-150 ms after the action (Luu & Pederson, 2004; Luu, Tucker & Makeig, 2004). This response is called the "error related negativity" or ERN response. Research has shown that this response does not seem to follow deliberately committed errors (Dehaene, Posner & Tucker, 1994; Stemmer, Witzke & Schönle, 2001). Instead, it appears as if the ERN follows actions that are incongruent with cognitive expectancies (Luu & Pederson, 2004; Luu, Tucker & Makeig, 2004). In other words, this response appears to be an "Oops, that's not what I meant to do" signal, making it a candidate measure for discriminating between the two types of errors, "slips" and "mistakes." Similarly, ongoing research is converging on the finding that there are several indicators that systematically index the learning process, such as the lateral inferior frontal negativity (LIFN), medial-frontal negativity (MFN) and P300 (Luu, Tucker & Stripling, manuscript in preparation). These responses are candidates for distinguishing guesses from learned responses.

Knowing why a student requires feedback (or some form of follow-on training and/or practice) is a good first step in determining what that feedback should be. While any instructional system could be improved upon, a reasonable first approximation of design specifications might go something like this: guesses should be remediated with feedback designed to fill in missing KSAs; true mistakes should be remediated with feedback designed to correct faulty and/or incomplete KSAs; and slips should be remediated with more practice, designed to establish automated procedures. Note that neurophysiological data alone, however, are not sufficient to generate instructional content. Rather, they help us sort behaviors into "like" categories, in preparation for further analyses; and these further analyses are based on an understanding of the learning objectives, the task environment and objective measures of student performance.

This relationship can be illustrated by describing an ongoing effort to conduct an assessment of the potential value added of incorporating neurophysiological measures into a SBT system. Subjects will be trained to categorize objects within the context of a warfare-based simulation. For any given object, the information available to support the categorization may be incomplete and/or ambiguous. In some cases, the environment will eventually and naturally provide information about the accuracy of a prior categorization decision, but this will not always be the case. (These features are not uncommon in real world learning environments.) Mathematical techniques, such as regression or fuzzy logic, can be applied to a set of data containing a subject's categorization decisions for a number of objects and the information available to the subject about each object when the decision was made.

Campbell and colleagues (2006) have shown that it is possible to interpret the resulting mathematically-expressed decision rules, critique them by comparing them to rules derived from expert performance data, and generate qualitative feedback that, at least in some cases, leads to improved performance. They also showed, unfortunately, that error variance in the data set often posed a significant challenge to the modeling process. There were, of course, brute force approaches available to reduce this effect. First, they threw out a significant chunk of the data collected during the early learning trials, in order to reduce the "noise" generated by guesses and allow the "signal" to be detected by the algorithm. Even after taking that step, however, they had to have their participants complete many scenarios, and make many decisions, in order to avoid accidentally finding spurious patterns in the performance data. The fact that the some of the environmental cues were either ambiguous or correlated (or both) resulted in a situation in which a few data points representing slips had the potential to mislead the modeling process, unless they were outweighed by a very large number of intentional decisions.

If EEG indicators, such as the P300 and ERN, could have been used to separate intentional decisions from slips and guesses, it is possible that more accurate models of participants' decision making rules could have been built earlier in the training process, allowing tailored and adaptive feedback to be delivered to each participant more quickly. And it is just this hypothesis that is being tested under the current effort. Two, randomly assigned groups will complete the scenario-based training. One group will have their decision making data modeled following the techniques used in Campbell, et. al. (2006). The other group will have their decision making data filtered using EEG indicators, before applying the modeling algorithms. The efficiency of each technique will be evaluated based on the amount of performance data that must be collected before a reliable model can be built and model-based feedback can be delivered. The effectiveness of each technique will be evaluated based on the steepness of the learning curve across the course of the training. This is the first effort that we are aware of to investigate the capability of neurological data to help answer the feedback questions of "why?" and "what?".

3 Feedback: When and How?

There are a couple of efforts underway investigating whether or not neurophysiological measures should and could inform the feedback questions of "when?" and "how?" The basis for this research includes a recently completed investigation by Bolton (2006) and one that is underway (Van Buskirk, in preparation). In these initial studies, the research focused on determining, if one had an accurate diagnosis of trainee cognitive state (perhaps supported by neural and physiological data), when and how would one intervene with feedback? Therefore, in both of these investigations, training scenarios were explicitly designed a priori to elicit particular cognitive states from the trainee during a simulation based training exercise. The elicited cognitive states targeted by the scenario design were consistent with the hypotheses of each of the investigations. If this research proved promising, the next step would be to integrate measurement technologies and algorithms that could provide neural and physiological markers of cognitive state in real-time in order to drive the feedback timing and feedback methods.

In a doctoral dissertation, Bolton (2006) sought to provide empirical guidance for the optimal timing of feedback delivery (i.e., immediate vs. delayed) in a dynamic, scenario based training (SBT) computer simulation. As a basis for the investigation, the argument was presented that a general theory of feedback timing was likely not possible and that 50 years of literature on the topic was overly simplified. To deal with this presumed oversimplification, Bolton (2006) provided an integration of theoretical perspectives to provide a more detailed and sensitive feedback timing hypothesis. First, Bolton presented the premise underlying temporal contiguity, that contiguous feedback with performance encourages accelerated learning of cue-strategy associations (Guthrie, 1935). Second, the theory of transfer appropriate processing was presented that states that the more similar the conditions are between the training setting and the testing setting, the more positive transfer of training will be produced (Morris, Bransford, & Franks, 1977). Third, Bolton likened dynamic, SBT simulations to a complex, multi-tasking environments which suggested that care should be taken in understanding the cognitive demands placed on the trainee, consistent with the tenets of Cognitive Load Theory (CLT; Sweller, 1993; Sweller, Van Merrienboer, & Paas, 1998). Finally, the conclusion was drawn that the benefits of temporal contiguity of feedback should be balanced against the potential costs of changing the requirements of the task or disrupting task performance during training with the presentation of immediate feedback.

In other words, in a dynamic, SBT simulation system, temporal contiguity of feedback to decisions and actions is important. However, to prevent the feedback from serving as a task interruption, the cognitive load of the scenario could be used to indicate the appropriate timing of the feedback delivery. If the cognitive load was low enough, immediate feedback could and should be provided. If the cognitive load was too high, the delivery of feedback should be delayed until the end of the scenario. The hypotheses developed for the investigation specifically addressed expected variations in performance and instructional efficiency consistent with the above postulation.

In order to test the hypotheses, training scenarios were designed a priori to represent either low cognitive load or high cognitive load and feedback was delivered either immediately during a scenario or delayed until the end of a scenario. This created 10 experimental conditions (a partial factorial design) and 120 volunteers were randomly assigned to one of those conditions. After familiarization on the experimental testbed, participants completed a total of seven, 10-minute scenarios, which were divided across two training phases. During each training phase participants received either immediate or delayed feedback and performed either high or low cognitive load scenarios. Four subtask measures were recorded during test scenarios as well as subjective reports of mental demand, temporal demand and frustration.

A series of planned comparisons were conducted to investigate the training effectiveness of differing scenario cognitive loads (low vs. high), timing of feedback delivery (immediate vs. delayed), and sequencing the timing of feedback delivery and the cognitive load of the scenario. In fact, the data did not support the hypotheses as tested. However, through post hoc exploratory data analyses, some light was shed on the possibility that even the more detailed feedback timing statement, that immediate feedback should be provided during low cognitive load training scenarios and feedback should be delayed when the cognitive load of the training scenario is high, might have been over simplistic. The data seemed to suggest that the nature of the task, the phase of the training and the cognitive state of the trainee should be taken into consideration when considering effective feedback timing strategies. Specifically, different tasks imposed different cognitive demands and those demands changed with additional training as expertise was developed. Additionally, the a priori specification of scenario cognitive load is difficult to define. At any point in time during a single training or testing scenario, cognitive load demands likely vary. Different sub-tasks likely place different demands on the brain.

Based on this premise, Van Buskirk (in preparation) designed an investigation to determine if the delivery of real-time feedback could be optimized during scenario-based training so as not to place additional demands on areas of the brain that were already approaching overload – the "how" for the chosen "when". This is consistent with evidence of multiple resource pools and memory stores (Baddeley & Logie, 1999; Wickens & Holland, 2000). Considering the constructs of spatial working memory and verbal working memory, the question is if real-time feedback can be delivered in a way so that is does not interfere with resource pools involved in task execution and learning. For example, if one is performing a highly taxing visuo-spatial training task, could feedback provided in the auditory channel be more effective than feedback provided to the visual channel or no feedback provided at all. This investigation is still underway therefore the results are still "to be determined."

4 Summary

The literature and investigations discussed in this paper point to the assertion that to realize the vision of a closed-loop training system, the "why," "what," "when," and "how" of feedback delivery, would require a sensitive measure of varying cognitive demands and states in real-time during training. Neurophysiological measures of cognitive state assessment could potentially provide the solution needed to realize this vision. With a more sensitive measure of what the trainee has learned and hasn't learned and with a more sensitive measure of cognitive load as it changes over time, more sensitive training interventions could be researched and developed. The result of incorporating neurophysiological measures into a training system could be optimized, closed-loop training system that produces maximal training effectiveness and efficiency. At this time, the authors are aware of at least one ongoing effort at Clemson University that has the goal of including physiological measures in a replication of the experiment conducted by Bolton to gain a better understanding of how such measures may benefit training.

References

1. Bolton, A.E.: Immediate versus delayed feedback in simulation based training: Matching feedback delivery timing to the cognitive demands of the training exercise. Unpublished doctoral dissertation. University of Central Florida, Orlando, FL

2. Campbell, G.E., Buff, W.L., Bolton, A.E.: Viewing training through a fuzzy lens. In: Kirlik, A. (ed.) Adaptation in Human-Technology Interaction: Methods, Models and Measures, pp. 149–162. Oxford University Press, Oxford (2006)

3. Dehaene, S., Posner, M., Tucker, D.: Localization of a neural system for error detection and compensation. Psychological Science 5(5), 303–305 (1994)

4. Guthrie, E.R.: The Psychology of Learning. Harper, New York (1935)

5. Luu, P., Tucker, D., Makeig, S.: Frontal midline theta and the error-related negativity: Neurophysiological mechanisms of action regulation. Clinical Neurophysiology 115, 1821–1835 (2004)

6. Luu, P., Tucker, D.M., Stripling, R.: Neural mechanisms underlying the learning of actions in context (manuscript in preparation)

7. Luu, P., Pederson, S.: The anterior cingulate cortex: Regulating actions in context. In: Posner, M.I. (ed.) Cognitive neuroscience of attention, pp. 232–244. Guilford Publication, New York (2004)

8. Morris, C.D., Bransford, J.D., Franks, J.J.: Levels of processing versus transfer appropriate processing. Journal of Verbal Learning and Verbal Behavior 16, 519–533 (1977)

9. Norman, D.A.: Categorization of action slips. Psychological Review 88, 1–15 (1981)

10. Reason, J.: Human error. Cambridge University Press, Cambridge (1990)

11. Stemmer, B., Witzke, W., Schönle, P.W.: Losing the error related negativity (ERN): an indicator for willed action. Neuroscience Letters 308(1), 60–62 (2001)

12. Sweller, J.: Some cognitive processes and their consequences for the organisation and presentation of information. Australian Journal of Psychology 45, 1–8 (1993)

13. Sweller, J., Van Merrienboer, J.J.G., Paas, F.G.W.C.: Cognitive architecture and instructional design. Educational Psychology Review 10, 251–296 (1998)

14. Van Buskirk, W. L.: The use of feedback in simulation based training: Investigating the relationship between feedback timing, content, and modality under high cognitive workload. Unpublished doctoral dissertation. University of Central Florida, Orlando, FL (in preparation)

Aiding Tomorrow's Augmented Cognition Researchers Through Modeling and Simulation Curricula

Julie Drexler, Randall Shumaker, Denise Nicholson, and Cali Fidopiastis

Institute for Simulation and Training, University of Central Florida,
3100 Technology Drive, Orlando, FL 32826
{jdrexler, shumaker, dnichols, cfidopia}@ist.ucf.edu

Abstract. Research in the newly emerged field of Augmented Cognition (AugCog) has demonstrated great potential to develop more intelligent computational systems capable of monitoring and adapting the systems to the changing cognitive state of human operators in order to minimize cognitive bottlenecks and improve task performance. As the AugCog field rapidly expands, an increasing number of researchers will be needed to conduct basic and applied research in this burgeoning field. However, due to its multidisciplinary nature and cutting-edge technological applications, most traditional academic disciplines cannot support the training needs of future AugCog researchers. Accordingly, an established Modeling and Simulation (M&S) graduate curriculum is described, which provides a broad basis of interdisciplinary knowledge and skills as well as depth of knowledge within a specific area of the M&S field. Support for use of the flexible M&S curriculum to provide the requisite multifaceted foundational training in Augmented Cognition principles is also presented.

Keywords: Augmented Cognition, Modeling, Simulation, Cognitive Neuroscience, Adaptive Technology, Human-Computer Interaction, Curriculum Development.

1 Introduction

A global trend in 21st century corporate, military, healthcare, and educational settings is the demand to do more with less, which translates into requirements for more efficient selection and assessment of personnel, decreased training time, and reduced manpower. Technological advances have also caused a shift in the tasks of many system operators from primarily physical work to primarily mental work [11]. Moreover, advances in computational capabilities have dramatically increased the prevalence of computers in today's society by providing faster access to increased quantities and types of information available to users. Well-documented limitations in human information processing capabilities (e.g., attention, working memory, sensory input, comprehension, etc.), however, can influence human-system interaction and ultimately impede or even degrade performance [18]. Additionally, the cognitive demands imposed on system users varies as a function of task demands such as the number of tasks that must be simultaneously performed, time constraints

D.D. Schmorrow, L.M. Reeves (Eds.): Augmented Cognition, HCII 2007, LNAI 4565, pp. 415–423, 2007.

of the task(s), level of accuracy required, and even environmental factors such as noise level or temperature [16]. Consequently, there is tremendous need for *intelligent* technological solutions to improve human systems so that optimal performance can be achieved.

2 Augmented Cognition

As previously mentioned, the prevalence of computational systems and interface complexity have dramatically increased over the years, but limitations in the cognitive abilities of human users can impede optimal performance of these systems. In response to the need for more intelligent computational systems, research in the burgeoning field of Augmented Cognition (AugCog) is focused on investigating and developing computational methods, technologies, and non-invasive neurophysiological tools that can be used to accommodate the changing cognitive state of system users in order to improve their performance [18].   Specifically, research in the AugCog field has demonstrated great potential to develop the requisite advanced computational system technologies which can monitor and accommodate the cognitive state of system users by augmenting (i.e., adapting) the system interface to minimize or eliminate information processing bottlenecks inherent in human-system interactions.

2.1 Augmented Cognition Systems

Augmented Cognition systems typically function within a closed-loop to manage information processing workload and reduce cognitive bottlenecks associated with human-system interaction applications [4, 19]. A basic closed-loop augmented system contains at least four main components: an operational or simulated environment, automated physiological sensors to monitor and assess a user's cognitive state, an adaptive interface, and an underlying computational architecture which integrates the other three components [1, 3, 14]. Figure 1 presents a graphical representation of a closed-loop augmented cognition system.

Within the closed-loop system shown in Figure 1: (*a*) the user's senses are stimulated by content and an environment, either in an operational environment by real signals or in a virtual environment by simulated signals. The adaptive system interfaces (*b*) may be a simple, single audio or visual channel up to a full multimodal array of stimuli [21]. To measure the current state of the system user (*c*) conventional adaptive multimodal systems relied upon behavioral measures to drive system adaptation (c.f. [15]), whereas Augmented Cognition provides a deeper understanding of the user's cognitive state through the use of neurophysiological sensing techniques. Neurophysiological technologies typically used in Augmented Cognition research have included eye tracking, electroencephalographic (EEG) signals, and functional near-infrared (fNIR) imaging, which monitors blood oxygenation and volume changes in the brain [2, 5, 8, 10, 20].

The final step in completing the closed-loop augmented cognition system (cf. Figure 1) is to (*d*) adapt the environment and system interface based on the measured cognitive state to optimally support the user's performance. When an information processing (i.e., cognitive) bottleneck is detected by the neurophysiological sensors,

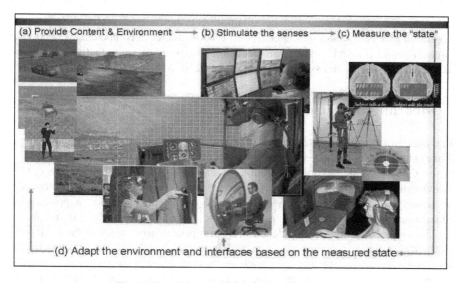

Fig. 1. Closed-loop augmented cognition system

they trigger the selection of mitigation strategies. A mitigation strategy is an intervention technique that leads into a corresponding set of concrete adaptive actions (e.g., attention management, multimodal interface adaptation, modality switching, operational performance support, task cooperation, dynamic task reallocation, and individualized embedded training strategies), which are then conveyed to the system user through an adapted interface [14, 17]. As the adaptation is applied to the interface, updated neurophysiological metrics of the operator's cognitive state become available. Thus, the Augmented Cognition system can iteratively evaluate the success of a given mitigation and initiate further mitigating actions if problems persist, and thus "close the loop" around the system user [14, 19].

2.2 Research in Augmented Cognition

The preceding discussion highlights the fact that the field of Augmented Cognition does not draw from one scientific discipline but, rather is an interaction and collaboration of multidisciplinary areas including cognitive science, neuroscience, cognitive psychology, human factors (engineering and psychology), systems engineering, and computer science. Over the past few years, the field has also been able to more solidly establish research methodologies that include state-of-the-art technologies such as functional near-infrared imaging (fNIR). Moreover, a closed-loop augmented cognition system could be beneficial for the design and/or evaluation of most any human-operated computational system which requires that the system be adaptable to the changing cognitive needs of the user [19]. Accordingly, the Augmented Cognition field is rapidly expanding and as a result, the demand for researchers qualified to conduct basic and applied research in this emergent field is expected to increase in the future. Due to its multidisciplinary nature and cutting-edge technological applications, however, most traditional academic disciplines cannot support the training needs of future Augmented Cognition researchers. In order to prevent what seems to be an imminent shortage of qualified Augmented Cognition professionals, it is imperative to identify the core competencies needed by future researchers and develop an academic program to provide the educational training these future professionals require to succeed in their careers.

3 Modeling and Simulation

The issues involving the preparation of future Augmented Cognition researchers are remarkably similar to the issues faced by the professional and academic members of the established Modeling and Simulation (M&S) community when it first emerged as a new multidisciplinary field. Specifically, the rapid advancement of computer-aided training systems in the early 1990's exposed the need to develop a professional educational training pathway for unskilled persons filling vacancies within the diverse simulation job market. Ensuing debates on appropriate curricula led to the creation of an interdisciplinary program of study, which exposed students to a cross-section of seemingly disparate subject matter such as Psychology, Engineering, and Computer Science. Although, when this information was applied collectively within an integrated curriculum, a graduate of this type of program was capable of flexibly solving problems within a multitude of occupations including those involving human-centered design.

3.1 Interdisciplinary Graduate Program in Modeling and Simulation

Over the years, academic institutions have progressed from providing certification level curricula to supporting accredited doctoral degree programs in Modeling and Simulation (M&S). The University of Central Florida (UCF) is one of the first universities to offer interdisciplinary graduate programs in Modeling and Simulation; other M&S graduate programs include the Naval Post-Graduate School, Old Dominion University, and Georgia Institute of Technology [9]. As with the field of Augmented Cognition, M&S practitioners require both generalized and specialized skills due to the size and complexity of the field [22]. Therefore, industry and government leaders in the M&S community actively participated in the design of the M&S curriculum and provided critical input regarding the broad foundation of interdisciplinary skills (i.e., the knowledge and relevant tools) that were needed by M&S practitioners as well as input on specific knowledge required to work within the various areas of the M&S field [9].

UCF's Modeling and Simulation curriculum for the master's degree is comprised of two main components. One component consists of a standardized set of courses designed to provide an interdisciplinary core body of knowledge in the fundamentals of M&S: Introduction to M&S, Quantitative Aspects of M&S, Engineering Statistics, Advanced Research Methodology, and Simulation Research Methods and Practicum. In addition to learning the M&S fundamentals, these courses are also intended to aid the development of a student's ability to critically review the scientific literature in the M&S field, solve complex problems through building simulation models, designing and carrying out experiments, analyzing data, communicating their findings, and manage M&S programs [22]. The other main curriculum component enables students to establish depth of knowledge within a specific area of the M&S field. UCF's interdisciplinary graduate program offers seven different M&S focus areas, which vary in terms of the required cornerstone courses and restricted electives in the curriculum. An overview of each focus area (brief description, cornerstone course, typical electives, and discipline areas from which the courses are drawn) is provided below [22].

Quantitative Aspects of Simulation: Focuses on applying advanced quantitative methods to modeling and simulation. Prepares graduates to apply mathematics and statistics to build multidisciplinary models and simulations. Cornerstone course: Mathematical Modeling. Typical electives: Statistical Aspects of Digital Simulation, Advanced Systems Simulation, Optimization Theory, and Data Fitting. Curriculum disciplines: Electrical Engineering, Mechanical Engineering, Industrial/Systems Engineering, Applied Mathematics, and Statistics.

Simulation Infrastructure: Focuses on an in-depth understanding of simulation systems' components and patterns of configuration and communication. Prepares graduates to develop and implement distributed simulation and training environments and/or manage a team developing these types of systems. Cornerstone course: Performance Models of Computers and Networks. Typical electives: High Performance Computer Architecture, Performance Analysis of Computer and Communication Systems, Computer Communication Networks Architecture. Curriculum disciplines: Computer Design/Architecture, Computer Programming, Computing Theory, Electrical Engineering, and Information Systems Management.

Simulation Managemen: Focuses on the management of modeling, simulation, and training (MS&T) projects. Prepares graduates to manage MS&T projects for military agencies or companies. Cornerstone course: The Environment of Technical Organizations; Typical electives: Simulation-Based Life cycle Engineering, Management Information Systems, Project Engineering, and Engineering Management. Curriculum disciplines: Industrial Engineering; Industrial/Systems Engineering; Electrical Engineering; and Mechanical Engineering.

Computer Visualization in M&S: Focuses on the technical aspects of computer graphic systems, virtual environments, and human-centered simulation systems. Prepares graduates to apply the state-of-the-art in computer graphics and other human-interface technologies. Cornerstone course: Computer Graphics. Typical electives: Computer Vision Systems, Engineering Applications of Computer Graphics, Machine Perception, and Human-Computer Interaction. Curriculum disciplines: Computer Applications for Computer Scientists, Electrical Engineering, and Industrial Engineering.

Simulation Modeling and Analysis: Focuses on the effective use of simulation as a tool for designing, planning, analysis, and decision making with an emphasis on problem definition, model formulation, design of simulation experiments, and model-based analysis. Prepares graduates to work with corporate and government decision makers in modeling and evaluating the impacts of proposed policies and system designs. Cornerstone course: Discrete Systems Simulation. Typical electives: Simulation Design and Analysis, Object-Oriented Simulation, Experimental Design, and Advanced Systems Simulation. Curriculum disciplines: Electrical Engineering, Industrial Engineering, and Industrial/Systems Engineering.

Interactive Simulation/Intelligent Systems: Focuses on the basic tools for creating designs for simulators and simulator-based training systems and the application of expert systems and other intelligent systems in a simulation setting. Prepares graduates for a career in the training simulation/simulator industries. Cornerstone course: Interactive Simulation. Typical electives: Training Systems Design, Intelligent Simulation, and Expert Systems and Knowledge Engineering. Curriculum disciplines: Computer Applications for Computer Scientists, Electrical Engineering, Industrial Engineering, Education: Technology and Media, and Transportation Engineering.

Human Systems in M&S: Focuses on the content and techniques of human behavior in simulation systems (e.g., human factors, human-computer interaction, virtual worlds, statistical and quantitative procedures, experimental design, and other research methodologies). Prepares graduates for research and development work on topics such as human-in-the-loop simulation and the use of various sensory input/output modalities to coordinate human-machine activities. Cornerstone course: Human Factors or Usability Engineering. Typical electives: Human-Computer Interaction, Human Performance, Advanced Research Methodology, Human Cognition and Learning. Curriculum disciplines: Industrial Engineering, Education: Technology and Media, Experimental Psychology, Industrial and Applied Psychology, Psychology; and Digital Media.

The curriculum for a doctoral degree expands on the master's degree requirements. In addition to adding Human-Computer Interaction to the set of required interdisciplinary core course, the Ph.D. curriculum incorporates a second set of standard interdisciplinary courses, called a "Restricted Core", which requires students to complete at least two courses from the following courses: Mathematical Modeling; Interactive Simulation or Continuous Simulation; and Discrete Systems Simulation or Object-Oriented Simulation [22]. The doctoral curriculum also requires students to complete at least three of the seven M&S focus area cornerstone courses.

Students in the M&S graduate program at UCF also have opportunities to obtain practical research and development (R&D) experience in any of the seven focus areas. One type of opportunity available to students is to work with members of the M&S faculty on R&D projects. Central Florida Research Park, located adjacent to UCF's main campus, is the hub of modeling, simulation and training research and acquisition for the Department of Defense [7]. Accordingly, other potential R&D opportunities include: The Naval Air Warfare Center, Training Systems Division (NAVAIR TSD); Air Force Agency for Modeling and Simulation; U.S. Army Program Executive Office for Simulation, Training and Instrumentation (PEO STRI); US Army Research Development and Engineering Command Simulation and Training Technology Center (RDECOM STTC); Marine Corps Program Manager for Training Systems (PMTRASYS), the Army Research Institute (ARI) Human Research and Engineering Directorate, and the Coast Guard Liaison Office; or at one of more than 140 M&S-related companies that have offices in the local area.

4 Applying an M&S Curriculum for Training Augmented Cognition Researchers

As discussed previously, the multi-disciplinary field of Augmented Cognition recently emerged in response to the need for computational systems that could monitor the cognitive state of human operators and adapt the system to their changing needs in order to minimize cognitive bottlenecks and improve task performance. To date, Augmented Cognition research has been primarily sponsored by military and defense agencies, but the commercial sector has shown interest in developing Augmented Cognition systems to manage information overload for non-military applications (e.g., air traffic control; [1]). Future applications of Augmented Cognition systems have also been proposed for education and training areas such as intelligent tutoring [13], synthetic learning environments [12], skills assessment (e.g., military selection and classification), and cognitive rehabilitation [6]. Consequently, as the Augmented Cognition field expands, an increasing number of researchers will be needed to work on basic and applied R&D projects.

The M&S graduate curriculum, described in the previous section, incorporates a broad basis of interdisciplinary knowledge and skills, many of which are also required to conduct effective research in the Augmented Cognition field. Accordingly, the

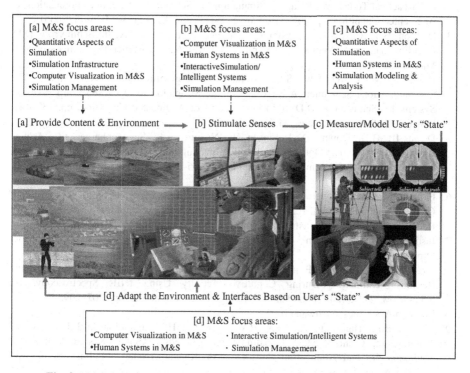

Fig. 2. M&S focus areas mapped to an augmented cognition closed-loop system

existing M&S graduate curriculum could be used to provide the foundation of diverse educational requirements that would enable future Augmented Cognition professionals to conduct basic and applied research in a variety of areas. Figure 2 provides a graphical representation of the relationship between the key components of an Augmented Cognition system and the various focus areas of the M&S curriculum.

The information shown in Figure 2 suggests that the various focus areas of the M&S curriculum provide the multifaceted approach necessary to train future augmented cognition researchers. Thus, the mature, yet flexible curriculum of a Modeling and Simulation program could offer the proper melding of psychology and technology-based coursework to support foundational training in Augmented Cognition principles as well as proving an opportunity for hands-on experience in research domains associated with the field.

References

1. Augmented Cognition International Society: What is augmented cognition? Retrieved January 30, 2007 from http://www.augmentedcognition.org/
2. Berka, C., Levendowski, D.J., Davis, G., Lumicao, M.N., Ramsey, C.K., Stanney, K., Reeves, L., Tremoulet, P.D., Harkness Regli, S.: EEG Indices Distinguish Spatial and Verbal Working Memory Processing: Implications for Real-Time Monitoring in a Closed-Loop Tactical Tomahawk Weapons Simulation. In: Schmorrow, D.D. (ed.) Foundations of Augmented Cognition, pp. 405–413. Lawrence Erlbaum Associates, Mahwah (2005)
3. Dickson, B.T.: Closed Loop Systems – Stability and Predictability. In: Schmorrow, D.D. (ed.) Foundations of Augmented Cognition, pp. 617–620. Lawrence Erlbaum Associates, Mahwah (2005)
4. Dorneich, M.C., Whitlow, S.D., Mathan, S., Carciofini, J., Ververs, P.M.: The Communications Scheduler: A Task Scheduling Mitigation for a Closed Loop Adaptive System. In: Schmorrow, D.D. (ed.) Foundations of Augmented Cognition, pp. 132–141. Lawrence Erlbaum Associates, Mahwah (2005)
5. Downs III, H.D., Downs, D., Robinson, W., Nishimura, E., Stautzenberger, J.P.: A New Approach to fNIR: The Optical Tomographic Imaging Spectrometer. In: Schmorrow, D.D. (ed.) Foundations of Augmented Cognition, pp. 205–206. Lawrence Erlbaum Associates, Mahwah (2005)
6. Fidopiastis, C.M., Stapleton, C.B., Whiteside, J.D., Hughes, C.E., Fiore, S.M., Martin, G.A, Rolland, J.P., Smith, E.M.: Human Experience Modeler: Context-Driven Cognitive Retraining to Facilitate Transfer of Learning. Cyberpsychol. Behav. 9, 183–187 (2006)
7. Institute for Simulation and Training. Retrieved February 6, 2007 from http://www.ist.ucf.edu
8. Izzetoglu, M., Shoko, N., Bunce, S., Izzetoglu, K., Onaral, B., Chance, B.: Hemodynamic Response Estimation During Cognitive Activity Using fNIR Spectroscopy. In: Schmorrow, D.D. (ed.) Foundations of Augmented Cognition, pp. 207–209. Lawrence Erlbaum Associates, Mahwah (2005)
9. Kincaid, J.P., Hamilton, R., Tarr, R.W., Sangani, H.: Simulation in Education and Training. In: Obaidat, M.S., Papadimitriou, G.I. (eds.) Applied System Simulation: Methodologies and Applications, pp. 437–456. Kluwer Academic Publishers, Norwell (2003)
10. May, J.G., Kennedy, R.S., Williams, M.C., Dunlap, W.P., Brannan, J.R.: Eye Movement Indices of Mental Workload. Acta Psychol. 75, 75–89 (1990)

11. Moroney, W.F., Bittner Jr., A.C.: Military Systems Techniques. In: Weimer, J. (ed.) Research Techniques in Human Engineering, pp. 363–438. Prentice Hall, Englewood Cliffs (1995)

12. Nasoz, F., Alvarez, K., Lisetti, C., Finkelstein, N.: Emotion Recognition from Physiological Signals for Presence Technologies. Int. J. Cogn. Technol. Work - Special Issue on Presence 6, 4–14 (2003)

13. Nicholson, D.M., Lackey, S.J., Arnold, R., Scott, K.: Augmented Cognition Technologies Applied to Training: A Roadmap for the Future. In: Schmorrow, D.D. (ed.) Foundations of Augmented Cognition, pp. 931–940. Lawrence Erlbaum Associates, Mahwah (2005)

14. Nicholson, D., Stanney, K., Fiore, S., Davis, L., Fidopiastis, C., Finkelstein, N., Arnold, R.: An Adaptive System for Improving and Augmenting Human Performance. In: Schmorrow, D.D., Stanney, K.M., Reeves, L.M. (eds.) Foundations of Augmented Cognition. 2nd edn. Strategic Analysis, Inc and the Augmented Cognition International Society, pp. 215–222. Arlington, Virginia (2006)

15. Osga, G.A.: 21st Century Workstations – Active Partners in Accomplishing Task Goals. In: Proceedings of the Human Factors and Ergonomics Society 44th Annual Meeting. Human Factors and Ergonomics Society, Santa Monica (2000)

16. Proctor, R.W., Van Zandt, T.: Human Factors in Simple and Complex Systems. Allyn and Bacon, Boston (1994)

17. Regli, S.H., Tremoulet, P., Hastie, H., Stibler, K.: Mitigation Strategy Design for Optimal Augmented Cognition Systems. In: Schmorrow, D.D., Stanney, K.M., Reeves, L.M. (eds.) Foundations of Augmented Cognition. 2nd edn. Strategic Analysis, Inc and the Augmented Cognition International Society, pp. 208–214. Arlington, Virginia (2006)

18. Schmorrow, D.D., Kruse, A.A.: Augmented Cognition. In: Bainbridge, W.S. (ed.) Berkshire Encyclopedia of Human-Computer Interaction, pp. 54–59. Berkshire Publishing, Great Barrington, Massachusetts (2004)

19. Schmorrow, D.S., Reeves, L.M., Bolton, A.: 21st Century Human Systems Integration: Augmented Cognition for Improved Defense Readiness. Paper presentation at The Technical Cooperation Program (TTCP) Human Resources and Performance Group (HUM) Human Systems Integration (HSI) Symposium on The Science and Practice of HIS for Defence Systems, Russell, Canberra (May 4-5, 2006)

20. St. John, M., Kobus, D.A., Morrison, J.G., Schmorrow, D.: Overview of the DARPA Augmented Cognition Technical Integration Experiment. Int. J. Hum. Comput. Interact. 17, 131–149 (2004)

21. Stanney, K., Samman, S., Reeves, L., Hale, K., Buff, W., Bowers, C., Goldiez, B., Nicholson, D., Lackey, S.: A Paradigm Shift in Interactive Computing: Deriving Multimodal Design Principles from Behavioral and Neurological Foundations. Int. J. Hum. Comput. Interact. 17, 229–257 (2004)

22. University of Central Florida: Graduate Catalog (2006-2007) [On-line]. Available: http://graduate.ucf.edu/catalog/

Designing for Augmented Cognition –
Problem Solving for Complex Environments

Joseph Juhnke, Timothy Mills, and Jennifer Hoppenrath

Tanagram Partners, 125 North Halsted Street, Suite 400
Chicago, Illinois 60661, USA
{jjuhnke, tmills, jhoppenrath}@tanagram.com

Abstract. The objective of this paper was to aggregate research done during several different Small Business Innovative Research (SBIR) grants as they apply to the design of complex environments and Augmented Cognition. This paper provides a high level exploration of the definition of situational awareness (SA), the action loop, an advanced mitigation framework, and a repeatable design methodology that was created to overcome several key mistakes made by UI designers. The discussion is illustrated using a recent user interface metaphor design project that maximizes information flow in a novel F-35 Joint Strike Fighter Cockpit. While testing is not complete on the resulting UI metaphor, initial observations indicate that the results of using these models and processes offer a significant improvement in performance and user acceptance appears to be high.

1 The Future of the Human-Computer Dyad

The user interface designer's job is becoming more difficult. Moore's law states the processing capabilities of computers will double every 18 months [1]. This has proven true for the last 40 years. It follows that as computers become more powerful the amount of information available in real-time will also increase. As complex domains such as the fighter cockpit continually increase the amount of data available to the user the inherent computer-to-human bottleneck will be aggravated at the expense of user efficiency. To this day computer applications have depended overwhelmingly on visual, verbal information, and have relied primarily on serial communication [5]. A properly designed complex application will overcome these limitations. Additionally, the downward pressure of ever-present budget cutbacks is making it essential to do more with fewer staff. Augmented Cognition (AugCog) seeks to revolutionize the way humans interact with computers by leveraging human physiological indicators to direct human-systems interaction [8]. This paper seeks to aid the UI designer when confronting the challenge of designing an AugCog application.

The human-computer dyad provides an interesting model. The human participant has the innate ability to assess complex situations, understand the context, and make appropriate decisions based on his or her aggregate situational awareness. Albers

D.D. Schmorrow, L.M. Reeves (Eds.): Augmented Cognition, HCII 2007, LNAI 4565, pp. 424–433, 2007.
© Springer-Verlag Berlin Heidelberg 2007

states people viewing information have a goal of locating the relevant information, mentally forming the relationships within the information, relating it to their real-world situations, and, most importantly, using it to perform a useful/correct action [1].

Unlike humans, the computer participant is particularly adept at processing large amounts of tabular data and summarizing it in more digestible forms. Neither participant shares the other's strengths. Together this complementary relationship has potential for significant increases in performance. As Benyon states, to accomplish this synergy "we must shift attention from humans, computers and tasks to communication, control and the distribution of domain knowledge" [2].

2   Defining Interaction Models

There are three models that must be considered when designing the user interface metaphor for the human-computer dyad: situational awareness, the action loop, and a mitigation framework.

2.1   Situational Awareness

Wickens defines situational awareness as "the continuous extraction of information about a dynamic system or environment, the integration of this information with previously acquired knowledge to form a coherent mental picture, and the use of that picture in directing further perception of, anticipation of, and attention to current events" [11]. The Air Force Research Laboratory similarly, and perhaps more simply, defines situational awareness as "how accurately a person perceives his current environment relative to the reality of that environment" [9]. Applying situational awareness to the goal of improving user interface, Davenport identifies three key areas of awareness encountered by the human participant: systems awareness, task awareness, and spatial awareness [3].

- *Systems Awareness* – This is the human participant's ability to understand the state of his or her equipment. In the cockpit, for example, systems awareness is often abstract and usually requires aggregation of various gauge indications. Knowing that the engine is running hot means nothing by itself, but combined with other systems indicators, may indicate a potential problem.
- *Task Awareness* – This is the human participant's ability to accurately obtain information relating to tasks relevant to his or her goals. Understanding the current state of all tasks that are underway is critical as poor task awareness increases cognitive load, diminishing overall situational awareness. Good task awareness also enables the human participant to make informed decisions when making changes to the planned task.
- *Spatial Awareness* – Spatial awareness can be broken into two sub-categories; global and local. Global spatial awareness is an understanding of the position of the human participant and his or her equipment in the world at that moment. It is the ability to accurately determine relative relationship and trajectory of objects within a global 360-degree sphere of influence and often pertains to the human participant's relation to a target destination, anticipation of upcoming objects, and other spatial directional judgments. Local spatial awareness pertains to the attitude

(vector and velocity) of the human participant's equipment. This is particularly important when dealing with moving platforms like aircraft. In observations of pilots using simulator software for the Information Flow SBIR, it was repeatedly noted that during increased times of cognitive load the first errors made were related to spatial awareness. As the local spatial orientation of aircraft changes rapidly and frequently, the related local spatial SA tended to be the first awareness lost. While further empirical evaluation is required, it quickly became apparent that designing an interface metaphor and mitigation plan that works to solve this tendency would be a high priority.

2.2 The Action Loop

We define the action loop as a cyclic process of actions taken by the human participant in response to the stimuli of an event. Stimuli may also come from the sensing of a missing but expected event. Based on Norman's stages of action [7] we have defined the action loop as a three-stage process: 1) perception, 2) evaluation, and 3) execution (Fig 1).

Norman's process begins with the formation of a goal (i.e. make the room brighter). Then follows with the formation of intention (i.e. I will turn the light on), then the specification of action (i.e. I will walk to the light switch and flip it). The resulting execution (i.e. executing the intended action) is then followed by the participant evaluating the effects of his or her action on the world. This is done in the perception (i.e. It's still dark in the room), interpretation (i.e. the light did not come on) and evaluation (i.e. the light must not work) stages of Norman's process. The process then begins again.

The action loop differs in that it begins with perception instead of goal forming because perception is a measurable state using an EEG type device. Accurate situational awareness is the aggregate result of a series of successful action loops.

1. *Perception* – Unlike Norman's model, the action loop begins with perception. This subtle shift in the entry point to Norman's cyclic process allows the beginning to be marked by a measurable event. This becomes important when designing the mitigation processes that will be discussed later. The action loop begins when the human participant first perceives an event (or missing event) that requires a response. An example of a perceived event might be the pilot observing a new target on the ground or observing a 1-degree heading deviation
2. *Evaluation* – The process continues with evaluation, where the human participant develops an understanding of the meaning of the event and considers possible responses. For evaluation to be successful a goal must result from the consideration. In the case of the 1-degree heading deviation, the pilot might consider first if the deviation requires a response and if so what input device should be used to correct the deviation.
3. *Execution* – Execution occurs when the response considered during evaluation is acted upon. If we continue with the heading deviation example, execution occurs after the pilot decides to apply slight pressure on the appropriate rudder pedal to correct the heading. Upon completion of the execution of an action the cycle begins again with perception of the response to the action and continues on.

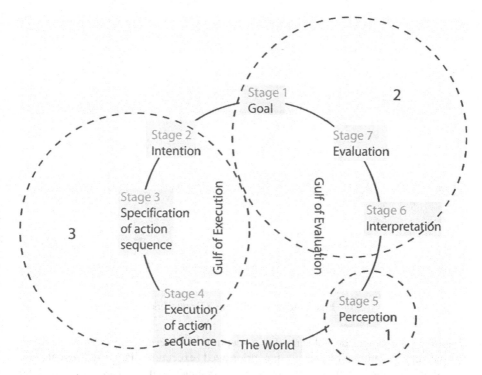

Fig. 1. Don Norman's Seven Stages of Action compared to an Action Loop

2.3 Mitigation Framework

As opposed to the permanent benefit of interface design improvements, mitigation strategies are temporary changes to the user interface, dynamically triggered at the appropriate moment to provide the greatest cognitive benefits precisely tailored to certain cognitive states [4]. A mitigation framework is a process by which the computer can determine whether the human participant is receiving information optimally, and, if not, what information must be mitigated, and how that information can be most effectively mitigated. During work on the enhancing mitigation SBIR we developed a dynamic mitigation framework that evaluates, prioritizes, and mitigates communication issues in real-time (Fig. 2).

The process is cyclic and spawns as many instances as there are events that need evaluation. Examples of events include a new track appearance, a user input, and the disappearance of an object to be resolved. As each event is triggered (for example a track displayed on a map enters a warning zone) the mitigation manager spawns a new process and determines if the event is already in one of the two mitigation queues: perception mitigation, and evaluation mitigation. The process was designed this way because each mitigation type requires a different set of interventions to be resolved. Based on an XML event classification schema, the system then determines whether or not the new event requires a response from the human participant. If not, the process ends and there is no event mitigation. If a response is desired, the system polls the cognitive sensing apparatus and waits to see if the event is perceived. If the

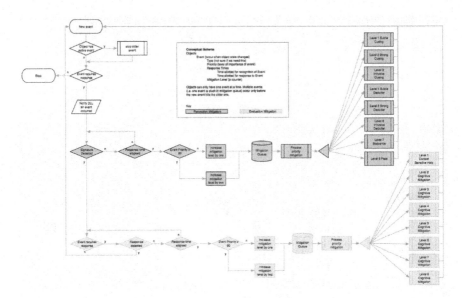

Fig. 2. Advance Mitigation Framework

cognitive state gauges do not sense the perception of the event, the event is placed in the perception mitigation queue for prioritized execution. Perceived events are monitored for understanding. If the pilot understands and evaluates the event no mitigation is triggered, otherwise the event is placed in the evaluation mitigation queue. Mitigations are resolved from either queue based on their priority one at a time so as not to overwhelm the human participant. The user input resulting from the response to the mitigation is considered a new event that deletes the prior event mitigation and requires no further action. The cycle is then completed. During subject testing of this framework for the first phase of the Shared Awareness SBIR, subjects became frustrated by some of the mitigations. When asked why they were frustrated, these subjects indicated that they were focusing on another issue and did not want to be distracted. Future versions of this framework will experiment with allowing the user to cancel or defer mitigations.

3   Designing for Augmented Cognition

The processes and models illustrated above are useful tools for the designer of complex applications. Applied within the bounds of a structured methodology, they become key to the navigation of the complex domain. The process of designing a complex application follows a process very similar to the process used for developing any application. The difference comes in the amount of documentation that must be generated. We use a modified iterative waterfall process that was initially derived from the Rational Unified Process. There are several steps that have been added that deal particularly with the Augmented Cognition domain. For the purposes of this paper we will focus on the Define phase of this process. The process is as follows:

1. Define the System Requirements
   - Define the System Actors
   - Define and Prioritize Communications
   - Define the Mitigation Plan
2. Plan the Application
3. Prototype the Application
4. Test the Prototype
   - Revise as necessary
5. Build the Application

3.1 Define the System Actors

An actor is any agent that is part of the interaction process. There are three main categories of actor: business, technical, and user. Business actors are stakeholders responsible for the development of the application. We use the term "business" because typically actors in this class represent some agency wishing to develop an application that serves a specific purpose. Technical actors include developers as well as the software and hardware products that will be used to build the final application. User actors are the end users of the product. They have specific needs that if not met, may result in their rejection of the final application. After determining who or what makes up the actor inventory it is important to understand how these actors interact. To do this one must begin with a requirements determination exercise.

3.2 Defining the Actor Requirements

When documenting requirements it is important to clearly define dependencies. This is done in a hierarchical map that illustrates the relationships between the overall goal and the communications that will help fulfill that goal. We know, for instance, that a pilot wishes to survive first, and complete missions successfully second. Continuing, we know that to complete a mission successfully, the pilot must maintain high levels of all four types of SA. The information required to maintain a high level of local spatial SA includes the vector and velocity of the craft in a 3-dimensional space. We can then subdivide the types of vector information by the typical aviation classifications (e.g.. pitch, roll, yaw, etc.). Figure 3 illustrates the beginning of what will ultimately become a requirements mind map, a visual representation of goals where the first node is the highest-level goal and the last defines the communications required to enable that specific branch of requirements.

3.3 Prioritizing and Maximizing Communications

Once all of the requirements are mapped as communications the next step is to prioritize them according to their ability to satisfy their associated goals. Prioritizing requirements provides a clear mapping of the communication needs of the interface. Modal representations that fulfill each requirement may vary in the prominence and/or the amount of "real estate" in the UI system they require to present effectively. Representations with higher priority should be more prominent (perhaps louder in an

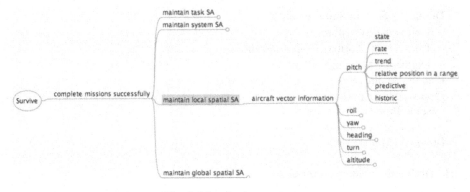

Fig. 3. Pilot requirements map

aural mode) and given higher value real estate. Improperly representing communication prioritization is probably the most common error made by UI designers.

The second most common mistake made by UI designers is not maximizing the density of displayed information. By looking at the action loop density, the designer can determine if the real estate is being used efficiently. Much like Tufte's ink-to-data ratio [10], one can determine how much information is being presented by a particular modal representation. During our work on the second phase of the Information Flow

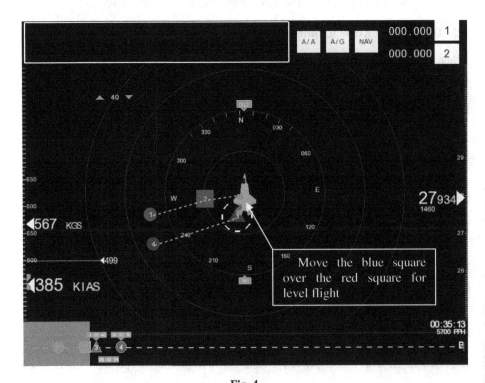

Fig. 4.

in Command and Control SBIR, we developed components for a novel F-35 cockpit design that will significantly improve the value of the data being presented by the computer participant(s). To maintain local spatial SA we created a 3-dimensional object that in addition to acting as a location marker on the moving map also provides the pilot with real-time attitude (vector) information (Fig. 4). This very simple addition to the UI metaphor adds pitch, roll, yaw, turn, heading and inversion (the 3-D object has a red belly to indicate when the plane is flying inverted) information; all in an extremely small amount of real estate. This allows the pilot to maintain local spatial SA while reviewing the moving map to improve global spatial SA. Human subject testing has shown that pilots, with little training, can adequately fly the plane using this the moving map screen and no other attitude information. While this screen was never designed to be a primary navigation device, these results are a powerful testament to its ability to allow the pilot to maintain local spatial SA while assessing the global spatial situation.

3.4 Mitigation Plan

During the requirements exercise it is important to go through a mitigation planning exercise. In the cockpit, many SA failures can result in death. Our challenge was to devise a viable mitigation for local spatial SA that is in no way a design improvement; in other words, a mitigation that would not benefit the user if it were to be enabled at all times.

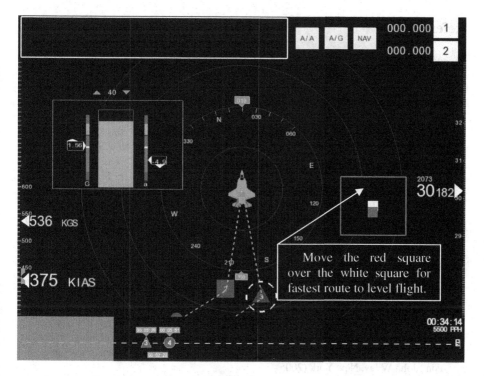

Fig. 5.

We developed the "puzzle piece," a visual element that appears next to the 3-dimensional plane and illustrates to the pilot the fastest control inputs to safely return the plane to level flight (Fig. 5). Currently the "puzzle piece" is triggered by rapid attitude changes above a set threshold, but could easily be triggered by confusion detected from the pilot in concert with rapid attitude changes. Pilots participating in human subject testing were very appreciative of the "puzzle piece", especially during unusual attitude recovery. One pilot commented that the computer showed him a faster way to level flight than he had considered, and he consistently relied on it to speed his recovery afterwards.

4 Conclusions

Designing complex mitigated applications that are perceived useful by users is challenging. Creating an environment that has a very high action loop density is a necessity when trying to implement a mitigation framework. Unless the information is already dense the mitigation will be seen as a design enhancement and not a true mitigation. Users will see mitigations that provide little value as intrusive and will likely reject them. Only planning the communications flow by defining the actors, thoroughly documenting and prioritizing requirements, and maximizing action loop density can establish an environment that both resonates with the goals of AugCog and is likely to be accepted by the user population.

References

1. Albers, M.E.: Information design considerations for improving situation awareness in complex problem-solving. In: Proceedings of the 17th annual international conference on Computer documentation, p.154–158, September 12-14, New Orleans, Louisiana, United States (1999)
2. David, B.: Communication and Shared Knowledge in Human-computer Systems. In: Smith, M., Salvendy, G., Koubek, R. (eds.) Proceedings of the 7th International Conference on Human- Computer Interaction, pp. 43–46. Elsevier, New York (1997)
3. Davenport, C.E.: Displays for Spatial Situational Awareness: The Use of Spatial Enhancements to Improve Global and Local Awareness. Air Force Institute of Technology, Wright-Patterson AFB, OH (1997)
4. Fuchs, S., Hale, K.S., Berka, C., Levendowski, D., Juhnke, J.: Physiological sensors cannot effectively drive system mitigation alone. In: Schmorrow, D.D., Stanney, K.M., Reeves, L.M. (eds.) Foundations of Augmented Cognition, 2nd edn. pp. 193–200. Arlington, VA: Strategic Analysis, Inc. (2006)
5. Jones, Marshall, Farquihar, J., Surry, D.: Using metacognitive theories to design user interfaces for computer-based learning. Educational Technology 35(4), 12–22 (1995)
6. Moore, G.: Nanometres and Gigabucks – Moore on Moore's Law. University Video Corporation Distinguished Lecture (1996) http://www.uvc.com
7. Norman, D.A.: The design of everyday things. New York: Doubleday. pp. 104–106 (1990)
8. Schmorrow, D., Stanney, K.M., Wilson, G., Young, P.: Augmented cognition in human-system interaction. In: Salvendy, G. (ed.) Handbook of human factors and ergonomics, 3rd edn., John Wiley, New York (2005)

9. Schutte, J.: Researchers benefit warfighters and air traffic controllers. Wright-Patterson AFB, Ohio (2006) http://www.afrl.af.mil/articles/040306_SAFE_Green.asp
10. Tufte, E.: The Visual Display of Quantitative Information. Graphics Press, Cheshire (1983)
11. Wickens, C.D.: The Tradeoff of Design and Unexpected Performance: Implications of Situational Awareness. In: Proceeding of the International Conference of Experimental Analysis and Measurement of Situational Awareness: Daytona Beach, Florida: Embry-Riddle Aeronautical University Press (1995)

Making the Giant Leap with Augmented Cognition Technologies: What Will Be the First "Killer App"?

Chris Forsythe[1], Chris Berka[2], Robert Matthews[3], and John Wagner[1]

[1] Sandia National Laboratories
MS1188, Albuquerque, NM, 87185-1188
{jcforsy, jswagne}@sandia.gov
[2] Advanced Brain Monitoring, Inc.
2850 Pio Pico drive, Suite A, Carlsbad, CA, 92008
chris@b-alert.com
[3] QUASAR
5764 Pacific Center Blvd., Suite 107, San Diego, CA, 92121
robm@quasarusa.com

Abstract. This paper highlights key topic areas to be discussed the authors in a panel format during the Augmented Cognition thematic area paper session: "Augmented Cognition Lessons Learned and Future Directions for Enabling 'Anyone, Anytime, Anywhere' Applications". The term "killer app" has been part of the vernacular in the commercial computer software and electronic devices industry to refer to breakthrough technologies [2]. A "killer app" generally emerges with the development of related technologies that extends over some time and involves numerous variations on a basic concept. Hypotheses may be offered with respect to the conditions that will be needed to enable a similar situation with augmented cognition technologies. This paper and resulting panel session will address the numerous concepts that have emerged from the augmented cognition field to date and postulate how and when this field's first "killer app" may emerge (e.g., 5, 10, 15, or more years from now).

Keywords: Augmented Cognition, human factors, ergonomics, design, computer science, neurotechnology, killer app.

1 Introduction

While the term "Augmented Cognition" may be loosely applied to a wide range of performance enhancing technologies [4], this paper focuses on the class of technologies that utilize physiological measures of cognitive state to accomplish closed-loop system adaptations to enhance the performance of operators. The term "killer app" has been part of the vernacular in the commercial computer software and electronic devices industry to refer to breakthrough technologies [2], [5]. With a "killer app," it is generally the case that there has been development of related technologies that extends over some time and involves numerous variations on a basic idea. However, none of the earlier efforts had been successful in gaining mass attention or

D.D. Schmorrow, L.M. Reeves (Eds.): Augmented Cognition, HCII 2007, LNAI 4565, pp. 434–438, 2007.
© Springer-Verlag Berlin Heidelberg 2007

developing a sustainable market and business model. In contrast, for any of a variety of reasons, the "killer app" is successful in generating broad interest and experiences great demand as a perception emerges that one "must have" the technology to be satisfied or to remain competitive. In the process, the "killer app" changes the way people think of the technology, and possibly also, their work, interactions with technology, relationships with other people and the potential opportunities available to them. This paper explores the speculative question, "What will be the first killer app for augmented cognition technologies?"

Through various efforts, numerous concepts have emerged for augmented cognition technologies. Many of these have been implemented in proof-of-principal demonstrations and their utility evaluated in laboratory and field settings [4]. Furthermore, there has been substantial progress in advancing the enabling technologies through capabilities such as wireless EEG monitoring, dry electrodes, cognitive state classification algorithms, etc. However, transition to operational environments or commercial applications has been limited and to date, there has been little impact of these technologies. Consequently, it is difficult to estimate whether the first "killer app" is 5, 10, or 15 years away, or longer.

Various characteristics may be proposed that contribute to the emergence of 'killer apps." Such characteristics may involve specific innovations (e.g. word processing for personal computers), availability of supporting infrastructure (e.g. cell phones) and viral social phenomena (e.g. internet blogs, MySpace, etc.) [2], [3]. Hypotheses may be offered with respect to the conditions that will be needed to enable a similar situation with augmented cognition technologies. Similarly, there are numerous practical limitations and technical hurdles that must be overcome, as well as social circumstances that could propel the adoption and demand for augmented cognition technologies. The following sections offer three perspectives concerning likely applications and contributory factors.

2 Interface of Brain, Mind and Machine

Contemporary humans are augmented by laptops, hand-helds and global satellite positioning and enchanted by engaging video games. The promise of expanding mental capacity and enhancing performance is driving cross-discipline teams of engineers, neuroscientists, cognitive psychologists and biophysicists to participate in this inevitable merging of man and machine.

It is now possible to routinely apply brain monitoring "electroencephalography or EEG" outside the laboratory making it feasible for use in education and training, human factors evaluations, military operations and market research. Although the relationships between specific mental states and EEG are just beginning to be understood, progress in detecting global state changes is sufficient to begin practical applications such as neurocognitive profiling, accomplished by integrating EEG with cognitive tests. These NeuroAssays can be used for diagnostic and treatment outcome evaluations, pharmaceutical investigations, and to identify potential biomarkers for specific diseases. For instance, technology may be posited that allows for real-time detection of factors predictive of an upcoming epileptic seizure [6].

Alternative applications of EEG include real-time assessment of drowsiness for truck drivers or airline pilots with the possibility of allocating tasks between machines and humans based on the operator status. For instance, EEG-based brain measures have been demonstrated as a basis for detecting varying levels of vigilance [11]. If computational systems can learn from and adapt to their human operators, a fundamental shift will be achieved in the way humans interact with technology.

3 Human-Human Interactions

Augmented Cognition is set to revolutionize the way we interact with computers and computerized systems. More importantly, however, Augmented Cognition has the capability to fundamentally alter interpersonal communication, which is often hampered by a lack of understanding regarding of what another person really is thinking or feeling. This point may be illustrated through the following scenario of the interaction between a teacher and a group of students. In a classroom full of their peers, a student will often hesitate to ask a question for fear of appearing foolish if the other students regard the question as too simple. This dynamic would, naturally, be different if each student had an anonymous readout of the mental state of the classroom; seeing that 90% of the class was also confused would make a student much more likely to raise their hand and ask a question. Furthermore, this classroom application would also improve the efficiency of the teacher through their ability to identify those areas of the course that caused most confusion amongst the students, or were distracted from their studies, and modify the course appropriately to improve the students' understanding and engagement with the topic. The data collected in the classroom would also be enormously useful to course administrators and writers of the curriculum, providing significant insight into those subjects that stimulate the students, which don't, and what is ultimately the most efficient way to teach students. As an extension of this idea, this concept may not only revolutionize the classroom but also many other areas of human-human interaction.

Today's technology allows for real-time estimates of the relative level of cognitive workload [1], [7], [10] with illustrative examples of applications with learning disorders [9]. The ability to detect cognitive phenomenon such as learning or confusion will require continuous monitoring with adaptation to the individual. However, the rudiments of such capabilities may be observed today within developments in the area of brain computer interfaces (e.g., [8]).

4 Ease and Enhancement

It will be asserted that here are two major application domains in which pervasive augmented cognition technologies are likely to emerge. The first domain consists of technologies that make life easier, and more fun. Here augmented cognition technologies would serve to reduce boredom and automate menial tasks. One may envision a cognitive beacon that knows an individual's cognitive state and adapts the environment to the individual in real time. It might open doors, perform redundant, boring tasks, interrupt activities before doing something foolish, or assist the individual in maintaining their health. This type technology has been demonstrated in automotive applications with drivers exhibiting enhanced capacity for processing information in multi-tasking situations [1]. It should be noted that there is a critical infrastructure component to this application similar to the IPod in that the IPod has been successful because there are mechanisms to easily download music/video. The proposed technology would require an infrastructure to adapt the world during real-time interactions.

The second domain concerns technologies that augment the individual to provide a competitive/economic advantage. Examples would include capabilities for enhancing memory, fostering appropriate social skills across different cultures, or enabling flawless navigation whether in a vehicle, on foot, in cyberspace or some form augmented reality. Such technologies might incorporate abilities to model and forecast the world based on the user's own hypotheses and warn them before problems develop. They could be used for training and rehearsal. These domains are proposed as two for which the opportunities are particularly good for a well-designed augmented cognition technology to penetrate existing markets and become generally pervasive.

5 Conclusion

While this paper has illustrated applications where the surrounding dynamics could create a compelling context for augmented cognition technologies, these are only speculations, and other equally viable proposals can be envisioned. It may be noted that the rudimentary technologies may already be found on many store shelves (e.g. heart rate monitors). However, no current technology has managed to approach any significant degree of pervasiveness. It may be argued that observations from the early days of web-based technologies may hold for augmented cognition technologies [4]. Specifically, the most successful early technologies had very successful non-web predecessors. If this proves to be the case, one should look to existing means by which people monitor and manipulate their cognitive state (e.g. caffeine use) to identify the prime candidates for the first pervasive augmented cognition technologies. However, as occurred with web-based technologies, with the passing from one generation to the next, there was a willingness to adopt technologies for which it is difficult to identify true technology predecessors (e.g. Slashdot, Flickr, YouTube).

References

1. Bruns, A., Hagemann, K., Schrauf, M., Kohlmorgen, J., Braun, M., Dornhege, G., Muller, K.R., Forsythe, C., Dixon, K.R., Lippitt, C.E., Balaban, C.D., Kincses, W.E.: EEG- and context-based cognitive-state classifications lead to improved cognitive performance while driving. In: Schmorrow, D.D. (ed.) Foundations of Augmented Cognition, 11th edn. pp. 1065–1066 (2005)
2. Clark, I.: The killer App: How to make millions with ground-breaking software. In: Proceedings of the APL Berlin 2000 Conference, Berlin, Germany, pp. 77–86 (2000)

3. Forsythe, C., Grose, E.: Predictive models of behavior with the internet. In: Proceedings of the Human Factors and Ergonomics Society 43rd Annual Meeting, Houston, TX, pp. 811–814 (1999)
4. Forsythe, C., Kruse, A., Schmorrow, D.: Augmented cognition. In: Forsythe, C., Bernard, M.L., Goldsmith, T.E. (eds.) Cognitive Systems: Human Cognitive Models in Systems Design, pp. 99–134. Earlbaum, Mahwah (2006)
5. Humphreys, P.: Is the 'killer app' an epidemic or will it make us stronger? Telecommunication Journal of Australia 56(2), 47–61 (2006)
6. Kiymik, M.K., Guler, I., Dizibuyuk, A., Akin, M.: Comparison of STFT and wavelet transform methods in determining epileptic seizure activity in EEG signals for real-time application. Computers in Biology and Medicine 35(7), 603–616 (2005)
7. Murata, A.: An attempt to evaluate mental workload using wavelet transform of EEG. Human Factors 47(3), 498–508 (2005)
8. Palaniappan, R.: Electroencephalogram signals from imagined activities: A novel biometric identifier for a small population. In: Corchado, E., Yin, H., Botti, V., Fyfe, C. (eds.) IDEAL 2006. LNCS, vol. 4224, pp. 604–611. Springer, Heidelberg (2006)
9. Rippon, G., Brunswick, N.: Trait and state EEG indices of information processing in developmental dyslexia. International Journal of Psychophysiology 36(3), 251–265 (2000)
10. Smith, M.E., Gevins, A., Brown, H., Karnik, A., Du, R.: Monitoring task loading with multivariate EEG measures during complex forms of human-computer interaction. Human Factors 43(3), 366–380 (2001)
11. Svoboda, P.: Detection of vigilance changes by linear and nonlinear EEG signal analysis. Neural Network World 16(1), 61–75 (2006)

Augmenting Cognition: Reviewing the Symbiotic Relation Between Man and Machine

Tjerk de Greef[1], Kees van Dongen[1], Marc Grootjen[2,3], and Jasper Lindenberg[4]

[1] Department of Human in Command, TNO Human Factors,
PO BOX 23, 3769 ZG Soesterberg, The Netherlands
[2] Defense Materiel Organization, Directorate Materiel Royal Netherlands Navy,
P.O. Box 20702, 2500 ES The Hague, The Netherlands
[3] Technical University of Delft,
P.O. Box 5031, 2628 CD Delft, The Netherlands
[4] Department of Human Interfaces, TNO Human Factors,
PO BOX 23, 3769 ZG Soesterberg, The Netherlands
{Tjerk.deGreef, Kees.vanDongen Jasper.Lindenberg}@tno.nl,
Marc@Grootjen.nl

Abstract. One of the goals of augmented cognition is creation of adaptive human-machine collaboration that continually optimizes performance of the human-machine system. Augmented Cognition aims to compensate for temporal limitations in human information processing, for instance in the case of overload, cognitive lockup, and underload. Adaptive behavior, however, may also have undesirable side effects. The dynamics of adaptive support may be unpredictable and may lead to human factors problems such as mode errors, 'out-of-the-loop' problems, and trust related issues. One of the most critical challenges in developing adaptive human-machine collaboration concerns system mitigations. A combination of performance, effort and task information should be taken into account for mitigation strategies. This paper concludes with the presentation of an iterative cognitive engineering framework, which addresses the adaptation strategy of the human and machine in an appropriate manner carefully weighing the costs and benefits.

1 Introduction

Since the industrial revolution, when men and machine started to work together, people aimed at an optimal performance of the human-machine system. Initially, during the first ages during and after the revolution, optimizing performance meant improving the machine or automated component. However, since the introduction of the personal computer and the turbulent developments in the decades afterwards, the human operators became the critical component in the human-computer system, leading to the comprehension that optimization of the interaction starts at design time. Literature describes different taxonomies which explain the *static* relation between an operator and a machine. For example, Fitts [1] was one of the first to acknowledge that both entities have different aptitudes. Fitts crafted a list describing where each entity

D.D. Schmorrow, L.M. Reeves (Eds.): Augmented Cognition, HCII 2007, LNAI 4565, pp. 439–448, 2007.
© Springer-Verlag Berlin Heidelberg 2007

excels. Following this approach, allocation is based on the aptitudes of each entity leading to categorized list of whether the human, machine, or a combination should implement this function [2].

The Fitts list provides an excelling insight into the aptitudes of each though it was not intended to incorporate *dynamic* situations and the list assumes the aptitudes to be static and other problems have been reported [3]. In reality the environment or context of the operator can change very rapidly creating a different demand for aptitudes. This leads the conception that function allocation should not be fixed at the design state, but should fluctuate over a continuum of levels. In the last couple of decades a number of different dynamic function allocation taxonomies have been proposed. Sheridan & Verplank [4] presented a ten-level taxonomy that explained the division of work between the human and machine, and how they collaborate. Endsley, on the other hand, [5] suggested a taxonomy in the context of expert systems to supplement human decision-making. Endsley [6] redefined their taxonomy since they required a model that was *"wider applicable to a range of cognitive and psychomotor tasks requiring real-time control within numerous domains"*. The latest and widely accepted taxonomy [7] suggests to apply automation to four broad classes of functions. Within each of these types, automation can be applied across a continuum of levels of automation (i.e. from fully manual to fully automatic) depending on the cognitive state of the operator.

Adaptive automation (AA) takes the dynamic division of labor between man and machine as a starting point. The term adaptive automation [8], dynamic task allocation, dynamic function allocation, or adaptive aiding [9] all reflect the real-time dynamic reallocation of work in order to optimize performance. It is based on the conception of actively aiding the operator only when human information processing limitations emerge and assistance is required in order overcome bottlenecks and to meet operational requirements. The concept of augmented cognition (AC) extends the AA paradigm by explicitly stating the symbolic integration of man and machines in a closed-loop system whereby the operator's cognitive state and the operational context are to be detected by the system [10].

Currently, a state-of-the-art document that highlights opportunities and possible pitfalls of AC lacks the scientific community. We strongly believe that it is important to evaluate the fast expanding ideas around the AC paradigm that compensates real-time for temporal limitations in human information processing. This paper reviews past and present research on the topic of the symbiotic relationship between man and machines starting with the static Fitts list, explaining the latest mitigation strategies, and finalizing with an iterative engineering methodology that takes into account the benefits and costs of the adaptation behavior of man and machine.

2 Potential Benefits and Risks of Augmented Cognition

For an effective and resilient human-machine system it is not wise to automate as many tasks as possible. Although machine performance is superior in some aspects; software and hardware is not always reliable (e.g. [11] [12]). Because of this, the human is often allocated the role of supervisor that can intervene when automation fails. This because humans are thought to learn more quickly and to out-perform machines in performing tasks in novel or unforeseen situations, e.g. intervening when machines do not function as intended. Unfortunately, humans demonstrate a degraded ability to intervene when kept out-of-the-loop too long: problems with vigilance, complacency, situation awareness, knowledge and skills-degradation may be observed [13]. To overcome these out-of-the-loop performance problems, a system that augments cognition is required to take the human in-the-loop. The human can be taken in-the-loop in situations of underload; when the additional demand for human attention does not exceed the resources the human has left available. Alternating high levels of automation in which the operator becomes a passive monitor with active involvement has shown to improve situation awareness and response to errors [14] [15].

Dynamically engaging humans may solve out-of-the-loop performance problems and may be useful in routine situations in which the demand for human attention is low. This solution is not desirable in all conditions: compared to alternating levels of automation, static automation of tasks frees-up more attention that can be allocated to concurrent tasks Kaber & Endsley [16]. Further, when multiple tasks demand human attention concurrently another problem becomes more urgent. In emergency situations, humans may become absorbed in some tasks, while ignoring others and performance on these latter tasks may degrade. For an effective and resilient human-machine system a decrease in human engagement needs to be compensated for by an increase in machine involvement. In the case of overload, when the demand for attention or speed exceeds the human ability, timely involvement of the machine in task execution is desirable. A number of studies [17] [18] [19] [20] or [21] have demonstrated beneficial effects.

The expected benefit of adaptive automation is that humans and machines can be taken in and out of the loop when needed. By dynamically allocating tasks to human or machine, the performance of the human-machine system is guaranteed despite disturbances in the ability of its components and despite changes in environmental demands. Unfortunately, there are also some risks associated with adaptive automation. A mayor risk is increased complexity combined with undesirable machine behavior. Although some of the complexity of adaptive automation may be hidden and not be a problem when the system always provides the right support at the right time in the right way, the potential benefits of adaptive automation turn into risks when the system wrongly concludes that support is or is not needed or when the timing of support is wrong (e.g. [22]). Unwanted interruptions, mode errors, or automation surprises may disrupt performance and may lead to errors of omission or commission, frustration, distrust, disuse, and rejection of the adaptive system. When the adaptive system is not reliable and the human has an additional layer of automation it has to monitor we create rather than solve problems. Whether this risk becomes real depends on the context-dependent ability of adaptive automation to make the decision *whether*, *when*, and *what* to automate. This will depend on the specific application and domain.

Another risk is that humans adapt to the new situation with adaptive automation in a way we do not expect or desire (e.g. [23]). Human may not use adaptive automation as intended. They may rely too much or too little on adaptive automation and for instance fool the system such that it mistakenly thinks that the human operator needs to be taken out or in-the loop. Thus also when the human shows unreliable behavior the potential benefit of adaptive automation may turn into an additional source of risk.

It is clear the potential benefits and risks of adaptive automation are context-dependent. It will depend on the specific implementation and context of use whether a system of human plus adaptive automation will be more or less effective or resilient than a system of human plus non-adaptive automation. Although it is too early to draw general conclusions, it is worth to investigate the conditions under which the potential benefits or risks of adaptive automation will be observed and to investigate how risks can be managed. One way to cope unreliable adaptive automation may be to make machine reasoning observable and adjustable. This would allow to human to understand the system and would enable him to give the system more or less room for intervention.

3 Mitigation Triggers

The basis for the AC argument is the real-time aiding of man to compensate for temporal limitations in the human information processing capacity. The previous section listed some studies that revealed beneficial effects of getting the operator out-of-the-loop in case a system augments an overloaded operators and involving the operator in the operational process when a state of underload is augmented. Assuming that machine assistance should be kept at lower levels unless high workload precludes effective human performance, AC will optimize the symbiotic relation between man and machine in an environment where the workload is varying [24]. One of the challenging factors in the development of a successful AC concept concerns the question of *when* changes in level of automation must be effectuated. Workload generally is the key concept to invoke such a change of authority, but most researchers agree that "*workload is a multidimensional, multifaceted concept that is difficult to define. It is generally agreed that attempts to measure workload relying on a single representative measure are unlikely to be of use*" [25]. Mental workload can be defined as an intervening variable similar to attention that modulates or indexes the tuning between the demands of the environment and the capacity of the operator [26]. This definition highlights the two main features of workload, which are the *capacity* of operators and the *task demands* made on them. Workload increases when the capacity decreases or the task demands increase. As stated, both the capacity and task demands are not fixed entities and are affected by many factors. Measurement workload is again much debated and we would like to elucidate the relationship between workload, task demands and performance. According to Fig. 1, an operator can experience different levels of workload dependent on the task-demands. It also shows that the performance does not necessarily decline as the operator experiences a high workload. One can keep performance on a maximum level by increasing effort. However, problems can arise when this effort is required for a prolonged period.

AC techniques describe various ways to estimate workload. According to Figure 1, we should measure performance, effort and task demands to get to an optimal mitigation strategy.

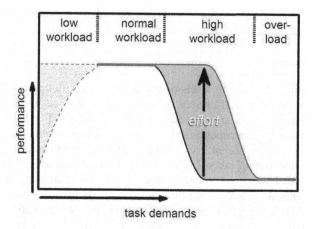

Fig. 1. The relation between task demands, performance, and workload (from [27])

3.1 Operator Performance

The *operator's own performance* could be used as a trigger. Using the operator's interactions with the system allows us to determine performance measurement. Side-stepping the discussion on how to create a performance model, which remains difficult, this candidate allows to trigger adaptive behavior in order to optimize human-computer cooperation. For example, Geddes [28] and Rouse, Geddes & Curry [29] apply adaptive automation based on the operator's intentions predicted from patterns of activity. Though successful, performance modeling have been criticized as being too information sensitive, requiring a massive database of operator performance [30].

3.2 Physiological Measurements

Besides performance measures to determine the effort, (neuro)physiological data to understand the effort from the operator are used in various studies as well (e.g. [31] [32] [33]) . Physiological measures can be recorded without respect to overt responses and provide an indication of cognitive activities. Specifically, pupillometry, heart rate variablility [17], and electroencephalographs [34] have been studied and have yielded a reliable description of cognitive state. Differences in state were used as triggers and yielded reductions in effort and/or improvements in operator performance. Today, the brain based electroencephalographs [30] demonstrate a reliable engagement index from a ratio of EEG power bands that can be used for triggering mechanisms.

   Various studies clearly demonstrate that physiological measures can measure the state of the operator. Although promising, there lingers one potential pitfall involving the usage of physiological measures to estimate effort. An operator continuously adapts to changes in workload, and physiological reactions are a sign of this adaptive behavior. If a system uses this information to reduce the workload, there are two adaptive systems that might work counterproductive as is demonstrated by Wilson [35]. On the other hand, when one expects an increase in physiological indicators due to excessive task demands and this increase is not reflected in the physiological data, one could draw the conclusion with respect to the state of the operator (i.e., is the operator still in command of the situation).

3.3 Task Demands

Another possibility to vary the levels of automation is to use the flow of the mission itself. Here, the occurrence of *critical events* can be used to change to a new level of automation. Critical events are defined as incidents that could endanger the goals of the mission. Scerbo [8] describes a model where the system continuously monitors the situation for the appearance of critical events and the occurrence of such an event triggers the reallocation of tasks. Inagaki [19] published a number of studies where a probabilistic model was used to decide who should have authority in the case of a critical event. Inagaki suggests that different time periods during the acceleration of an airplane for takeoff make it more or less important for automation to assume responsibility for a reject takeoff decision, should such a decision be required following an engine failure.

4 Cognitive Engineering for Adaptive Automation

Effective, efficient, and easy-to-learn operation support is crucial for joint human machine performance in complex task environments, such as ship control centers and process control rooms. An important aim of AC is to accommodate user characteristics, tasks, and contexts in order to provide the "right" information, services, and (support)functions at the *right* time and in the *right* way [36]. The previous sections provided an overview of both the opportunities and pitfalls of AC. Also different types of triggers were discussed including the difficulties that occur in identification, selection, and calibration of appropriate triggers. It turns out that due to the adaptive nature of both the human and machine, it is difficult to provide generic and detailed predictions on the overall human-machine performance at design time. Therefore, a new type of iterative methodology is needed that guides the development process. This method should enable us to address the mutual adaptation in an appropriate manner carefully weighing the costs and benefits at each iteration.

Cognitive engineering (CE) approaches originated in the 1980s to improve computer-supported task performance by increasing insight in the cognitive factors of human-machine interaction (e.g., [37] [38]). These approaches guide the iterative process of development in which an artefact is specified in detail, and specifications are regularly assessed to refine the specification. For adaptive systems, the "classical" methods have to be extended with an explicit technology input for two reasons. First, the technological design space sets a focus in the process of specification and generation of ideas. Second, the reciprocal effects of technology and human factors are made explicit and are integrated in the development process. Also, the technology might not be mature at design time which prevents accurate performance predictions, an effect which is leveraged by the reciprocal effects. Finally, not a single mode of operation is chosen but a range of HMC modes. This range, its dynamics and triggers are guided by current en predicted technology. So, we propose a CE+ method, adding a technology perspective into common human factors (HF) engineering practices [39]. In addition to the added focus on the technology we propose to develop practical theories and methods that are *situated* in the domain. This is important to be able to assure an accurate weighing of costs and benefits within a specific domain while designing and developing adaptive systems.

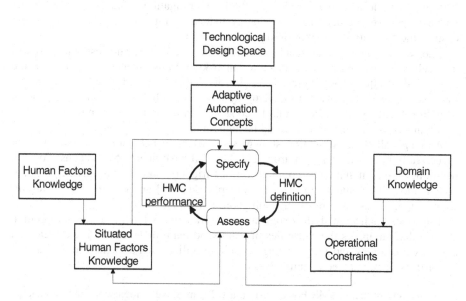

Fig. 2. The situated CE+ method for optimizing human-machine co-operation using adaptive automation. The iteration stops if a suitable HMC definition is reached.

The situated CE+ method is shown in Figure 2. Generic human factors knowledge is contextualized into situated HF-knowledge (instantiated practical theories, guidelines, and methods for the specification and assessment). Adaptive automation concepts, triggers and ranges are derived from the technological design space. An analysis of the domain provides operational constraints. During HMC specification of the situated HF knowledge, the AC concepts and the operational constraints must be addressed concurrently resulting in a preliminary HMC definition. During the assessment it is checked whether the definition actually agrees with operational constraints and HF predictions. An assessment will provide qualitative or quantitative results in terms of effectiveness, efficiency, satisfaction, learnability, and trust which are used to refine, adjust or extend the specification. Eventually, the process of iteration stops when the assessment shows that the overall HMC system satisfies the requirements (as far as the resources and completion date allow). The situated CE+ framework has been developed and applied for the design of cognitive support that augments the capacities of teams and team-members during critical and complex operations (e.g., to improve task load management, trouble-shooting and situation awareness). It is based on experiences with previous and current (space, navy) missions and based on practical theories on the object of support (e.g. cognitive task load [40]).

5 Conclusion

This paper reviews past and present research on the topic of the symbiotic relationship between man and machines, explaining the latest mitigation strategies, and finalizing with an iterative engineering methodology that takes into account the benefits and costs of the adaptation behavior of man and machine.

One way to make human-machine systems more effective and resilient is by dynamically engaging humans and machines in tasks. With augmented cognition it is the machine that adjusts the way activities are divided and shared between human and machine. Investigating ways to develop systems that reliably augment cognition in operational settings and allows one to cope with unreliability and knowledge about how humans use these systems should be high on the research agenda.

Although all three mitigation strategies for adaptive behavior have been proven successfully in experimental environments, they all have their pros and cons. To date, no studies have attempted to combine various triggers, and we strongly believe that combination of techniques prove very valuable [41] [42] and that the combining information might assist in resolving ambiguous situations.

The paper finalizes with the explanation of a framework for the design of cognitive support that augments the capacities of teams and team-members during critical and complex operations and we encourage people to utilize such a method in the designing process of augmented cognition systems.

Acknowledgements. CAMS-Force Vision, a software development company associated with the Royal Netherlands Navy, funded this research. The authors especially want to thank the anonymous reviewers for their useful comments.

References

1. Fitts, P.M.: Human engineering for an effective air navigation and traffic control system. Ohio State Univeristy Foundation Repor, Columbus, OH (1951)
2. Sheridan, T.B.: Function allocation: algorithm, alchemy or apostasy. ALLFN'97, pp. 307–316 (1997)
3. Dongen, K., Maanen, P.P.: Design for dynamic task allocation. In: Proceedings of the 7th International Conference on Naturalistic Decision Making (2005)
4. Sheridan, T.B., Verplank, W L.: Human and Computer Control of Undersea Teleoperators, MIT Man-Machine Systems Laboratory, Cambridge, MA, Tech.Rep. (1978)
5. Endsley, M.: The application of human factors to the development of expert systems for advanced cockpits. In: Proceedings of the Human Factors Society 31st Annual Meeting, pp. 1388–1392 (1987)
6. Endsley, M.R., Kaber, D.B.: Level of automation effects on performance, situation awareness and workload in a dynamic control task. Ergonomics, 462–492 (1999)

7. Parasuraman, R., Sheridan, T., Wickens, C.: A Model for Types and Levels of Human Interaction with Automation. IEEE transactions on systems, man and cybernetics, 286–297 (2000)
8. Scerbo, M.: Theoretical perspectives on adaptive automation. In: Parasuraman, R., Mouloua, M. (eds.) Automation and human performance: theory and applications, pp. 37–63. Lawrence Erlbaum Assiciated, Mahwah (1996)
9. Rouse, W.B.: Adaptive aiding for Human/Computer Control. Human factors, 431–443 (1988)
10. Kruse, A.A., Schmorrow, D.D.: Session overview: Foundations of augmented cognition. In: Schmorrow, D.D. (ed.) Foundations of Augmented Cognition, pp. 441–445. Lawrence Erlbaum Associates, Mawah (2005)
11. Lützhöft, M.H., Dekker, S.W.A.: On your watch: automation on the bridge. The Journal of Navigation, 83–96 (2002)
12. Parasuraman, R., Miller, C.: Trust and Etiquette in High-Criticality Automated Systems. Communications of the ACM, 51–55 (2004)
13. Endsley, M., Kiris, E.: The Out-of-the-Loop Performance Problem and Level of Control in Automation. Human factors: the journal of the Human Factors Society, 381–394 (1995)
14. Parasuraman, R., Mouloua, M., Molloy, R.: Effects of adaptive task allocation on monitoring of automated systems. Human factors, 665–679 (1996)
15. Kaber, D.B., Wright, M.C., Prinzel, L.P., Clamann, M.P.: Adaptive automation of human-machine system information processing functions. Human factors, 50–66 (2005)
16. Kaber, B., Endsley, M.R.: The effect of level of automation and adaptive automation on human performance, Situation Awareness and Workload in a dynamic control task (2004) (in press)
17. Hilburn, B., Jorna, P., Byrne, E., Parasuraman, R.: The effect of adaptive air traffic control (ATC) decision aiding on controller mental workload. In: Mouloua, M., Koonce, J.M. (eds.) Human-automation interaction: research and practice, pp. 84–91. Lawrence Erlbaum Associates, Mahwah (1997)
18. Scallen, S., Hancock, P., Duley, J.: Pilot performance and preference for short cycles of automation in adaptive function allocation. Applied ergonomics, 397–404 (1995)
19. Inagaki, T.: Situation-adaptive Autonomy for Time-critical Takeoff Decisions. International journal of modelling and simulation, 175–180 (2000)
20. Moray, N., Inagaki, T., Itoh, M.: Adaptive Automation, Trust, and Self-Confidence in Fault Management of Time-Critical Tasks. Journal of experimental psychology 6(1), 44–58 (2000)
21. Scott, W.B.: Automatic GCAS: 'You can't fly any lower'. Aviation Week & Space Technology, 76–79 (1999)
22. Parasuraman, R., Mouloua, M., Hilburn, B.: Adaptive aiding and adaptive task allocation enhance human machine interaction. In: Scerbo, M., Mouloua, M. (eds.) Automation technology and human performance:Current research and trends, pp. 119–123. Erlbaum, Mahwah (1999)
23. Zaslow, J.: My Tivo Thinks I'm Gay. Wall Street Journal (2002)
24. Wickens, C., Hollands, J.: Engineering psychology and human performance. Prentice-Hall, Upper Saddle River, New Jersey (2000)
25. Gopher, D., Donchin, E.: Workload - An examination of the concept. In: Boff, K., Kaufman, L., Thomas, J. (eds.) Handbook of Perception and Human Performance (chapter 41), pp. 1–49. Wiley, New York (1986)
26. Kantowitz, B.H.: Mental Workload. In: Hancock, P. A. (ed.) Human factors psychology. North-Holland, New York, pp. 81–121 (1987)

27. Veltman, J.A., Jansen, C.: The role of operator state assessment in adaptive automation, TNO Human Factors Research Institute (2006)

28. Geddes, N.D.: Intent Inferencing using scripts and plans. In: Proceedings of the First Annual Aerospace Applications of Artificial Intelligence Conference, pp. 160–172. Wright-Patterson Air Force Base, U.S. Air Force (1985)

29. Rouse, W.B., Geddes, N.D., Curry, R.E.: An architecture for intelligent interfaces: Outline of an approach to supporting operators of complex systems. Human Computer Interaction, 87–122 (1986)

30. Bailey, R.B., Scerbo, M.W., Freeman, F.G., Mikulka, P.J., Scott, A.S.: Comparison of a Brain-Based Adaptive System and a Manual Adaptable System for Involking Automation. Human Factors, 693–709 (2006)

31. Pope, A.T., Comstick, R.J., Bartolome, D.S., Bogart, E.H., Burdette, D.W.: Biocybernetic system validates index of operator engagement in automated task. In: Mouloua, M., Parasuraman, R. (eds.) Human performance in automated systems: Current research and trends, pp. 300–306. Lawrence Erlbaum, Hillsdale (1994)

32. Byrne, E.A., Parasuraman, R.: Psychophysiology and adaptive automation. Biological Psychology, 249–268 (1996)

33. Veltman, J.A., Gaillard, A.W.K.: Physiological workload reactions to increasing levels of task difficulty. Ergonomics, 656–669 (1998)

34. Prinzel, L.J., Freeman, F.G., Scerbo, M.W., Mikulka, P.J., Pope, A.T.: A Closed-loop system for examining Psychophysiological Measures for Adaptive Task allocation. International Journal of Aviation Psychology, 393–410 (1999)

35. Wilson, G.F., Russel, C A.: Psychophysiologically Versus Task Determined Adaptive Aiding Accomplishment. In: Schmorrow, D. D., Stanney, K. M., Reeves, L.M. Foundations of Augmented Cognition. 2nd edn. pp. 201–207 (2006)

36. Fischer, G.: User modeling in Human-Computer Interaction. User Modeling and User-Adapted Interaction, 65–68 (2001)

37. Rasmussen, J.: Information processing and human-machine interaction: an approach to cognitive engineering. North-Holland, Amsterdam (1986)

38. Norman, D.A.: Cognitive engineering. In: Norman, D.A., Draper, S.W. (eds.) User-Centered System Design: New perspectives on human-computer interaction, Erlbaum, Hillsdale (1986)

39. Maanen, P.P., Lindenberg, J., Neerincx, M.A.: Integrating Human Factors and Artificial Intelligence in the Development of Human-Machine Cooperation. In: Arabnia, H.R., Joshua, R. (eds.) Proceedings of the 2005 International Conference on Artificial Intelligence (ICAI'05), CSREA Press, Las Vegas (2005)

40. Neerincx, M.: Cognitive task load analysis: allocating tasks and designing support. In: Hollnagel, E. (ed.) Handbook of cognitive task design, pp. 283–305. Erlbaum, Mahwah (2003)

41. Grootjen, M., Bierman, E.P.B., Neerincx, M.A.: Optimizing cognitive task load in naval ship control centres: Design of an adaptive interface, IEA 16th World Congress on Ergonomics (2006)

42. Fuchs, S., Hale, K.S., Berka, C., Levendowski, D., Juhnke, J.: Physiological Sensors cannot Effectively Drive System Mitigation Alone. In: Schmorrow, D. D., Stanney, K. M., Reeves, L. M (eds.) Augmented Cognition: Past, present & Future, 193–200 (2006)

Author Index

Lecture Notes in Artificial Intelligence (LNAI)

Vol. 4293: A. Gelbukh, C.A. Reyes-Garcia (Eds.), MI-CAI 2006: Advances in Artificial Intelligence. XXVIII, 1232 pages. 2006.

Vol. 4289: M. Ackermann, B. Berendt, M. Grobelnik, A. Hotho, D. Mladenič, G. Semeraro, M. Spiliopoulou, G. Stumme, V. Svátek, M. van Someren (Eds.), Semantics, Web and Mining. X, 197 pages. 2006.

Vol. 4285: Y. Matsumoto, R.W. Sproat, K.-F. Wong, M. Zhang (Eds.), Computer Processing of Oriental Languages. XVII, 544 pages. 2006.

Vol. 4274: Q. Huo, B. Ma, E.-S. Chng, H. Li (Eds.), Chinese Spoken Language Processing. XXIV, 805 pages. 2006.

Vol. 4265: L. Todorovski, N. Lavrač, K.P. Jantke (Eds.), Discovery Science. XIV, 384 pages. 2006.

Vol. 4264: J.L. Balcázar, P.M. Long, F. Stephan (Eds.), Algorithmic Learning Theory. XIII, 393 pages. 2006.

Vol. 4259: S. Greco, Y. Hata, S. Hirano, M. Inuiguchi, S. Miyamoto, H.S. Nguyen, R. Słowiński (Eds.), Rough Sets and Current Trends in Computing. XXII, 951 pages. 2006.

Vol. 4253: B. Gabrys, R.J. Howlett, L.C. Jain (Eds.), Knowledge-Based Intelligent Information and Engineering Systems, Part III. XXXII, 1301 pages. 2006.

Vol. 4252: B. Gabrys, R.J. Howlett, L.C. Jain (Eds.), Knowledge-Based Intelligent Information and Engineering Systems, Part II. XXXIII, 1335 pages. 2006.

Vol. 4251: B. Gabrys, R.J. Howlett, L.C. Jain (Eds.), Knowledge-Based Intelligent Information and Engineering Systems, Part I. LXVI, 1297 pages. 2006.

Vol. 4248: S. Staab, V. Svátek (Eds.), Managing Knowledge in a World of Networks. XIV, 400 pages. 2006.

Vol. 4246: M. Hermann, A. Voronkov (Eds.), Logic for Programming, Artificial Intelligence, and Reasoning. XIII, 588 pages. 2006.

Vol. 4223: L. Wang, L. Jiao, G. Shi, X. Li, J. Liu (Eds.), Fuzzy Systems and Knowledge Discovery. XXVIII, 1335 pages. 2006.

Vol. 4213: J. Fürnkranz, T. Scheffer, M. Spiliopoulou (Eds.), Knowledge Discovery in Databases: PKDD 2006. XXII, 660 pages. 2006.

Vol. 4212: J. Fürnkranz, T. Scheffer, M. Spiliopoulou (Eds.), Machine Learning: ECML 2006. XXIII, 851 pages. 2006.

Vol. 4211: P. Vogt, Y. Sugita, E. Tuci, C.L. Nehaniv (Eds.), Symbol Grounding and Beyond. VIII, 237 pages. 2006.

Vol. 4203: F. Esposito, Z.W. Raś, D. Malerba, G. Semeraro (Eds.), Foundations of Intelligent Systems. XVIII, 767 pages. 2006.

Vol. 4201: Y. Sakakibara, S. Kobayashi, K. Sato, T. Nishino, E. Tomita (Eds.), Grammatical Inference: Algorithms and Applications. XII, 359 pages. 2006.

Vol. 4200: I.F.C. Smith (Ed.), Intelligent Computing in Engineering and Architecture. XIII, 692 pages. 2006.

Vol. 4198: O. Nasraoui, O. Zaïane, M. Spiliopoulou, B. Mobasher, B. Masand, P.S. Yu (Eds.), Advances in Web Mining and Web Usage Analysis. IX, 177 pages. 2006.

Vol. 4196: K. Fischer, I.J. Timm, E. André, N. Zhong (Eds.), Multiagent System Technologies. X, 185 pages. 2006.

Vol. 4188: P. Sojka, I. Kopeček, K. Pala (Eds.), Text, Speech and Dialogue. XV, 721 pages. 2006.

Vol. 4183: J. Euzenat, J. Domingue (Eds.), Artificial Intelligence: Methodology, Systems, and Applications. XIII, 291 pages. 2006.

Vol. 4180: M. Kohlhase, OMDoc – An Open Markup Format for Mathematical Documents [version 1.2]. XIX, 428 pages. 2006.

Vol. 4177: R. Marín, E. Onaindía, A. Bugarín, J. Santos (Eds.), Current Topics in Artificial Intelligence. XV, 482 pages. 2006.

Vol. 4160: M. Fisher, W. van der Hoek, B. Konev, A. Lisitsa (Eds.), Logics in Artificial Intelligence. XII, 516 pages. 2006.

Vol. 4155: O. Stock, M. Schaerf (Eds.), Reasoning, Action and Interaction in AI Theories and Systems. XVIII, 343 pages. 2006.

Vol. 4149: M. Klusch, M. Rovatsos, T.R. Payne (Eds.), Cooperative Information Agents X. XII, 477 pages. 2006.

Vol. 4140: J.S. Sichman, H. Coelho, S.O. Rezende (Eds.), Advances in Artificial Intelligence - IBERAMIA-SBIA 2006. XXIII, 635 pages. 2006.

Vol. 4139: T. Salakoski, F. Ginter, S. Pyysalo, T. Pahikkala (Eds.), Advances in Natural Language Processing. XVI, 771 pages. 2006.

Vol. 4133: J. Gratch, M. Young, R. Aylett, D. Ballin, P. Olivier (Eds.), Intelligent Virtual Agents. XIV, 472 pages. 2006.

Vol. 4130: U. Furbach, N. Shankar (Eds.), Automated Reasoning. XV, 680 pages. 2006.

Vol. 4120: J. Calmet, T. Ida, D. Wang (Eds.), Artificial Intelligence and Symbolic Computation. XIII, 269 pages. 2006.

Vol. 4118: Z. Despotovic, S. Joseph, C. Sartori (Eds.), Agents and Peer-to-Peer Computing. XIV, 173 pages. 2006.

Vol. 4114: D.-S. Huang, K. Li, G.W. Irwin (Eds.), Computational Intelligence, Part II. XXVII, 1337 pages. 2006.

Vol. 4108: J.M. Borwein, W.M. Farmer (Eds.), Mathematical Knowledge Management. VIII, 295 pages. 2006.

Vol. 4106: T.R. Roth-Berghofer, M.H. Göker, H.A. Güvenir (Eds.), Advances in Case-Based Reasoning. XIV, 566 pages. 2006.

Vol. 4099: Q. Yang, G. Webb (Eds.), PRICAI 2006: Trends in Artificial Intelligence. XXVIII, 1263 pages. 2006.

Vol. 4095: S. Nolfi, G. Baldassarre, R. Calabretta, J.C.T. Hallam, D. Marocco, J.-A. Meyer, O. Miglino, D. Parisi (Eds.), From Animals to Animats 9. XV, 869 pages. 2006.

Vol. 4093: X. Li, O.R. Zaïane, Z. Li (Eds.), Advanced Data Mining and Applications. XXI, 1110 pages. 2006.

Vol. 4092: J. Lang, F. Lin, J. Wang (Eds.), Knowledge Science, Engineering and Management. XV, 664 pages. 2006.